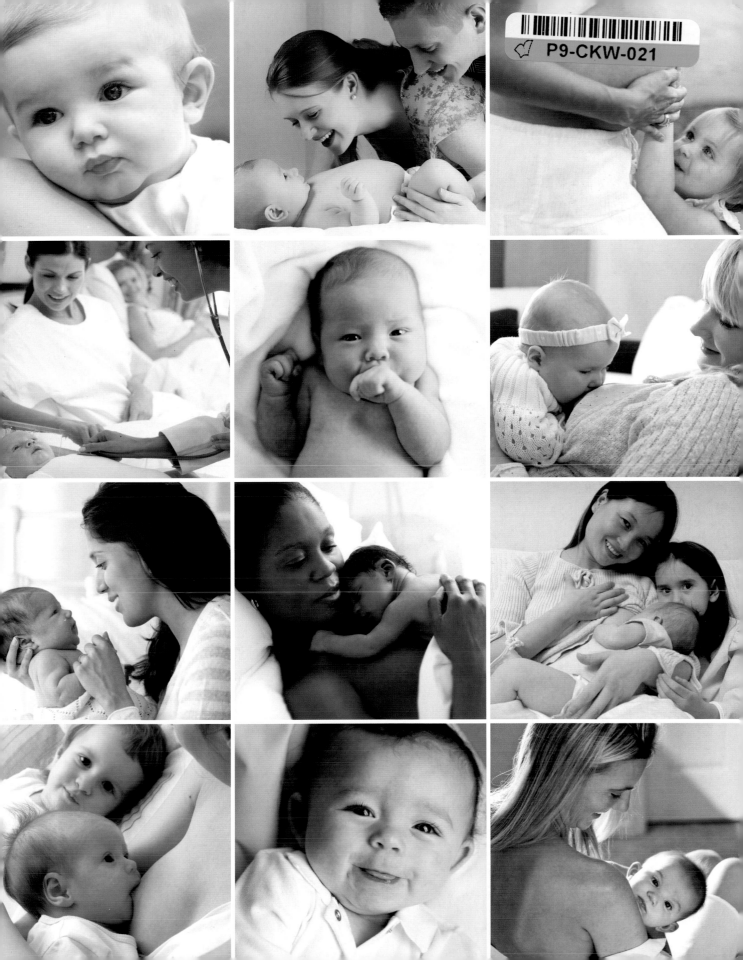

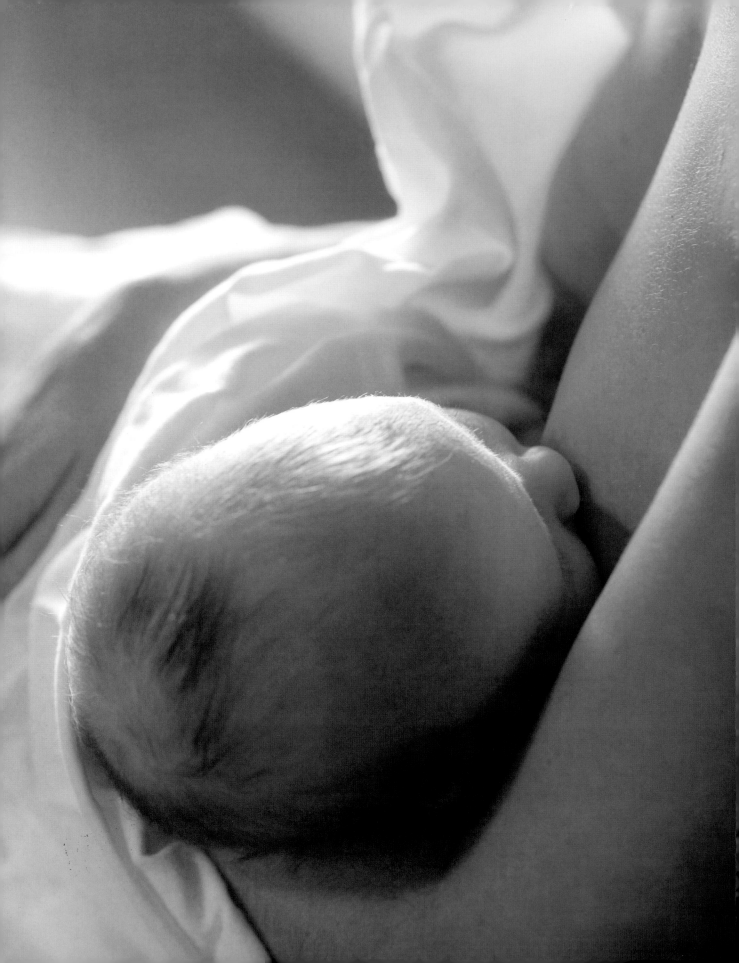

the better way to breastfeed

The Latest, Most Effective Ways
to Feed and Nurture Your Baby
with Comfort and Ease

Robin Elise Weiss
L.C.C.E., C.L.C

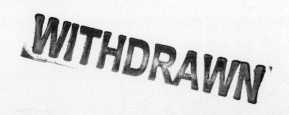

FAIR WINDS
PRESS
BEVERLY, MASSACHUSETTS

Text © Robin Elise Weiss

First published in the USA in 2010 by
Fair Winds Press, a member of
Quayside Publishing Group
100 Cummings Center
Suite 406-L
Beverly, MA 01915-6101
www.fairwindspress.com

14 13 12 11 10   1 2 3 4 5

ISBN-13: 978-1-59233-422-3
ISBN-10: 1-59233-422-9

Library of Congress Cataloging-in-Publication Data

Weiss, Robin Elise.
  The better way to breastfeed : the latest, most effective ways to feed and
nurture your baby with comfort and ease / Robin Elise Weiss.
      p. cm.
  Includes index.
  ISBN-13: 978-1-59233-422-3
  ISBN-10: 1-59233-422-9
  1. Breastfeeding--Popular works. I. Title.
  RJ216.W44 2010
  649'.33--dc22

                                                    2009052497
                                                       CIP

Cover design: Carol Holtz
Book design: Laura H. Couallier, Laura Herrmann Design
Editor: Andrea Mattei
Technical Edit: Denise Punger, M.D., F.A.A.F.P., I.B.C.L.C.
Photo Research: Daryl Gammons-Jones
Illustrations: Robert Brandt
Cover images: JGI/gettyimages.com, (left); iStockphoto.com, (second, left & middle);
    fotolia.com, (second, right); LWA/gettyimages.com, (right); © Kablonk!/agefotostock.com,
    (bottom)

Printed and bound in China

The information in this book is for educational purposes only. It is not intended to replace
the advice of a physician or medical practitioner. Please see your health care provider before
beginning any new health program.

DEDICATION

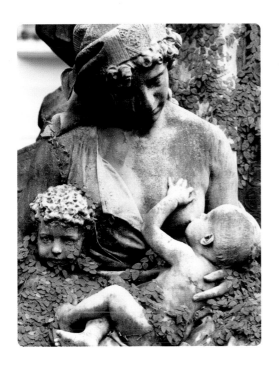

This book is dedicated to my grandmother, Carolyn Rose Horrar. She shared with me many great stories of parenting, and she taught me a lot about breastfeeding myths and how to be a great mother. Not a day goes by that I do not recall a gem of wisdom she passed down to me and, therefore, my children.

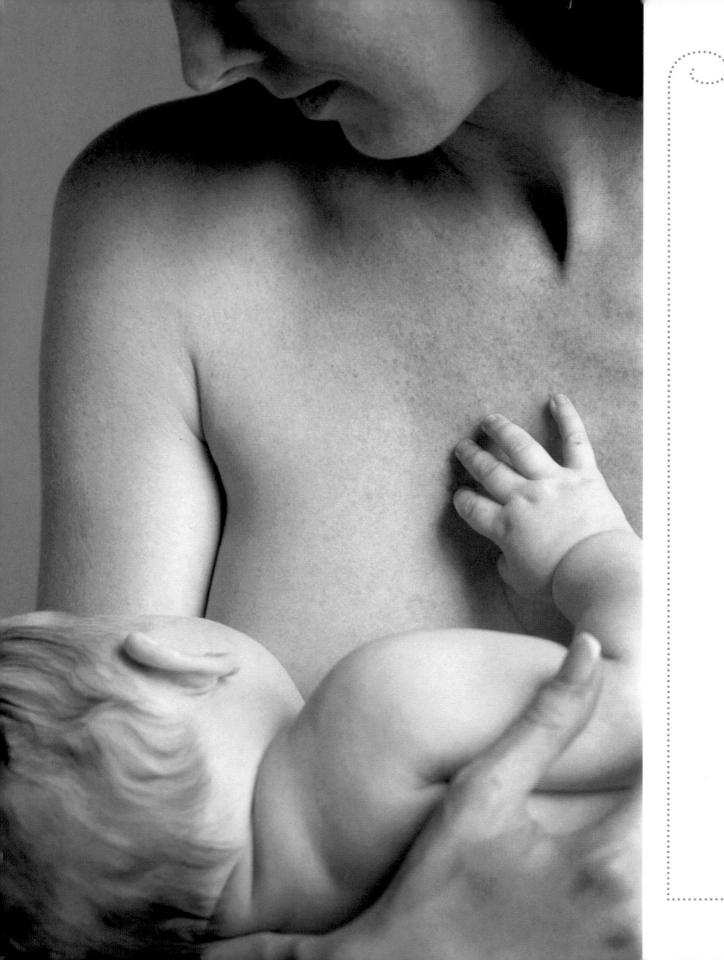

Contents

FOREWORD

The *Better Way to Breastfeed* by Robin Elise Weiss is a source for all mothers who want to succeed in breastfeeding, no matter what the goals look like for each individual family.

Robin has written an easy-to-understand breastfeeding guide for new mothers who are planning to have their first breastfeeding experiences, as well as experienced mothers who need to refresh their minds about breastfeeding. Robin is a certified lactation counselor, doula, childbirth educator, and published author on related mothering topics. Most importantly, she is a mother of eight children, including twins.

Being a mother and working with new mothers for more than twenty years, Robin understands the information a new mother needs. Her experiences included breastfeeding her singleton children for varying lengths of time. She breastfed her twins until they were older than two. And one of her babies, like many, refused to take the breast, but she provided breast milk for more than eighteen months via a breast pump. Robin's wide range of experiences helps her to understand the unique needs of mothers, babies, and families.

Robin is an advocate for breastfeeding. Her book is organized by chapters and topics, making it very easy to find information. She then applies her years of professional and mothering experiences to provide a wealth of practical tips as she discusses each topic. In each section, when appropriate, she also presents the American Academy of Pediatrics (AAP) formal position. She chose this point of reference because it is the one new moms trust the most.

As a family physician enthusiastically dedicated to prioritizing successful lactation even in the most extraordinary situations, I don't always agree with how the AAP dilutes the knowledge and wisdom I have acquired after years of clinical and personal experience to a one-size-fits-all approach to breastfeeding. Breastfeeding might not always come easy, yet a mother's determination and intuition, along with access to correct information, are most important for reaching her goals. Robin connects the more formal medical-opinion papers with sound information from the lactation community, and then ties it in to real mothering experience.

I am fortunate these days to have built up a mothering community. I am surrounded by circles of women who understand before they come to me how important nursing is to their child. And they have confidence in child-led weaning. Women referred to my office have often met with their local International Board-Certified Lactation Consult (IBCLC), La Leche League Leaders, or WIC office first, and have read a few books about breastfeeding.

But most women have not been surrounded by breastfeeding support. They go into breastfeed-

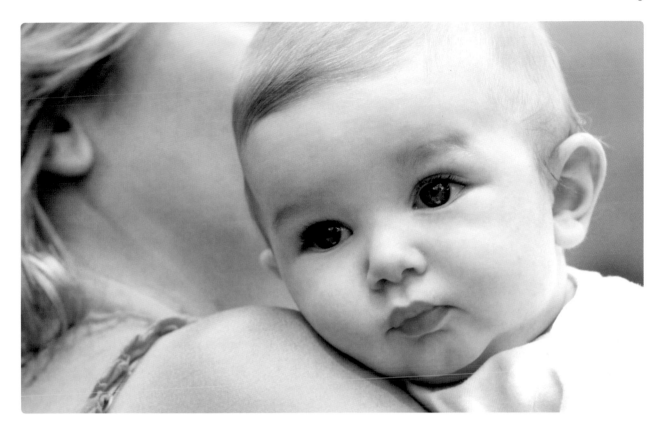

ing blindly, never having been around any other breastfeeding mothers and instead having been influenced by our bottle-feeding culture throughout their lives. This can pose many problems for them when it comes to meeting their breastfeeding goals. This book starts right at the beginning to fill in those gaps.

Despite being a family physician with a core in obstetrics and pediatrics, my formal education provided me with little useful information to impart breastfeeding knowledge to my patients. For similar reasons, your physician (pediatrician, OB, or family doctor) might not be the best medical professional to rely on when it comes to getting solid breastfeeding information. The little bit of feeding information

I did recall from my training did not seem to apply to me once my little one was in my arms. In many cases, it even seemed at odds with what I was now experiencing as a new breastfeeding mother.

Robin's book brings me back to where I was as a brand-new mother, wondering, with my first baby at my engorged breast, whether the effort to breastfeed was worth it. Her book is *the* book for soon-to-be moms who are anticipating the birth of their babies and the new experience of breastfeeding. Happy breastfeeding! May you and your baby fully enjoy all the benefits!

—Denise Punger M.D., F.A.A.F.P., I.B.C.L.C.
Private Practice Family and Breastfeeding Medicine,
Mother to three breastfed boys and Author of
Permission to Mother, www.permissiontomother.com

INTRODUCTION

Breastfeeding is a special, but
sometimes challenging, commitment.

Breastfeeding is a special but sometimes challenging commitment. However, science is showing that it is one that has numerous physical and emotional benefits for you and your baby. The specifics of how you choose to breastfeed will ultimately reflect what works for you, your family, your lifestyle, and your baby. To be successful at breastfeeding you need a solid foundation of commitment, knowledge, and support. My objective in writing this book is to help you to be successful in your breastfeeding practice, no matter what your personal goals are.

Belief in the process is important. Believing that breastfeeding is a good choice for your baby and belief that you can surmount any bumps in the road is important in staying dedicated to your breastfeeding practice. You probably already believe in breastfeeding or you wouldn't have picked up this book. That said, you are probably hoping to learn the little things that make breastfeeding go more smoothly—the tips and techniques from personal and professional experience that will help ease you into being a breastfeeding mom. This book will keep you committed to your breastfeeding choice by giving you the most up-to-date

and effective information on the topic as well as step-by-step photos that will show you how to troubleshoot issues.

Two of your biggest obstacles to successful breastfeeding are lack of information as well as misinformation. As a breastfeeding mom you will encounter volumes of outdated breastfeeding information from many sources—including your pediatrician. While your pediatrician means well, he or she probably lacks the most up-to-date medical training in regard to breastfeeding because medical schools don't cover it comprehensively, and also because the amazing things we are learning about breastfeeding occur rapidly.

This means that your pediatrician's knowledge is probably limited to the children that they have at home or what they were taught several years ago. This is when a lactation professional should be your primary source of information. While it may seem contrary, there are times within these pages that I'll advise you to seek the advice of your lactation professionals over, or in addition to, your pediatrician. This is because it is a lactation professional's job to stay on top of the most current medical information as well as the best practical information that will help mothers breastfeed easily and with comfort. A lactation professional has one focus—breastfeeding. Your pediatrician has a broader area of expertise that can be consulted for other issues concerning your baby's health. Ultimately, the two of them working as a team form the best knowledge base and resource for you and your baby.

Rallying support is critical in your desire to be successful. Perhaps you've heard from friends that breastfeeding is hard. It can be for some women, but, from what those who have had trouble and still succeeded tell us is, that the support from others really made the difference. Having your husband, your friends, your parents, and your in-laws behind you can make all the difference in the world when it comes to making breastfeeding work for you and your family. I promise to give you all the tools that you, as well as your support system, will need to be educated in your choice to breastfeed.

Most importantly, have faith. You will have good days, and you will have challenging days. The ups and downs that come with breastfeeding are just part of the experience. Do your best—surround yourself with a team of experts, starring you and your baby as their "most valuable players."

— Robin Elise Weiss

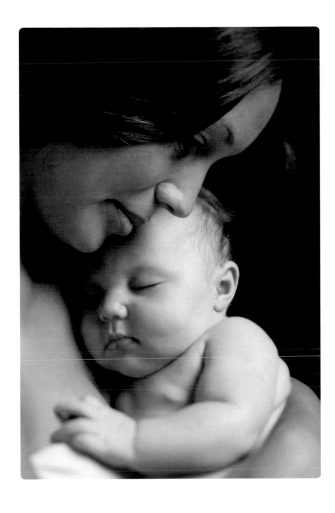

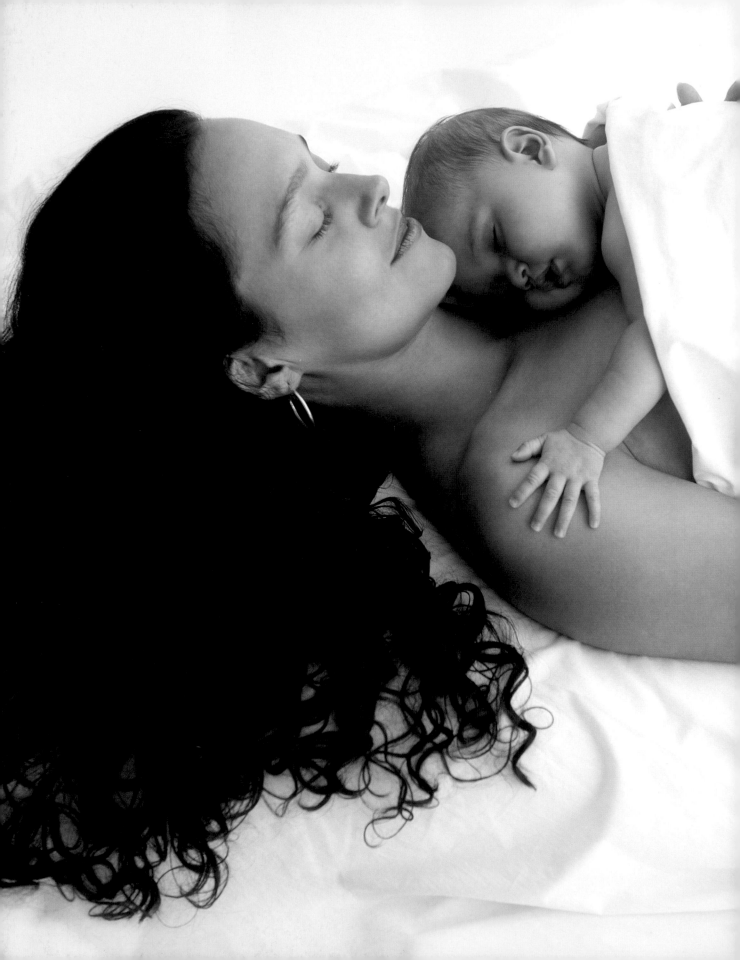

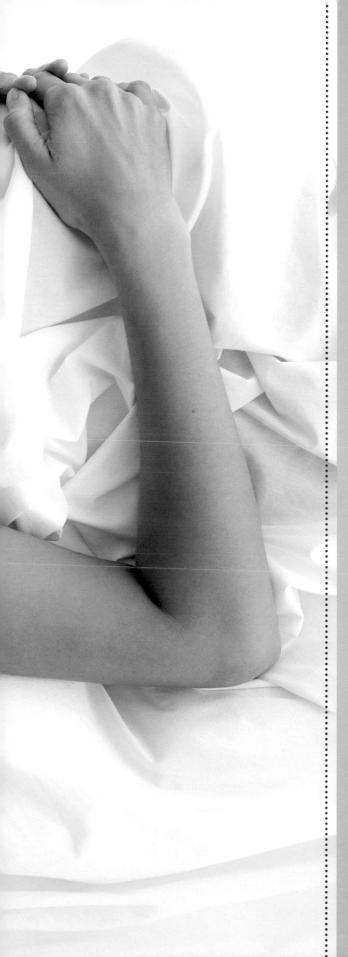

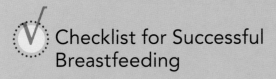
Before You Breastfeed

✓ Checklist for Successful Breastfeeding

- ☐ Know the benefits of breastfeeding.
- ☐ Prepare your body for breastfeeding.
- ☐ Learn how your birth choices affect breastfeeding.
- ☐ Take a breastfeeding class.
- ☐ Purchase a nursing bra.
- ☐ Write your newborn care plan for your birth.
- ☐ Define your breastfeeding goals.
- ☐ Build confidence in breastfeeding.

Breastfeeding is one of the most natural and wonderful things you can do for your baby, yourself, and your family. As breastfeeding is a natural process, a section on how to prepare to breastfeed might seem unnecessary. In some cases that might be true. But just because breastfeeding is natural doesn't mean new mothers automatically know how to do it. Like many other aspects of parenting, breastfeeding is a learned skill.

Part of the reason that a section on preparing to breastfeed is needed in this book is because of the lack of breastfeeding knowledge we have grown up with in our lives. In generations past, breastfeeding was a common part of everyday life, and young women were quite familiar with the process. In many instances, the naturalness of breastfeeding has largely been lost. We see images of formula-feeding babies on a daily basis, and many of us seldom—if ever—saw babies being breastfed as we were growing up.

This lack of breastfeeding education as a part of daily life means we have lost a valuable opportunity to see how breastfeeding works and to incorporate it into our mindset. You probably did not see your mother breastfeeding your siblings. The few women who breastfed when you were younger probably did not do so at the neighborhood block party.

This chapter is about building your confidence: not only in the process of breastfeeding, but also in your body's abilities. You will also learn how to prevent some socially induced barriers to successful breastfeeding. By combining all of this information, your breastfeeding plans and goals will be clear to you and to those around you. In addition, you will have the skills you need to put those plans into place with the help of the other chapters in this book.

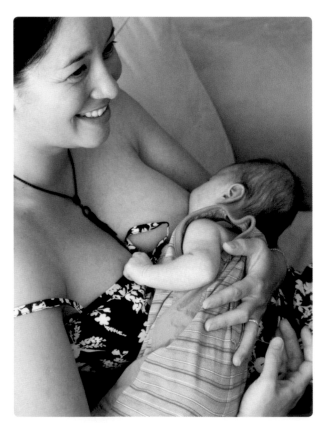

One of the many benefits of breastfeeding is the relaxing, enjoyable experience for both mom and baby.

KNOW THE BENEFITS OF BREASTFEEDING

Breastfeeding has many benefits. In most places you might be told only about the benefits for your baby. There are also benefits to you, your family, and even society. Some of the benefits to your baby include:

- Decrease in the risk of sudden infant death syndrome (SIDS)

- Decrease in childhood leukemias
- Fewer ear infections and respiratory infections
- Lower risk of obesity
- Fewer stomach viruses
- Less incidence of diarrhea
- Lowered risk of types 1 and 2 diabetes
- Less atopic dermatitis
- Less risk of asthma
- Less necrotizing enterocolitis (NEC) in preemies
- Minor increase in IQ

- Lower risk of developing type 2 diabetes
- Decreased risk of postpartum depression (PPD)
- Fewer incidences of breast cancer
- Lower incidence of ovarian cancer

This is an amazing list of benefits for your baby. There are also some additional benefits that do not fit neatly in a list. These benefits summarize some of the reasons breast milk is such an amazing food.

For example, your breast milk changes. It is different at one day and at one month after giving birth. The breast milk you make at one o'clock in the morning is different from the milk you make at one o'clock in the afternoon. Your body knows exactly where you were in your pregnancy at the time you gave birth, providing extra protection and nutrition for babies who were born early. And your body and breast milk make adjustments as you encounter germs in your environment to help your baby receive immunities through your breast milk. Nothing is as perfect for your baby as your breast milk.

While the benefits to the baby are often extolled, the benefits to the mother might not be as obvious. Recent studies are showing us more and more benefits breastfeeding mothers receive every day. Some of the major benefits to your health can include:

But if you talk to a breastfeeding mother, she probably won't tell you about the health benefits. Instead, you'll likely hear how convenient it is to breastfeed. Your breast milk is always ready, so mom and baby don't have to suffer through crying as bottles are prepared. Breast milk is always the right temperature. You do not need to lug around additional equipment or sterilize your nipples. Breastfed babies tend to spit up less, and therefore there is less laundry to do and there are fewer stains to scrub out. These practical aspects are the things mothers will tell you about breastfeeding.

Breastfeeding can also save your family time and money. As stated in *Pediatrics,* in February of 2005, infants who are breastfed typically have fewer doctor visits for illness; you or your partner will miss fewer days at work from having to stay home with your baby or go to doctor appointments. This also means less money spent on copayments to the baby's doctor.

Society also benefits from breastfeeding, in that breastfeeding results in a more productive workforce because parents miss fewer workdays staying home with sick children. This translates to lower health care bills as well. In addition, breastfeeding does not require the equipment that bottle feeding does, so fewer products end up in landfills, which is better for our environment.

The most important benefit of breastfeeding is likely to be personal. There are certainly people who will cite research or one of the aforementioned benefits as the reason they believe breastfeeding is best for their baby, but the personal reasons are often the ones that really matter. Now, your reason for breastfeeding might be that you want to reduce the chances of illness for your baby, or it may be that you want to feed your baby in a more natural manner. There is not a single right answer to the question of what is the biggest benefit of breastfeeding—there are many benefits, and they are all important. But more often than not, the unique and close bond that breastfeeding creates brings the greatest benefits for both mother and baby.

PREPARE YOUR BODY FOR BREASTFEEDING

You need to do very little to prepare your body for breastfeeding. From the moment of conception, your body has been preparing to breastfeed. You might have noticed that your breasts have gotten larger. Your nipples may have increased in size or become darker in preparation for breastfeeding. You might even notice at some point during pregnancy that your breasts have begun to leak a sticky yellow substance called colostrum, a pre-milk substance that is rich in antibodies and helps your baby to move meconium through her body.

These changes happen without you having to think about them. Nature knows what is best for your baby and helps you out. But what nature cannot do is to overcome the mind. This is why mental and emotional preparation is so important when getting ready for the gift of breastfeeding.

During pregnancy, you might hear stories of breastfeeding successes and failures. You might hear lots of myths and fabrications regarding breastfeeding, particularly when it comes to your body. Many of these tales have to do with your breasts. Read on, and we'll dispel many of these untruths.

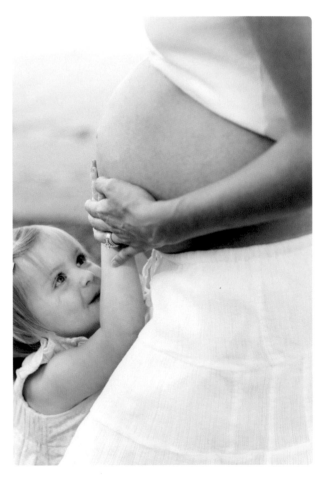

In addition to preparing for childbirth, it is important to research the information you need to know about breastfeeding. Besides nutrition basics, become familiar with your own body.

Breast Shape and Size

Breasts come in many different shapes and sizes. This is simply a natural variation. How large or small your breasts are has a lot to do with your family's genetics, your health, and your overall body shape. Overly large or small breasts do not mean you cannot breastfeed. This is a common myth. Breast size is not about the ability to make or hold breast milk. It is merely due to the amount and placement of fat deposits around the breast.

Large Breasts

Large-breasted women are often left alone in the "breast tissue being appropriate to breastfeed" argument. The assumption is that if you have large breasts, you have enough space to hold the milk or adequate tissue to make the milk. Since breast tissue and milk production are not related, you know this is a myth.

What large-breasted women can have trouble with is positioning their baby well at the very beginning. Having a lot of breast tissue can make it harder to hold your baby and your breast, especially if you are engorged in the early days of breastfeeding. Usually you can easily overcome this by using pillows, or extra hands when possible, to help hold your breast and your baby. Once your baby gets the hang of latching on, it is usually not a problem for either one of you.

Small Breasts

If you have smaller breasts, you might worry about making enough breast milk for your baby. In fact, if you start out with smaller breasts before pregnancy, you might be surprised at the amount of growth pregnancy can bring to some women, though not all. The size or shape of your breasts does not matter when it comes to producing breast milk.

Small breasts are just as capable of breastfeeding a baby as large breasts are. It is easy to believe that the size of the "container" will represent how much storage capacity is available. This is not so when it comes to breasts and breast milk. The amount of milk you produce is very different from the concept of how much milk your body will store at one time. You can produce plenty of milk; your breast might simply need to empty and refill more frequently. (This doesn't necessarily mean you'll have to nurse your baby more frequently if you have smaller breasts. It just means milk will continue to flow into your breasts as needed when your baby is nursing.)

Nipple Piercings

There is no reason to believe that the average nipple piercing will affect your ability to breastfeed, although it is generally recommended that you do

Adoptive Breastfeeding

The AAP now recommends that adoptive mothers breastfeed when possible. For more on adoptive breastfeeding, refer to page 217.

Inverted and Flat Nipples

You usually can't tell if you have inverted nipples simply by looking at your breasts or nipples, although there is a simple test you can do to check. With your shirt off, stand in front of a mirror, facing toward it. Using your forefinger and thumb, gently compress or pinch your breast about 1 inch (2.5 cm) away from the nipple on the dark portion of your breast, the areola.

If your nipple becomes erect, your nipple is fine. If your nipple goes inside the breast tissue, this is called an inverted nipple. If your nipple remains flat against the breast tissue,

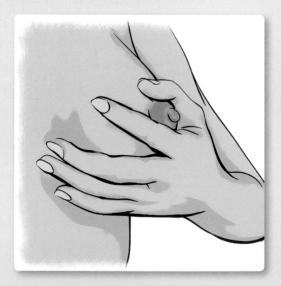

Using your thumb and forefinger, gently pinch the areola about one inch (2.5 cm) behind the nipple. If the nipple is inverted, it will pull inward.

it is said to be a flat nipple. Once you have tested one side, test the other side as well. It is possible to have nipples that respond differently. Inverted nipples are a variation of normal. In fact, flat or inverted nipples are very common in girls prior to puberty. The fact that your nipples are inverted is not a huge issue. You should talk to your lactation consultant or practitioner about his or her opinion on trying to treat inverted nipples prior to birth.

Some practitioners believe you can train the nipple to cease being inverted before your baby arrives. Others believe the baby is the best cure for inverted nipples. The hormones pregnancy produces are also great for helping the nipples prepare for birth and breastfeeding. You will have to decide which method you prefer for your body if you have this issue.

Treatment for flat or inverted nipples varies among practitioners. Some recommend that you use a special tool that is basically a miniature breast pump. You use this small, hand-held suction device to pull out the nipple. One such item on the market is called the Evert-It.

You can also practice the Hoffman Technique. It is possible to use this technique during pregnancy. It is based on the theory that flat or inverted nipples occur because

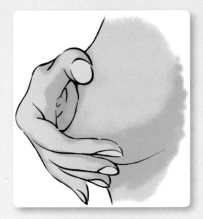
Flat nipple

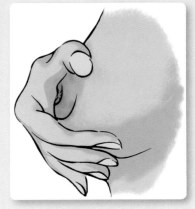
Inverted nipple

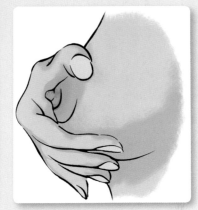
Normal nipple

tissue near the base of the nipple is adhering to itself and preventing the nipple from becoming erect. To implement this technique, place both of your thumbs at the base of your nipple. Press inward and then pull each thumb outward in the opposite direction. This is meant to loosen any tissue that is tight and is preventing your nipple from becoming erect. You can do this twice per day, but no more than five times per day, on each inverted nipple.

The use of breast shells is another method some practitioners recommend. These are two-part, hard plastic shells worn over the breast. The bottom piece goes over the top of the areola and the hole is placed over the nipple area. The top portion connects to the bottom, allowing for a slight space around the nipple. You can wear these during pregnancy, inside your bra. The hope is that the steady but gentle pressure will help draw out the nipple. You should discard any colostrum that collects in the breast shell, and wash and air-dry the shells before each use.

Other methods for dealing with inverted or flat nipples are best suited for after the birth of your baby. The key here is that by achieving a good, deep latch when your baby is born, you can resolve most of these issues with no problems.

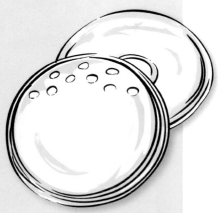

Breast shells are a two-part system worn over the breast during pregnancy in an attempt to draw out the nipple in preparation for breastfeeding.

not get your nipple(s) pierced while you are pregnant, and that once you have your nipple pierced,
you leave the jewelry in for many months before
you remove it. To safely breastfeed, you should
remove your nipple jewelry to prevent your baby
from choking on it or getting a soft tissue injury in
his mouth from sucking with the jewelry in place.
When you are in between feedings you can replace
the jewelry if you are able to do so yourself. Otherwise, you will have to wait until your baby has
weaned before replacing the nipple jewelry.

Nipple Size

The average nipple—not the areola, but the nipple
itself—is about the size of a dime. Nipple size is
typically not an issue when you get your baby to
open his mouth wide during the latch. Though you
might hear mothers complain about their babies
not latching well, this inability to latch properly
can be due to many other reasons, including the
baby not opening his mouth wide enough, improper

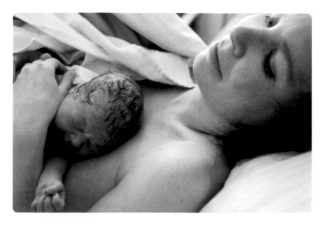

*Skin-to-skin contact as soon after birth as pos-
sible is the best thing that you can do to help
breastfeeding get off to a good start.*

positioning, and so on. During the early days of
breastfeeding, engorgement can make your nipple
seem larger than it is normally. This typically
passes in a few days.

LEARN HOW YOUR BIRTH CHOICES AFFECT BREASTFEEDING

You will make many choices during the course of
your labor, birth, and postpartum period. Some of
these you will make out of medical need, and others
you will make based on your preferences. As you
read through this section, you will see recurring
themes on making sure you and your baby get off
to the best start possible. Trust your instincts to do
what is best for you and your baby.

Induction of Labor

You might be wondering what the induction of labor
has to do with breastfeeding. Actually, it can play a
big role in how well breastfeeding starts. One of the
biggest problems with induction is the risk of prematurity. This risk comes from a variety of reasons,
including the fact that simply being thirty-seven
weeks pregnant, or even thirty-nine weeks pregnant, does not mean your baby is ready to be born.
Some babies simply need more time in utero. There
can also be variances in your due date calculation.

Currently, it is recommended that no one be induced prior to thirty-nine weeks' gestation, without
medical reason, to help lower the risk of giving birth
to a premature infant. However, even this thirty-
nine-week cutoff is not going to guarantee that your
baby is ready to be born. The problems associated

WOMEN'S WISDOM:

Be mindful of people who are eager to tell you horror stories. Breastfeeding, like pregnancy and childbirth, seems to be a topic that everyone—even strangers—will feel they can ramble on about to you. Tune out any negativity you hear from those who were not as successful with breastfeeding as you intend to be. Read, take a class, and talk to friends and family members who have been successful at breastfeeding. If you are prepared, it will make a world of difference.

with even slight prematurity fall into the category of the late preterm infant.

Babies born with the late preterm status have subtle issues. They might be a bit sleepier. They might not nurse as well. They might need to be prompted to feed. They might be more likely to have jaundice. All of these small things can add up to babies who do not thrive at the breast as they should. And nearly all of these problems can be traced back to the induction of labor.

When you remove the prematurity risks, there are still plenty of reasons that an induction for medical or nonmedical grounds will affect breastfeeding. These can include the added interventions in labor, such as IV fluids or the increased risks of cesarean section that come with the induction of labor, particularly for first-time mothers. Each of these interventions can create trauma for the baby or increase the likelihood that the baby will need to be in the neonatal intensive care unit (NICU). They might also make the postpartum period more difficult and painful, meaning that breastfeeding can suffer as well. This is not to say that plenty of women do not successfully breastfeed through these types of circumstances, but simply that it can be more difficult to do so.

Medications in Labor

Medications used in labor can help you diminish your pain quite effectively. But these medications, even the epidural, can affect how your newborn breastfeeds. Some of the effects of various medications are better known than others. In fact, some studies including the prospective, "Intrapartum Epidural Analgesia and Breastfeeding," conducted in 2006 show that the effects of the medications can last for weeks or lead to the discontinuation of breastfeeding earlier than you may have intended.

Choosing medications wisely and knowing all the risks and benefits involved is important. This goes for all medications used in labor and birth, including those that are not directly for pain in labor.

You might be able to lessen the effects of some of the medications. For example, this might involve smaller doses, better timing in labor, and potentially less time spent with medications such as the epidural.

Effects that can be seen in the newborn will vary based on the medication used, the length of time the medication was in use, and when it was used in relation to the birth. Here are some things you might notice:

- Sleepy baby
- Discordant suck
- Sleepy mom
- Disinterested baby

Fortunately, you can overcome most of these problems with planning and work. One of the best things you can do is to have uninterrupted skin-to-skin contact with your baby immediately after birth to encourage your baby to nurse, as the AAP recommends. Even if your baby does not choose to nurse at this point, studies find that these babies still have greater success at breastfeeding in the long term.

IV Fluids in Labor

Women might commonly receive fluids through an IV during labor. This might be to deliver antibiotics or even pain medication. An IV is also routinely used with epidural anesthesia, even though it is not the route of pain medications for the epidural.

These fluids will gather in a new mother's tissues, making her feel swollen and uncomfortable. This is true even of her breast tissue. Sometimes this can make it difficult for the baby to latch on until the fluid has left the mother's system, usually in the first week of the postpartum period.

Cesarean or Instrumental Delivery

Today, more women are having cesarean sections. This means the recovery that goes along with this will impact breastfeeding. Now that hospitals are becoming more aware of the effects of cesareans on breastfeeding, more can be done to help prevent negative effects from the surgery. One example is to have the baby breastfeeding or at least offered the breast immediately after birth, while still in the operating room. Breastfeeding should also be encouraged and supported beyond that time period. The recovery room is a great place to ensure that mom and baby are skin to skin and nursing. Be sure to ask for this if you are having a cesarean birth.

Your baby might also have some issues after a cesarean birth which will make him less likely to want to nurse. This is particularly true if there was no labor prior to the cesarean. Your baby might have more fluid and breathing issues, making it difficult to nurse or requiring special care in the nursery. Being with your baby as much as you can, even having dad have skin-to-skin contact with baby if you are unable to, is beneficial to the baby.

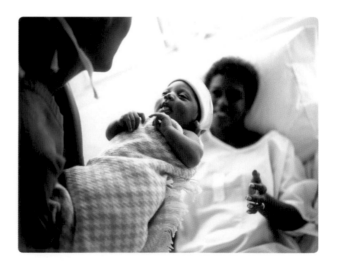

If your baby is handed to you bundled up, undress him to his diaper and hold him skin-to-skin and cover both of you with a blanket.

Infants who are born with the use of forceps and vacuum extraction might also have issues with breastfeeding. They might be unwilling to nurse due to pain from the procedure. Or they might fall into a deep sleep after the birth.

Immediate and Uninterrupted Contact after Birth

Immediate and uninterrupted skin-to-skin contact after birth is one of the best things you can do for your baby and for your breastfeeding relationship. This is part of the normal birth cycle and can be done for almost any birth, including babies who are born via cesarean section.

It is a natural instinct for mothers to want to be close to their babies. By holding your baby skin to skin, your body will produce more endorphins and oxytocin. This is designed to help you to feel more "motherly." The Cochrane Collaboration analyzed thirty medical studies and determined that mothers who experience this tend to make more breast milk, have an easier time responding to their babies, and are better able to establish breastfeeding. Babies who stay in close contact with their mothers after birth tend to cry less, breathe more easily, have better blood sugar levels, and stay warmer than their counterparts.

Immediate means your baby is handed directly to you after birth. Your baby should not go to the warmer, even for a minute, barring medical complications. No routine procedures should be performed, such as weight checks, length checks, or vitamin K or other injections. The baby should simply come to mom. If that is not the policy at the place where you have chosen to give birth, you will need to work to ensure that this is what you get for your baby's best chance at a great start with breastfeeding as well as the best milk supply.

Swaddling

Swaddling has its place in newborn care. However, according to "Breast and Infant Temperatures with Twins during Shared Kangaroo Care," published in the *Journal of Obstetric, Gynecologic, and Neonatal Nursing,* swaddling is not encouraged because of its direct impact on the skin-to-skin placement in the first few hours of life. All of the blankets and the lack of skin-to-skin contact can interfere with breastfeeding by making it physically hard to reach the baby through all of those layers. It can also lead to a baby having a lower body temperature and requiring time in the nursery to warm up, since the mother's body is the best place to keep baby warm. This is because the mother's body actually acts as a radiant warmer, warming and cooling in direct response to the baby's body temperature.

If your baby is swaddled in blankets when he is given to you to feed, you should remove the blankets. Sometimes parents get it in their heads that whatever the hospital staff has done must not be undone. The staff is merely doing what they do for every single baby; there is no magic involved. Unwrap your baby for feedings. This will ensure better feedings now, for a more successful breastfeeding relationship later.

Bathing

Bathing is frequently done within the first few hours of life. However, bathing not only takes the baby away from the mother, but it can also have other negative effects. Many hospitals will want a newly bathed baby to spend time in the nursery under warming lamps to ensure that the baby stays warm. Babies do not require bathing. You can ask that any meconium or blood be removed from both you and your baby, and then that both of you be covered with warm blankets so that your body temperature will keep the baby warm. Studies have examined the smell of amniotic fluid, nearly imperceptible to you, and how it enhances your baby's ability to find and latch onto the breast and, thus, its effects on your maternal hormone production. To learn more about this natural phenomenon, reference the book, *Your Amazing Newborn* by Marshall H. Klaus, M.D., and Phyllis Klaus, M.F.T.

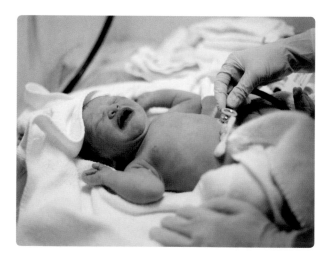

Any medical procedures that can be delayed shortly after birth will help to get a breastfeeding connection for mother and baby established first.

Other Routine Procedures

Many other procedures can take place in the first hour after birth. These include, but are not limited to, the following:

- Weight measurement
- Height measurement
- Cord blood retrieval
- Heel stick test (for metabolic, genetic, and blood sugar testing)
- Immunizations (hepatitis B)
- Vitamin K injection
- Eye prophylaxis
- Newborn exam

If your baby is doing well, he can be observed, monitored, and given injections and other tests while he is resting with you. Many hospitals do this, particularly those with the World Health Organization's Baby-Friendly Hospital designation. Alternatively, these procedures can be delayed, allowing you the time you need to be with your baby. Rarely do these procedures need to be performed on a stable newborn at the moment of birth. Do not be talked into having these things done and getting your baby back later, as this is frequently only for the hospital's preference and not for true medical need.

Extra People in the Room

Another subtle issue in the delivery room that might cause problems with breastfeeding is visitors. For most families, your stay in the labor and birth room will typically be only about an hour. During

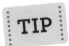

Baby-Friendly Hospitals

Is your hospital baby friendly? Check the list at www.babyfriendlyusa.org. Be sure to ask your hospital about its policies and philosophy regarding breastfeeding.

that time, you'll be having postpartum uterine checks, and the medical staff will be attending to various other tasks, while your sole job should be to hold, love, and offer the breast to your new baby.

Having other family members who want to come and greet the new baby can make your job very difficult for a variety of reasons. For one thing, they will all want their turn holding the new baby. It can be difficult for many mothers to say no to this. If you do manage to hang on to your baby and you are holding him skin to skin, you might be hampered in feeding him because you are not yet ready to nurse in public.

A more basic reason is simply that other people are a distraction. You need to focus only on your baby and perhaps on your partner as well. Adding a bunch of visitors is typically not the best idea at this point.

If you are worried about how the people in the waiting room will feel, ask for help. The nurses and other medical staff members are usually happy to help you explain that you are not yet ready for visitors. They can put a sign on the door asking visitors to come back later. You can also send your doula out to talk to the family with a message from you. Some new parents provide visitors with a few newborn snapshots and requests for food. This can give visitors tasks to perform in the short time until you get to your postpartum room and they can join you.

Artificial Nipples

Artificial nipples—pacifiers and bottle nipples—can be a huge problem for some babies. While not every baby will suffer from nipple confusion, some will. Nipple confusion occurs when a baby has been introduced to an artificial nipple and then becomes confused or upset when offered the breast. Often, this can result in the baby refusing the breast. While most babies can be retrained, it is not pleasant and should not be necessary when artificial nipples can be avoided in all cases.

Pacifiers and baby bottles are the most common artificial nipples that are introduced in the postpartum stay. Occasionally, however, medication will be administered in this manner. To avoid the use of artificial nipples, you should request that your baby not be given any type of artificial nipple for any reason.

Should a medical staff member wish to give your baby any oral medication, a syringe can be used. If a procedure needs to be performed on your baby, you can ask that the procedure be performed while the baby nurses. This works very well for keeping your baby calm. As cited in the journal, *Ambulatory Pediatrics,* it is recommended by health care practitioners for all types of procedures, including injections.

Pacifiers are also problematic for another reason. When your baby sucks on a pacifier to help him calm down, he is not nursing. Nursing in the first few weeks of life is key to building your milk supply, even when the sucking or nursing is for comfort. When your baby uses a pacifier, your breasts do not get that stimulation, and this can negatively affect your milk supply.

In the rare event that it is determined you must supplement your baby with your expressed breast milk, breast milk from the milk bank, sugar water, or other liquids, you can ask that alternatives to artificial nipples are used. This might be a special cup designed to feed newborns. You could also do finger feedings. Ask your local lactation professional to help you decide which type of feeding device will be the best choice for your baby in these rare instances.

Nursery Stays

Nursery stays for healthy newborns are really not recommended by lactation professionals and many pediatricians since you are unable to respond to your baby's cues for feeding and the nursery staff is not always able to see these cues and return your baby to you. All newborn procedures and checks can be done at your bedside. Some family physicians and pediatricians will request that the baby be sent to the nursery for well-being checks, but if you talk to the medical staff beforehand, you can usually get around this typical scenario.

One big issue with babies going into the hospital nursery is that frequently the nurses are too busy to return your baby quickly. While in the nursery, your baby might receive treatment—either by accident or intentionally—that you do not want him to have. He might be given a pacifier or be made to wait longer for a feeding than if he were in your room, for instance. While you are separated from your baby, you will also have trouble learning your baby's cues. Do not be fooled by the "you'll get rest if the baby is in the nursery" routine. It simply does not really work that way.

Mothers report that they often feel anxious by having their baby away from them in the nursery, worried about the baby being brought when he or she is hungry or needy. Nurses are often busy, and while their intentions are well meaning they simply can't watch every baby that closely nor are they always able to leave the nursery when your baby or you are ready. Hospitals in general are not places of rest for new mothers, as they will be having physical assessments every few hours, medications, shift changes, and so on.

Pain

Let's face it, giving birth can leave you feeling tired and in pain. You've used muscles you didn't even know you had. Running a marathon would probably be easier! If you have had a difficult birth or a cesarean, you might experience even more pain. Pain might make you feel reluctant to interact with anyone, including your baby.

If this is the case, try to deal with the pain you're experiencing to help you be with your baby. This might mean taking pain medications or using other helpful aids such as sitz baths to ease discomfort. You might, at some point, require narcotics or strong pain medications. If this is what it takes to be comfortable, do not hesitate to take it. When you are in pain you are not able to care for your baby.

That being said, all prescription as well as over-the-counter pain medications will get through your breast milk into your baby in small amounts. The most common problem is that this can make your baby a bit sleepy as well, which can lead to decreased breastfeeding or poor latch. In other words, if a mother is given inordinate amounts of medication, she may suffer some serious side effects such as decreased respiration. So the best option is to use stronger medications at first, and then once you are up and mobile, switch to non-narcotic pain medications as quickly as you can. This will benefit

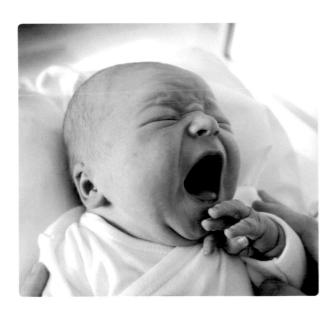

Crying is a late sign of hunger in a baby. Missing the early signs, or attempting to use a scheduled feeding system, is not optimal for mom or baby.

both you and your baby. Be careful not to overdo it! You might find that if you get too ambitious with your activities too quickly, you might once again require a dose or two of the narcotic medication even after you thought you didn't need it anymore. Don't worry, unless the pain remains at that more intense level despite medications. If this happens, be sure to call your midwife or doctor. While all medications will wind up in your breast milk, they do so in a much lower concentration than those given directly to your baby or even many of the medications used commonly in labor and delivery.

Scheduled or Timed Feedings

Once you give birth, your body is set to provide your baby with a full supply of breast milk. To make sure your body does its job, you need to have access to your baby. By allowing your baby free access to the breast in these first days and weeks after birth, you will set your body up to establish the best milk supply possible.

Remember, the more a baby sucks at your breast, the more milk your body will make. This means you need to allow your baby to nurse as often as his cues say that he wants to eat. Frequently, a newborn will eat eight to twelve times per day in the first weeks—sometimes even more. Keep in mind that these feedings are not necessarily evenly spaced throughout the day. Cluster feeding occurs when your baby seems to take only short breaks away from the breast and then wants to return. This is normal and is not a sign that your baby is not getting enough breast milk.

Also avoid limiting the amount of time your baby spends on each breast. Some well-meaning, but misinformed, nurses might try to encourage you to put a time limit on a breastfeeding session, often citing sore nipples. But time on the breast does not cause sore nipples. Sore nipples are most frequently caused by poor latching. Other causes may include yeast infections and Raynaud's Phenomenon (a blanching of the nipple).

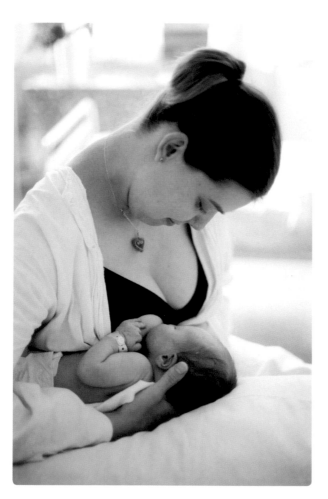

Allowing your baby to end the breastfeeding session on his own will ensure that he has the best feeding possible. Your baby should decide how long to nurse.

Keep this timing issue in mind when deciding how you wish to write your newborn care plan. (For more on writing a newborn care plan, see page 34.) Many hospitals offer rooming in for new mothers and babies. Take advantage of this time to get to know your baby and learn to read his feeding cues.

Misinformation

One thing that surprises many people is that most newborn and postpartum nurses do not have formal training in breastfeeding or caring for breastfeeding mothers and newborns. Their knowledge of breastfeeding might be limited to what they learned in nursing school, which may not be much at all. Nurses might also sometimes receive information on how to breastfeed from pharmaceutical/formula companies (and clearly, the formula companies' goals are at odds with breastfeeding goals). Sometimes nurses' breastfeeding training is composed of only what they have picked up while working over the years, which may not be accurate.

These busy but caring nurses really mean well when they're helping you, and they might even have great advice. The problems arise when you have three nurses per day and each one tells you to do something differently. This can be a real drain on your confidence as a newly nursing mother.

This is one reason why it's best to take a breastfeeding class before you have your baby. Be sure to pack this book in your hospital bag so that you have some ready references should you need clarification. Other than that, simply smile and thank nurses for their kind advice, and then do what you think is best for you and your baby.

Breastfeeding Discharge Packs

Depending on the hospital, free breastfeeding discharge packs can consist of a cute bag, breastfeeding advice from a formula company, and sometimes a bottle or bottle nipple for the samples, and they always include free formula and coupons for future formula purchases. While that might seem harmless enough, studies published in Pediatrics and by the Cochrane Collaboration have shown that the simple act of taking such a discharge pack home, with or without formula, undermines breastfeeding because it reduces the amount of time a mother breastfeeds by sabotaging her confidence and providing misinformation. Use the money you save by breastfeeding to buy yourself a really neat diaper bag. Also ask nurses if they can instead send you home with a baby-friendly discharge pack from your local breastfeeding support group or birth network. When available, these usually have water bottles, a variety of snacks, local coupons, breastfeeding-friendly samples, and/or breastfeeding information inside. This might be more likely to happen at a hospital designated by the World Health Organization (WHO) as a baby-friendly hospital.

TAKE A BREASTFEEDING CLASS

A breastfeeding class is a great option for most first-time mothers. Not only is it a place to learn the basics of breastfeeding, but it is also a chance for you to meet like-minded people who might be of support at a later date, should you need help or want to feel a part of a breastfeeding community.

Breastfeeding classes are typically taught by women who hold an International Board-Certified Lactation Consultant (IBCLC) or Certified Lactation Counselor (CLC) credential. They may or may not have ever breastfed a baby. These classes can be taught in hospitals, clinics, private practitioner offices, community centers, and homes. Remember, not all lactation professionals are great teachers, even if they are amazing in the one-on-one support setting. You are the consumer and you have choices in the classes you pick. Be sure to find a class that is right for you.

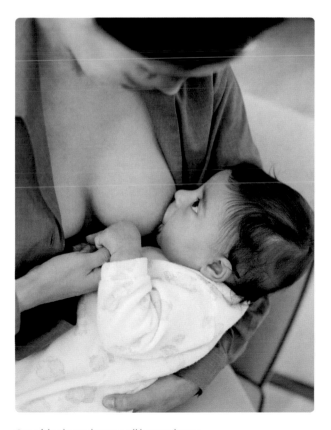

One of the things that you will learn in breastfeeding class is to notice what looks and feels right as far as your baby latches. A shallow latch will result in sore nipples and a baby who doesn't gain weight well.

When investigating your options, ask each instructor what will be covered in the breastfeeding class. Some classes are very basic, whereas others go into more detail. Here are some examples of what might be taught:

- Learning the benefits of breastfeeding
- Getting started with breastfeeding
- Latching your baby on
- Identifying when you need help
- Finding help
- Understanding common birth practices that might influence breastfeeding
- Reviewing hospital or birth-center policies for breastfeeding infants
- Getting support from your family while breastfeeding
- Working and breastfeeding
- Reviewing breast pump basics

A good breastfeeding class is not necessarily one that gives you more information. It can be a class that gives you enough of the right information in a manner in which you can learn it or understand it. Some women decide to take multiple breastfeeding classes.

Also consider attending free local La Leche League meetings. These are taught by volunteers who are trained to provide breastfeeding support. Leaders are mothers who have had firsthand experience nursing their own children. These meetings usually run once a month with a different topic. While the topics discussed will vary, they are centered on four basic themes:

- Advantages of breastfeeding
- Adjusting to life with a new baby
- Overcoming difficulties
- Nutrition and weaning

At La Leche League meetings, not only will you increase your knowledge of breastfeeding, but you will also learn from other mothers, both the leaders and the other participants. Some of these women are actively nursing and do so often at meetings. Watching other mothers breastfeeding their babies does wonders to help boost your confidence. You will also establish a rapport with the group so that when you return with your baby you will already feel comfortable.

Consider taking advantage of both classes and support groups. Sometimes taking the breastfeeding class at your hospital or birth center might have benefits for you. For instance, the class might entitle you to certain coupons or rights to see the lactation professional on duty when you give birth.

You might also get to hear how your place of birth feels about breastfeeding. For example, you might hear about birth practices, such as routinely separating the mother and baby after birth, which can hamper breastfeeding. This will give you time to see what you would need to do to get a pass on that routine. You may also hear some things that make you feel that your place of birth is not as friendly to breastfeeding mothers and babies as you might like them to be. Do not despair. While having a friendly hospital or birth center is preferable, it is not the only piece to the puzzle.

PURCHASE A NURSING BRA

A great nursing bra can be your best friend! It will help you feel more comfortable and well supported as you nurse your baby. Some women might advise you to save your money and just pull up the cup on an old bra, but once you have experienced the feel and convenience of a good nursing bra, you will never want to cut corners.

You might have a local maternity and nursing store that offers a selection of maternity and nursing bras. You might also have to go online to find bras that work for you and your preferences. Fortunately, many stores carry a wide variety of nursing bras, particularly in harder-to-find bra sizes. This might be a hassle if you need to return a bra, so be sure to check out the measurement charts clearly, and be aware of the return policy.

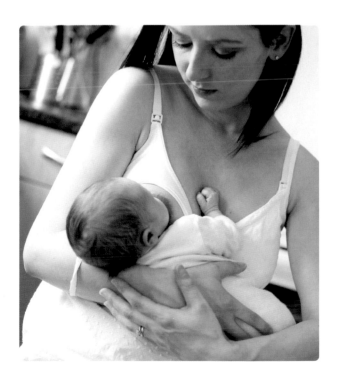

Nursing Bra Styles

Nursing bras come in several different styles. Your main concern should be how the cup attaches to the base bra. There are a couple of different options.

The most common type of nursing bra has a cup that fastens to the strap via hooks, snaps, or clips. You simply unhook the bra cup and it comes down, allowing you to expose your breast for a feeding. These are relatively easy to find and your dominant hand does not seem to matter when using this style of nursing bra.

When trying to decide which type of closure you want, you might be confused. Snaps are probably not as common in this location, but you can find them. Some women find that snaps are a bit too difficult to undo easily, quickly, or quietly. Snaps also have a tendency to quickly become loose, making them open at the most inopportune times.

Some nursing bras have cups that are designed to fold over to expose the breast for nursing. Typically, these bras can also be worn while sleeping. They tend to not be the best choice for women who are large breasted due to the lack of support.

Now, with all this talk of functionality, do not think that you have to give up fashion. Plenty of fancy nursing bras are available. They also come in great fabrics, including bamboo, silk, and other luxurious fabrics.

A nursing bra is an invaluable asset to the breastfeeding mother, making feeding times easier.

While a nursing bra might scream functional in your mind, this does not mean it has to be uncomfortable or even ugly. In fact, some nursing bras are downright sexy. Anytime you shop for a bra, you have to wade through the "strictly business" bras to get to the luxury or fashionable bras. Why would you think breastfeeding would be any different? Sure, you can't buy a nursing bra at Victoria's Secret, but then again Victoria's Secret does not make a bra with easy-access panels.

Other types of bras are available for nursing, such as the hands-free pumping bra. These are specialty bras and most mothers don't need them. The hands-free pumping bra has two cups in place of the regular cup. Both hook to the base of the bra, but the inner cup has an additional vertical slit through the middle of the cup. This is where you will place the horn of the breast pump, and then hook the bra cup to the base. Attach the pump to the outside of the horn and you can then pump without your hands.

Washing your bras should not be a problem. Be sure to check the care instructions before purchasing a bra to ensure that you can handle the care that it requires. Most nursing bras are machine washable, though some request that you use the delicate cycle.

Purchase three or four bras with which to begin your postpartum period. This can help to ensure that you always have a clean, dry bra available to wear. You might also wish to add to your bra collection as you figure out what works well for you.

Getting Fitted for a Nursing Bra

Getting the right fit is important when it comes to bras. Most women simply start guessing when they are buying a bra. During pregnancy and into your nursing experience, you will want to take the time to be sure that you are wearing well-fitting bras. An improper fit might actually cause you pain and potentially affect your milk supply.

Consider looking for the right bra for you in the third trimester of pregnancy. At this point, your breasts have seen the majority of their growth. Some pregnant women also find that nursing bras are more comfortable, and they begin to wear them immediately. There is no harm in this practice.

If you were to try to select a bra prior to your third trimester you may find yourself purchasing another set of bras as your breasts grow. You should also be dissuaded from waiting until after your

Underwire Nursing Bras

Underwires in nursing bras have been considered something to avoid for a while. They can increase your pain level and might cause plugged ducts. There are some alternatives to underwires, such as styles that feature extra padding or underbraiding for support. It is possible to find nursing bras with underwires. If you find you are not irritated or bothered, then by all means, try it!

Proper Fitting of a Nursing Bra

You will take two measurements. The first measurement is going to be where the band will sit, under your breasts. Be sure that the measuring tape is flat against your skin. Write this number down: It is your band size. Now you will want to measure yourself across the fullest part of your breasts, near your nipples. Remember not to measure too tightly! Write this number down. The difference between your band size and the other number is what will determine your cup size according to this chart:

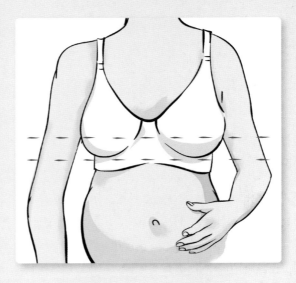

½" to 1" (1.3 to 2.5 cm)	=	**AA** cup
1" to 1½" (2.5 to 3.8 cm)	=	**A** cup
1½" to 2½" (3.8 to 6.4 cm)	=	**B** cup
2½" to 3½" (6.4 to 8.9 cm)	=	**C** cup
3½" to 4" (8.9 to 10.2 cm)	=	**D** cup
4" to 5" (10.2 to 12.7 cm)	=	**DD/E** cup
5" to 6" (12.7 to 15.2 cm)	=	**DDD/F** cup
6" to 7" (15.2 to 17.8 cm)	=	**G** cup
7" to 8" (17.8 to 20.3 cm)	=	**H** cup
8" to 9" (20.3 to 22.9 cm)	=	**I** cup
9" to 10" (22.9 to 25.4 cm)	=	**J** cup

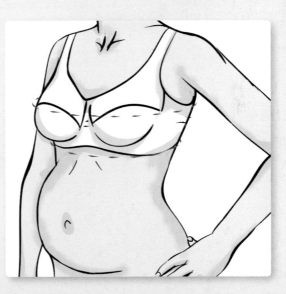

baby is born. During the first couple of weeks your breasts might go up as much as one full cup size due to breast engorgement. Purchasing a bra at this point would also lead you to buy more bras down the road as your breast milk supply regulates itself.

Getting fitted is a simple thing to do. Many maternity and nursing stores or boutiques have women who are trained to fit you for a bra. This can be helpful for many women, while others prefer to do it at home, alone. If you will be shopping at a larger store that does not have fitting assistance or if you prefer to do it at home by yourself, all you will need is a measuring tape (see page 33).

WRITE YOUR NEWBORN CARE PLAN FOR YOUR BIRTH

A newborn care plan is much like a birth plan for your new baby. You will need a newborn care plan no matter where you intend to give birth or with whom. This can be a part of your birth plan or it can be separate.

Your newborn care plan should detail the basics and specifics of the care you need for your newborn. This will also include your breastfeeding preferences. Consider adding the following:

- Where will your baby go immediately after birth?
- How long will your baby stay with you after birth?
- Where will your baby stay while you are at the hospital?

- How do you want baby care done and where?
- Are there any procedures or practices that you do not want or wish to have delayed?
- Who can hold your baby?
- What is your plan should your baby require extra medical attention?
- Do you want your baby to be given a pacifier for any reason?
- If it is deemed medically necessary for your baby to have sugar water or expressed breast milk, do you prefer that it be done via finger feeding or a cup?
- What did you learn at your breastfeeding class or on your hospital tour that might be an issue for you and your baby?

You will learn about these options and which choices you would want to make in your breastfeeding class, from other friends, and from your own experiences. There is no one right plan for every family, although certain choices are more breastfeeding friendly.

No matter what you have put into your newborn care plan, make it easy to read and friendly for your practitioners. It is best to keep your newborn care plan to one page. It should be typed if at all possible, not handwritten. Consider using bullet points to help you simplify what you have to say. This allows those reading the document to get what they need from it quickly.

Do not use a variety of fonts and colors. This can make your newborn care plan difficult to read. Some families might choose to personalize their plan with the style or color paper that it is printed on.

If you are having your baby at a hospital or birth center, find out whether you need to have your baby's care provider sign your care plan and enter it into your hospital record. Also ask to whom the care plan should be given. It is a good idea to have multiple copies made of the signed original. You might need to give it to several different staff members

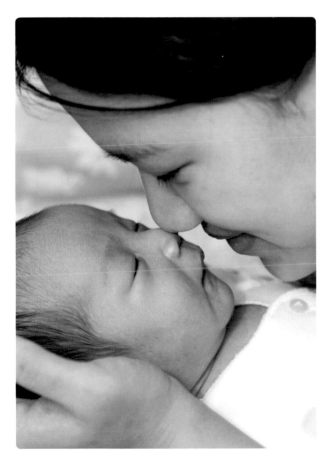

You've waited and thought about the moment you'd meet your baby for so long—enjoy it and soak it all in! Try to spend some quiet, alone time as a family before inviting visitors.

and nurses during your stay. For example, you will want someone in the labor and birth area to have a copy as well as the postpartum team who is caring for you and your baby.

If the hospital is not sure what to do with your newborn care plan, ask to give it to the head of the department. Many women will include newborn care plans with their birth plan. Some hospitals might not recognize this the same way. Simply explain what the care plan is and how it works.

DEFINE YOUR BREASTFEEDING GOALS

Breastfeeding goals are personal. There is no one right answer for anyone, but there are benchmarks. The AAP recommends that your baby receive breast milk and no other liquids or foods until the age of six months, at which point you may start solid foods if your baby is showing signs of readiness. The AAP also recommends breastfeeding for until at least one year of age, and beyond one year if that is what is comfortable for you and your family.

You might also have a personal goal that might have nothing to do with what medical professionals say about breastfeeding and its benefits. This might be related to something you saw growing up, or a personal experience. For example, if you felt like you were encouraged to wean prematurely in a previous breastfeeding experience, you may want to choose your original goal. Or perhaps you feel like your previous standards were too high and you want to choose a lower goal to help ensure that you are successful.

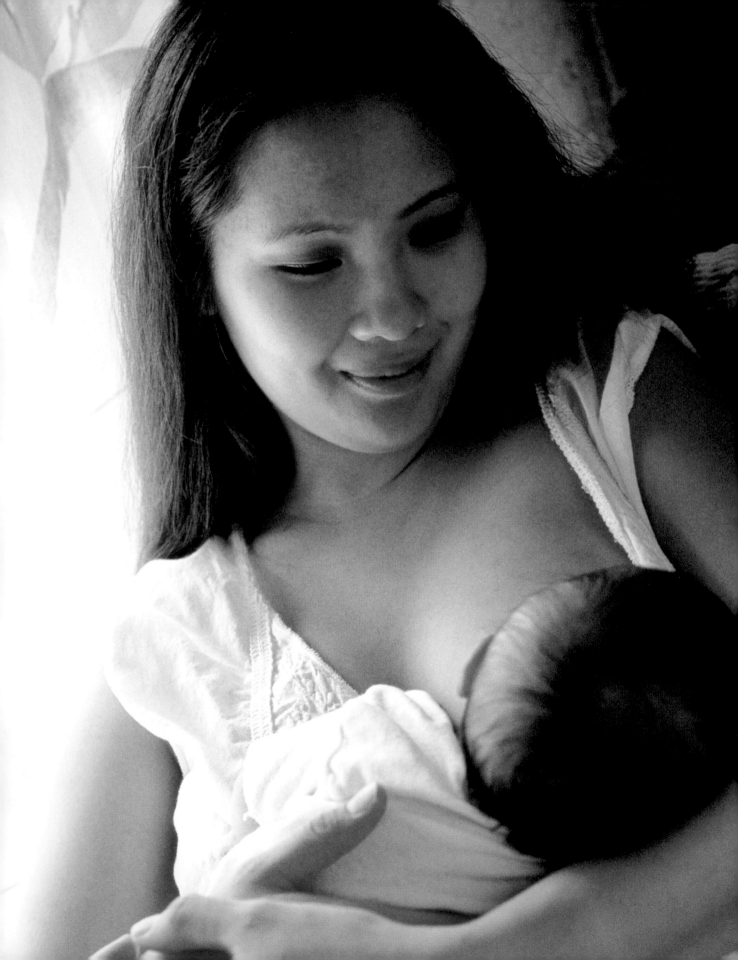

Sometimes thinking of breastfeeding in terms of a year can feel overwhelming; other times it's not a big deal. One recommendation that you might try is to take a larger goal and break it down into smaller goals. So, for example, if your goal is to breastfeed exclusively for six months, celebrate at the end of every month for a job well done!

You might even set short-term and long-term goals. Sometimes the long-term goals are a bit harder to see. Certainly, nursing a newborn is vastly different from nursing a one-year-old or toddler. You might not be able to envision what it will be like to eventually nurse an older baby or toddler, because those differences are incredibly difficult to see when you are first cradling a new baby. Take each progression in small stages and things will not feel so overwhelming. Eventually, you will get to each new step naturally, in due time.

It is also important to note that breastfeeding takes work. As someone once said to me, "I wish I would have known it wasn't peaceful and easy at first; a moonbeam from above that came down and made it all work." You and your baby have to take

Breastfeeding goals are personal, but you should go all out to reach yours and not give up. Have confidence in yourself and your baby.

CONFIDENCE CUE

It might be hard to anticipate what breastfeeding will be like as you're pregnant, if this is your first child. Of course, it's customary to be apprehensive of the unknown. But if you prepare yourself well and commit to your goal, you will be able to handle whatever comes your way. Your commitment to your choice to breastfeed is what will give you confidence in the early days, even if it takes a while to feel like you're sure of what you're doing. Get your facts straight and try to figure out where your stumbling blocks are early on. Make sure you have a support team in mind ahead of time—these people will help to make your breastfeeding experience easier for you and your baby.

the time to get to know one another, to hang out together, and to watch each other. Just as it would if you were entering into any other new relationship, this will take time and effort. You and your baby are worth it. And the effort you put in at first will pay off in spades later on. As you become a more experienced nursing mother, you will reap the benefits more clearly, and that is when you will find nursing to be easier, more enjoyable, and peaceful.

When trying to decide which goal or goals are right for you, talk to other mothers who have successful breastfeeding relationships that you would like to emulate. They can usually offer good advice that will boost and motivate you. This can help you as you formulate your plan and goals.

Once you have set your goals, you will need to find out what it will take to make them a reality. Will you need help? If so, from whom? Have you shared your goals with someone? It is particularly important to share your goals with those in your support system. This will also help guide them in the advice that they offer you when you are in need. Have you written your goals down? This can make them feel more concrete. While your goals should always be flexible, seeing them in writing might make you feel like you have more ownership over them. Know that whether your goal is to simply make it past the first feeding or the first year, you will need support.

BUILD CONFIDENCE IN BREASTFEEDING

Breastfeeding can be hard work. You really need to have a commitment to breastfeeding to make breastfeeding work for you. Can you imagine saying, "I think I will try to graduate from college." That is probably not something you would ever say. Instead, you would move forward with college, excited and filled with anticipation. And even when things got tough, you would persevere. The same holds true for breastfeeding.

To prepare for college you would study. You would look at a variety of schools. You would visit campuses. You would pick the college that fit your needs. You would look into meal plans and classes. If you ran into a problem, you would know to whom you should turn.

Self-Care Tips

Remember to take some time for yourself before your baby is born. Babies are wonderful, but they change your life in every way. Enjoy these last few months of being able to come and go as you please. And perhaps carve out some time to get away with your husband or partner, so the two of you can spend some alone time before officially beginning your new roles as parents!

Your commitment to breastfeeding is no less important. You should prepare for breastfeeding by reading books, talking to other mothers, and exploring your breastfeeding options. You should figure out ahead of time whom to turn to if you encounter difficulty. Perhaps you would even visit with lactation counselor or consultant prior to the birth of your baby. You would find social support groups for breastfeeding as well.

Saying that you will try to breastfeed undermines your confidence. It says you are worried. While it is fine and natural to be worried, take it a step further and be proactive. Surround yourself with supportive professionals such as your baby's doctor, your obstetrician or midwife, and even a lactation specialist. And just like college, building a social support network is also important. Figure out which of your friends are supportive and can offer advice to you if you hit a rough spot.

Hopefully, breastfeeding will be the equivalent of a bunny slope or easy A class for you and your baby, but if it isn't you will feel prepared to handle it. You will already have your support system in place so that you can immediately get support. You will have the confidence that you need to succeed in making the best decision for you and your baby, whether that is jumping in with both feet and signing up for the honors courses or dropping a course along the way.

Breastfeeding Affirmation

I am prepared with the confidence and knowledge to breastfeed my baby.

CHAPTER 1

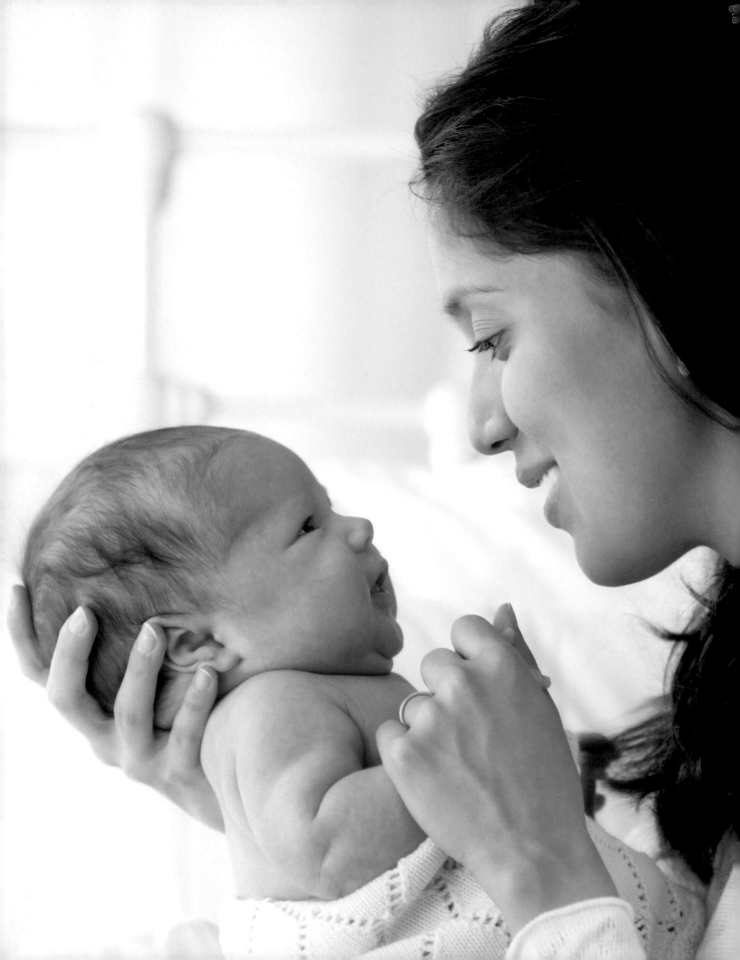

First Feedings

 ## Checklist for Successful Breastfeeding

- ☐ Discover how your breasts make milk.
- ☐ Understand how letdown occurs.
- ☐ Realize the importance of skin-to-skin contact.
- ☐ Learn to read your baby's hunger cues.
- ☐ Get a good latch with your baby.
- ☐ Watch for the elements of a good feeding.
- ☐ Recognize and deal with barriers to good feedings.
- ☐ Figure out whether your baby is getting enough breast milk.
- ☐ Learn how to tell your baby is well nourished.
- ☐ Wake a sleepy baby.
- ☐ Learn to burp a baby.
- ☐ Know how to end a feeding.
- ☐ Discover alternative feeding methods if your baby can't nurse at first.

The first feedings you have with your baby should be easy and relaxed. Think of your early moments of breastfeeding as an enjoyable learning experience rather than a "do or die" task. And don't let anyone put undue pressure on you—least of all yourself. Your ability to breastfeed will develop with patience and care. Enjoy these early moments with your baby!

Before diving into some basic tips to help you as you begin nursing your baby, read the next few sections to learn a quick lesson about the fascinating process of how your body makes milk. The various parts of your body work in a complex interplay with your hormones to create a perfect system that benefits both you and your baby. Following is your crash course Breast Milk Making 101.

DISCOVER HOW YOUR BREASTS MAKE MILK

Just as your body prepares in a variety of ways to care for and nurture your growing child when you are pregnant, so too are your breasts preparing to do their job. Regardless of whether you notice changes occurring in your breasts during pregnancy, you can be sure that your body will know what to do when the time comes! By the time you go through labor and deliver your baby, your body will send signals that trigger your breasts to begin lactation. Your baby will then take the lead, encouraging colostrum, and eventually full milk production, as she nurses at the breast.

Pregnancy

The process of milk production actually begins during pregnancy. The breast changes that are noticeable in the earliest days of gestation are actually your body prepping to breastfeed. All of these changes signal pregnancy and the impending ability to feed your baby.

During pregnancy, you might notice that your breasts are enlarging. They might be tender to the touch. You might also notice that the areola, the dark circle on your breast, is getting larger and darker. This is all due to hormonal changes.

Some of the changes are thought to be of benefit to the baby. For example, a larger and darker areola can be visually attractive to the newborn. Remember, your baby sees contrasting colors more readily than anything else. Montgomery's tubercles, or glands of Montgomery, are small white bumps that appear on your areola. These are designed to help lubricate and cleanse your nipple during pregnancy and breastfeeding.

Once you hit puberty, your mammary glands became activated by the production of estrogen. This is when you noticed that your breasts began to grow. During pregnancy, the placenta stimulates the breast tissue by producing estrogen and progesterone. The tissue in your breasts is made up of fat padding (which is why breasts come in different shapes and sizes) and a standard number of milk ducts. During pregnancy, the glandular tissue begins to replace the fatty tissue, and you can see an impressive 1 to 1.5 lb. (0.45 to 0.68 kg) gain per breast in pregnancy.

At this point, your breasts are made up of fatty tissue, glandular tissue, and milk ducts. Milk ducts are a series of pathways that increase during pregnancy in number and size. Toward the end of this channel is a ductule, connected to alveoli, which is like a small bag. This is where breast milk is actually made. A group of the alveoli is called a lobule. A group of lobules is called a lobe. There are between fifteen and twenty lobes, and each connects to a milk duct. Each duct has a tiny opening in your nipple, like multiple little channels ending at the tip. So when your baby nurses, she gets multiple small

Anatomy of a Breast

The breast is located between the second and sixth rib, with tissue extending to the *axilla*, or armpit. The breast is on top of the *pectoralis major* and *pectoralis minor* chest muscles and consists of fatty tissue, connective tissue, lymphatics, nerves, and blood vessels.

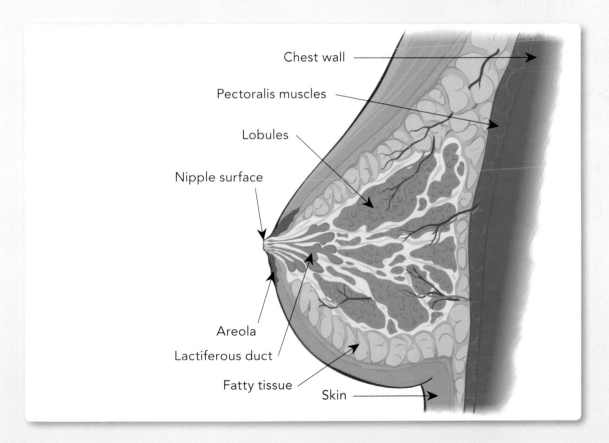

Chest wall

Pectoralis muscles

Lobules

Nipple surface

Areola

Lactiferous duct

Fatty tissue

Skin

streams of milk all at once. This intricate system matures during pregnancy. The pathways are completed by the time you are well into your second trimester. That way, should your baby be born early, your body is ready to breastfeed.

Birth

When you give birth, the placenta, which has been secreting estrogen and progesterone, is expelled. This causes your levels of estrogen and progesterone to drop suddenly. Your body responds with the production of prolactin. This motherly hormone helps your body to begin milk production usually within three days of expelling the placenta. Even a fragment of placenta left in place can hinder milk production.

UNDERSTAND HOW LETDOWN OCCURS

The term *letdown* refers to the hormonal dance that happens as milk is released for suckling. It typically starts when your baby begins to nurse. The stimulation of the areola tells the pituitary gland to release oxytocin as well as prolactin. These hormones cause the milk to be ejected, known as the milk ejection reflex (MER) or letdown.

During letdown, a mother might notice that her breasts feel odd. Some women describe it as a prickly or tingly feeling. Other mothers say they feel warmth on their breasts and can feel the milk releasing. Sometimes you might notice letdown if you hear your baby crying, you think about your baby, or you are due for a feeding. This is why thinking of

your baby can sometimes help with milk production when using a breast pump. One breast often leaks when you are feeding on the other side. Sometimes you might even notice a forceful spray, depending on the force of the letdown.

Don't worry if you don't feel your milk let down, however. It is also normal not to notice the letdowns at all. Sensations vary greatly among women, and just because you don't feel your milk letting down doesn't mean you are not producing plenty of it!

REALIZE THE IMPORTANCE OF SKIN-TO-SKIN CONTACT

Now that you know about the physical process of breastfeeding, it's time to dive into how to get started with your baby. Perhaps most importantly,

Good News about Breastfeeding and Postpartum Cramping

The oxytocin that is released while you are nursing might cause you to notice some cramping or even a slight increase in your postpartum bleeding for a few days. That is because oxytocin also contracts the uterus. This is perfectly normal, even healthy, as the cramping that breastfeeding sparks helps your uterus to shrink back to its normal prepregnancy size and placement.

this involves, quite literally, getting close and staying close with your baby.

Skin-to-skin contact has many benefits, but the one mothers talk about over and over is simply the joy of the physical experience of holding your newborn close to your body. You have waited a long time to hold your baby on the outside, and that time has come. Merely holding your baby does a lot for breastfeeding. Holding your baby leads to earlier and more frequent breastfeeding, which can lead to a better milk supply. In addition to stimulating milk production and encouraging your baby to nurse, you will also see some of the following benefits from skin-to-skin contact:

- Babies stay warmer skin to skin with mom than anywhere else.
- Close contact helps to facilitate early bonding between mother and baby.
- It can help with physical healing for mother.
- It will calm the baby.

The American Academy of Pediatrics (AAP) recommends that babies and mothers be together in the first hour after birth to promote early breastfeeding. Babies who latch on during this period often latch on much better than babies who did not latch during this period. Although unhurried time to latch, nurse, and get to know one another is optimal, breastfeeding can still be successful without this time; it is simply more of an uphill battle for some mother/infant couples.

How you set up skin-to-skin time is what will help you to make breastfeeding successful. First of all, you should have your shirt open or off. Your baby should be naked or be wearing only a diaper. (This also means no mittens, as your baby will orient herself with her hands, as well as no headbands because they can be in the way.) A hat is a good idea for newborns, however, since they lose a lot of body heat through their heads. Once your baby is resting on your body, cover yourself and your baby with a blanket or towel. Do not wrap it too tightly around either of you; simply lay it on top. Give your baby room to move and wiggle.

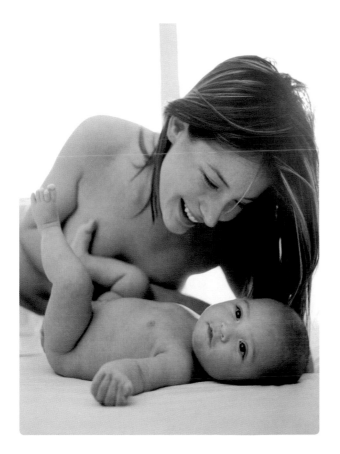

After giving birth, skin-to-skin contact is so important. It not only helps with bonding but can help you with breastfeeding.

LEARN TO READ YOUR BABY'S HUNGER CUES

While it is easy to believe that we do not know much about babies, the truth is that babies actually give us a lot of information that we need to help them thrive. Your baby's feeding cues are some of the first and most important things you will need to learn as a parent. The feeding cues your baby will display fall into two categories: early feeding cues and late feeding cues.

Early Feeding Cues

Being able to respond to early feeding cues will help to ensure that your baby is best able to respond to you and to latch well to your breast. These cues are often the same for most infants.

- Hands come to baby's mouth.
- Baby might suck on hand, tongue, lip, and so forth.
- Eyes might flutter if closed or dart around if open.
- Baby might flex arms.
- Baby's body might be rigid.
- Baby might bob head and root with an open mouth on mom's arm, shoulder, and so on.

You might also notice that your baby makes certain noises when he is hungry. Or if you touch your baby's cheek and he "attacks," he might be looking for your breast.

Responding to these cues as soon as you notice them is optimal. This is one of the many reasons why being physically close to your baby in the first weeks is key to breastfeeding success.

Late Feeding Cues

The one feeding cue that people typically recognize is a baby crying. While most people believe this to be an early sign of hunger, it is not at all. It is actually a very late feeding cue. What starts as a whimper can quickly turn into screaming. As your baby's crying escalates, it is almost impossible to quickly and easily calm him down to get a feeding going.

If your baby has already started to cry and needs to be calmed, do that before trying to feed him. Hold your baby skin to skin to see if that will calm him. Also offer a clean finger to allow your baby to calm down that way. Some babies will prefer

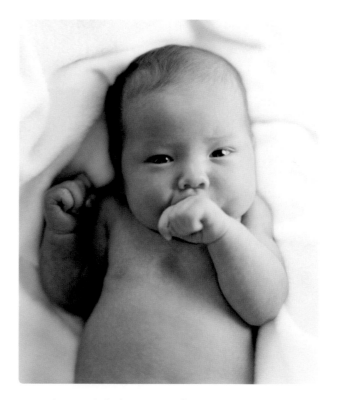

Responding to early feeding cues provides the best opportunity for you and your baby to have a relaxed breastfeeding experience.

to be swaddled, at least for the time during which they are trying to calm themselves down with your help. Once your baby has calmed down, you can begin the feeding.

It is important to remember that all babies cry, and that they cry for many reasons. One of the following just might be the reason:

- Overstimulated
- Tired
- Bored
- In pain
- Soiled
- Lonely

As you pay attention to your baby's mannerisms, you will soon be able to tell what your baby needs. Some parents do this by the sound or tone of the baby's cry. Other parents figure it out based on their history with the baby. Either way, you will soon understand more of what your baby needs.

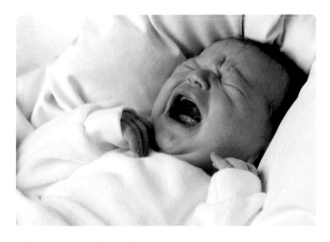

Calm your baby and consider the reasons he may have gotten to the point of crying. Try comforting and swaddling him before beginning a feeding.

Cue Feeding

Cue feeding is a method whereby your baby and your body work together to create a harmonious relationship between the breast milk your baby needs to thrive and the breast milk your body produces. By following your baby's lead and listening to your body, you are more likely to have the best milk supply possible, particularly in the early days of nursing. If you try to schedule feedings, particularly now, you will find that both your baby and your milk supply can be in trouble.

Babies fed according to a clock, rather than their innate needs, are more likely to suffer from failure to thrive, an inability to gain weight appropriately, or even loss of weight. It is important to remember that the basis of your milk supply starts now, and your baby is designed to set that system up. There will be plenty of time later when your baby's feeding demands are not so great, but for now, during the newborn period, that is not the case.

Remember, your baby's body is made to take in smaller, frequent feedings, which is why it is so critical that he nurses frequently, without adhering to a set schedule. The first feedings your body makes, your colostrum, fit that bill perfectly. The colostrum is rich in protein and antibodies and helps ready your baby for the next feeding. Even if your breasts don't feel full of milk, you will have colostrum. Your baby needs this precious liquid in only small doses. Remember, your baby has never been hungry before birth. Your body nourished your baby around the clock. So the concept of needing to eat is new for your baby. Consuming just a little bit at each feeding will go a long way.

WOMEN'S WISDOM:

Getting the baby to the breast early and often can solve almost any problem. Be sure to have plenty of undisturbed time just to hold your baby skin to skin as you learn to nurse. To get the best possible breastfeeding outcome, forget the clock, and just tune in to your baby. Work toward being calm together before attempting to nurse, and remember that crying is a late sign of hunger. Catch your baby before he gets to that point. Tips for a smooth feeding:

- Get anything you need ahead of time (pillow, drink, etc.).
- Calm yourself.
- Calm your baby.
- Remember, the first weeks of feeding might require quiet or alone time.
- Let your baby lead the feeding.
- Enjoy this time with your baby!

A good latch is the key to success in your breastfeeding connection. Your baby will nurse successfully and you will avoid soreness.

GET A GOOD LATCH WITH YOUR BABY

A good latch is a key to success in your breastfeeding relationship. It will be your clue to how well your baby is nursing, which will also speak to how much breast milk your baby is getting. Your baby's latch can also cause you a lot of pain if it is not done correctly. That being said, sometimes latch is over-analyzed. Your baby really does have an instinct to latch on and to do it well. You just need the tools to help your baby latch effectively.

Your First Feeding

Skin-to-skin time right after birth is the ideal time to get your baby to latch on. Placing her between your breasts provides the best chance for her to try to nurse. This is because your baby will instinctively try to find your breast from this position. Talk to your baby and stroke her back. This will probably come very naturally. As you are doing so, watch your baby. At first you might notice that your baby just lies on your chest. Then you might notice that she is wiggling and moving.

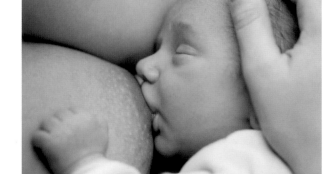

Latch a Calm Baby, Not a Crying One

Latching is always easiest and best when you start with a baby who is calm. Look for your baby's early feeding cues, and get her to the breast before she is crying or upset.

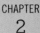

CHAPTER 2

Give your baby as much freedom to move and wiggle as possible. Often, when we try to "help" we mess up a good thing. Your baby will typically wiggle or even drop down toward a breast. Support your baby as she searches for your breast, but do not be tempted to take the lead. Your job is to keep your baby warm and safe. Do not let her fall, but do allow her to move downward.

Babies might find the nipple all by themselves. Let your baby explore. You can move your arms so that they are out of the way. This might help your baby. Your baby might open and close her mouth. You might hear her lips smacking. These are all normal behaviors as your baby prepares to latch on.

Your baby's head might begin to bob as she looks for your breast. This is normal. If you are holding your baby too tightly or not allowing her head to move, she might have trouble finding your breast. As your baby starts to choose a side, you can follow her, but do not lead her to one side or the other. Help her to stay calm by supporting her bottom with your

arm tucked around it. Place your hand lightly on the center of her back. Do not apply so much pressure that you prevent her from moving; apply just enough to keep her neck safe.

Your baby will most likely approach your breast chin first. Your baby will know your breast by feel. Do not panic; both of you need to be calm and unrushed.

Your baby's nose will be at your nipple. Her mouth should open wide, to latch onto the areola, not just the tip of your nipple. You can gently help your baby if she is not taking your nipple into her mouth, but be careful to let her have enough freedom to move. Just make sure she can still be safe. You should never force your baby onto your breast. There should be no sudden or forced movements.

Sometimes your baby will get fussy. This can be because you missed feeding cues and your baby is now really hungry. It can also be because your baby feels cold, frightened, or rushed, or it can be due to any number of other reasons. For your baby to associate your breast with only positive experiences, promptly remove her if she is crying at the breast. Bring her back to an upright position so that you are heart to heart with your baby.

You can calm a fussy baby in a number of ways. You can talk to her in a calm voice, stroke her, and offer a calm presence. You might also offer a clean finger for your baby to suck on for a minute. This is often all it takes for a baby to calm down. Then allow the baby to find the breast again.

This method of latching on will work for any feeding. As you and your baby become more comfortable with breastfeeding, it will not take any time

A Good Latch

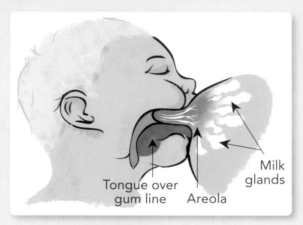

Tongue over gum line   Areola   Milk glands

A Perfect Latch

The perfect latch is not painful. You can see that your baby has a good seal around the breast and it should be fairly quiet, with only the sound of swallowing possibly being heard—no slurping or clicking. You may also notice that your baby's ears move as he nurses.

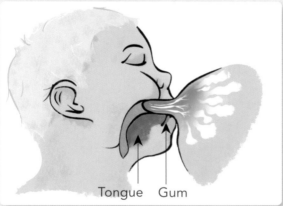

Tongue   Gum

Too Little

You will often hear people mistakenly say that your baby needs to get the whole areola in his mouth. The truth is that there are some women who have very large areolas that don't fit inside the baby's mouth. What is behind this is that your baby needs to have the entire nipple and a good bit of tissue from the areola in his mouth to adequately receive breast milk.

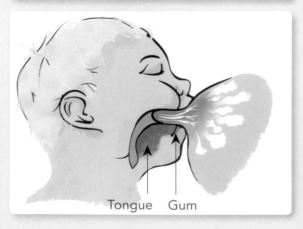

Tongue   Gum

Tongue Not Over the Gum Line

Your baby needs to stick his tongue out over the gum line. This helps him get breast milk, but it also protects your breast tissue form rubbing on the gum line, which can make your breast very sore.

at all. And soon you will be able to just offer your baby the breast, without repeating the other steps. You can deal with many breastfeeding problems by heading back to these basics.

What a Good Latch Feels Like and Looks Like

A good latch is not painful. Some mothers will describe a good latch as a rhythmic tugging as the baby nurses. Your breasts might tingle as your breast milk lets down.

If you feel pain, burning, piercing, or anything that is painful, stop. Break the baby's suction carefully by popping your little finger into the corner of your baby's mouth, as you would to end a feeding. Start the process over again. How well your baby breastfeeds in general will determine where you start the process, from the beginning of the previous description, or just at the point of trying to relatch. Let your baby's skills be your guide.

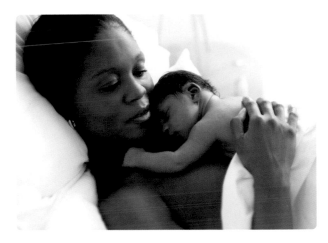

Take your time when feeding your newborn. Relaxation sends a positive message to your baby and will ensure success as you become more confident in your role as a breastfeeding mother.

A proper latch means your baby has a good portion of the areola in her mouth. The amount might look lopsided because of an asymmetrical latch. You will also notice that your areola is larger or smaller than other women's areolas. This will affect how much of the areola the baby takes into her mouth.

You should not hear any slurping or clicking, as such sounds are a sign that your baby has a potentially painful or ineffective latch. If you do hear these noises, you will want to break the suction and try to relatch your baby into a better latch. Sometimes you can hear a baby swallow; that is not a problem. If you have a question, ask your lactation professional.

As your baby nurses, you should be able to see her ear wiggle from the proper movement of the jaw. You might notice she will take breaks in the nursing. This is normal and to be expected. As your baby first latches on she might suck very quickly, and after a minute or so her sucks might turn into a longer, more drawn-out pattern. This has to do with your breast milk and how it lets down. You should hear your baby swallow every few sucks. In this way, you'll be able to recognize that she is getting a good amount of milk.

WATCH FOR THE ELEMENTS OF A GOOD FEEDING

A good feeding will be an unhurried affair. Ideally, both mother and baby should be as relaxed as possible. But not every feeding will always be like this for every mother and baby, particularly if there is a learning curve at first or a breastfeeding issue that complicates matters.

Growth Spurts

During a growth spurt, your baby will experience a large amount of growth in a short period of time. This growth can be developmental, such as when he is mastering a new skill, or it can be weight or length related. You will typically know that a growth spurt is coming because for forty-eight to seventy-two hours your baby will nurse more frequently. Remember, nursing more frequently is how your baby regulates your breast milk supply. More frequent nursing tells your body that you need to increase your production of breast milk. After those time periods, your breasts have responded with more milk and your baby eases back, typically into the previous habits that had been established.

Growth spurts are more common at three weeks, six weeks, three months, and six months of age. Obviously, some babies will be a bit ahead or behind this schedule. If it feels as though your baby is nursing all the time and you can't figure out why, a growth spurt might be the culprit.

When nursing your baby, don't watch the clock! Your baby should decide how long to nurse. You should offer both breasts at every feeding. Most babies will nurse from both breasts at every feeding, although some babies prefer to feed from a single breast at each feeding.

Cluster Feeding

Since newborns eat often at first, you will have plenty of time to practice. Remember, as a new mom your first and most important job is to feed your baby! Granted, it can be hard not to stress about other things—such as cleaning the house, doing the laundry, figuring out dinner, and so on. But try to let that slide a bit—at least for a little while. During your baby's first month (or more), he'll need to eat at least eight to twelve times in a twenty-four hour period. Neither your baby nor your breasts can read a clock, so don't agonize over whether your baby is eating in evenly spaced intervals, because that's not how breastfeeding works.

Instead of nursing according to a set pattern, your baby might do what is known as cluster feeding. This means you might find your baby will want to eat at more frequent intervals for part of the day. This can last for a few days or simply be the feeding pattern that works with your baby's growth pattern. These frequent feedings are not a sign that your baby is not getting enough breast milk. In fact, cluster-feeding periods usually mean your baby is fueling up on a lot of milk. Then, all of those back-to-back feedings are typically followed by a longer period of rest for the baby.

RECOGNIZE AND DEAL WITH BARRIERS TO GOOD FEEDINGS

Certain things can make breastfeeding more difficult. To begin to address the issues, you need to be aware of them:

- Pain from giving birth or breastfeeding
- Tension or being upset (meaning either mother or baby is upset or tense)
- Too many other people in the room
- Uncomfortable surroundings (e.g., the temperature is too hot or cold, the room isn't relaxing or comforting, the furniture is too hard, etc.)
- Physical problem with the baby (e.g., tongue tie, cleft lip, etc.)
- Physical problem with the mother (thrush, blocked ducts, mastitis, etc.)
- Sleepy baby
- Improper latch
- Lack of support

Preparing for breastfeeding can help you overcome these barriers. When you are in the middle of breastfeeding it can seem a bit harder to deal with everything that is thrown at you. These feelings are fairly normal in the early postpartum days, which is why you'll need good support. (Read on in chapter 4 for detailed guidance on finding and building your support system!) Try to plan ahead when possible, although, of course, you won't be able to anticipate

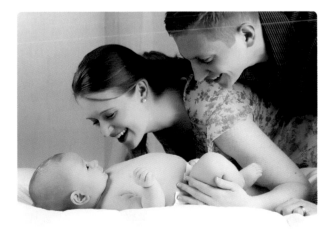

Breastfeeding is a family affair. Although only mom can breastfeed, the support and love she gets from her partner is crucial to the success of breastfeeding.

Release Tension

If you are tense when trying to nurse, it can become an obstacle for you and your baby. Your baby will pick up on your tension and, in turn, will not feel comfortable or be able to relax while nursing. Try these techniques to enhance your nursing sessions: First, make sure you are sitting in a comfortable place. Be aware of your body positioning—relax your neck and shoulders. Sit back, and don't hunch forward. Try setting up a nursing station in your home, with a comfortable chair, a small table, and some favorite items to pass the time, such as books or magazines. You'll feel like you have a space of your own to go to when nursing.

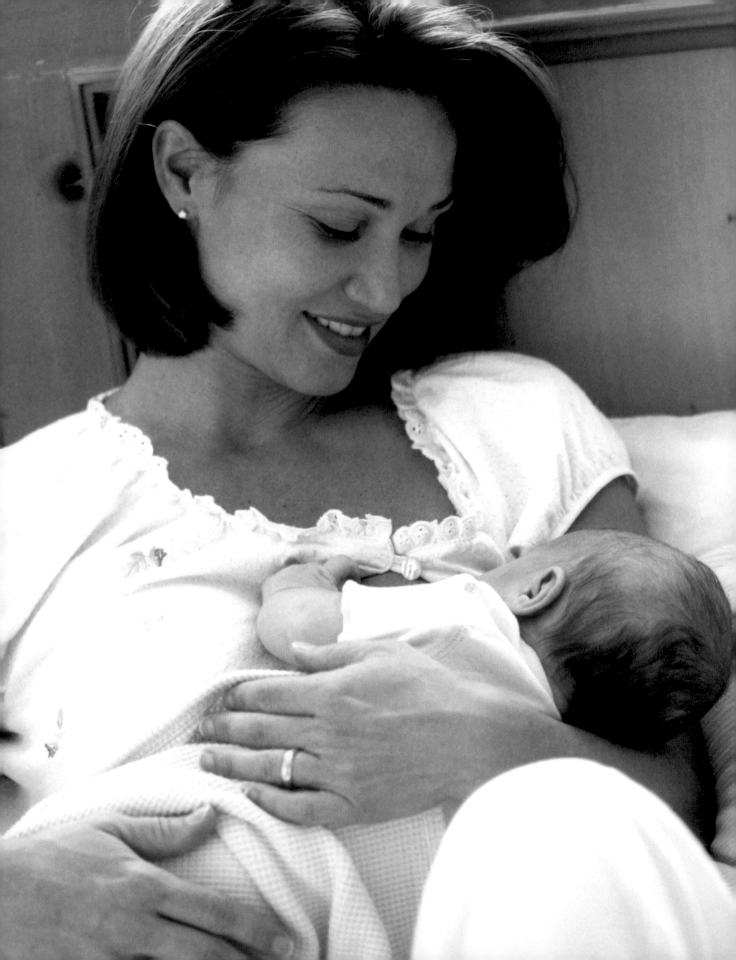

everything that will come your way in these early days of breastfeeding. The key is to recognize a barrier as early as possible, and then do what you can to overcome it.

So, for example, if you're in pain after giving birth, be sure to address that with medication or in some other way. This might mean taking the time to create a medication schedule that keeps you pain free and reminds you to take your medication on time. It might mean taking time to have a sitz bath every day.

If your baby is having problems, seek help from others who are knowledgeable. This might mean seeking support from a specialist or simply talking to another mother who had a baby with a similar difficulty. Sometimes just getting a bit of validation and knowing that others have thrived in your situation, can make all the difference in the world.

Remember, most of these barriers are temporary. You can work toward a solution with help from others. Patience and time are key ingredients in your breastfeeding relationship.

Be Gentle with Yourself and Your Baby

Your breastfeeding expectations might or might not match what your breastfeeding experience actually turns out to be. You might be recovering from a rough birth physically or emotionally. This can make breastfeeding more difficult. Perhaps you and your baby were separated after birth. Even if this was medically necessary, it can start your breastfeeding experience off on the wrong foot. If this has been your experience, don't despair! You can still get breastfeeding back on track—but it just might take more work than you had hoped it would.

Whatever the issues you're dealing with, the key is to be gentle with yourself and your baby. Remind yourself of your breastfeeding goals. Remind yourself that road bumps can happen. Remember that people are available to help you. Most breastfeeding problems can be resolved quickly with professional help and patience.

Once you and your baby get the hang of good feeding techniques, life will get a lot easier for both of you. When your baby starts to show signs of hunger, you'll be able to respond rapidly. This will decrease the time it takes to feed your baby, and it will also boost your confidence in both your breastfeeding and your mothering ability.

FIGURE OUT WHETHER YOUR BABY IS GETTING ENOUGH BREAST MILK

Measuring things seems to be human nature. One thing that breastfeeding mothers repeatedly wonder is how much milk is going into their baby's stomach. While the exact number of ounces is not easy to discern, there are ways you can tell whether your baby is getting enough breast milk.

The First Few Days

Your baby's true need for breast milk in the first few days is minimal. The colostrum that is present in your breasts is adequate for your baby's nutritional needs. In addition, this thick, golden substance can help your baby with a boost in immunities. It will also help your baby to pass meconium.

Meconium is a thick, dark, tarry substance that has lined your baby's intestines in utero. After birth, the meconium will begin to pass. As your baby drinks more and more breast milk, the meconium will pass more quickly. You will notice that the color of your baby's stool goes from black to green to mustard yellow. The consistency of the stool will also become looser. Don't worry; these stools are not diarrhea. These lighter-colored stools should begin by day three. This passing of meconium and change in stool color and consistency is a good indicator that your baby is getting ample amounts of breast milk.

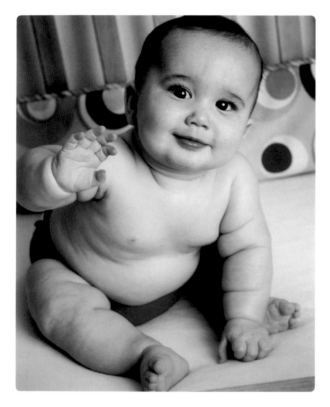

Weight gain is one way to tell if your baby is getting enough breast milk. Remember that all babies gain differently—some babies look plump, while others do not—yet both are well-fed.

At the end of the first week, your baby should be having two or three dirty diapers per day. The rest of the diapers should be wet. Your baby will be having two to three wet diapers at the beginning of the week, and more later. It can be more difficult to tell whether disposable diapers are wet, even if they're the fancy ones with wetness indicators built in. If the diaper does not feel wet, the best way to tell is to squeeze the disposable material between your fingers. If it feels squishy, you know it's saturated with urine.

The First Few Weeks

As weeks pass, your baby might go down to one large bowel movement per day or you might see your baby pass stool at every feeding. If your baby does not have a bowel movement on a near-daily basis, that can be a sign that he is not getting enough milk.

Your baby should also have six to eight wet cloth diapers per day or five to six wet disposable diapers per day. If you have trouble telling whether your baby is wet or whether a diaper is wet enough to count as a wet diaper, pour 3 tablespoons (45 ml) of water into a clean diaper. Feel the weight of the diaper, and then you can learn to compare that weight to your baby's subsequent diapers.

Questions to Ask Yourself

You will also want to assess your baby's milk intake by asking yourself the following questions:

- Does my baby nurse eight to twelve times per day?

- Does my baby spend at least twenty minutes at each feeding?
- Do I let my baby decide how long to nurse?
- Is my baby gaining 4 to 7 ounces (0.11 to 0.2 kg) per week after the first few days of life?
- Does my baby have an adequate diaper pattern?

The following methods are not good ways to tell whether your baby is getting enough milk:

- Feeling your breasts to determine how "full" they are (just because your breasts don't feel full does not mean your baby is not getting milk; once your baby begins nursing, he will stimulate your breasts to let down more milk)

- Watching how much you can or can't hand-express or pump (babies are naturally more effective at drawing milk from the breast and, therefore, drink more than you might see from a pump session)
- Relying on how much or how little your baby sleeps (often, a baby who sleeps too much is actually becoming lethargic and not drinking enough milk)
- Observing baby's behavior (changes in your baby's behavior—e.g., baby is sleepier, is not sleeping enough, is suddenly always awake and alert, or is crying a lot and is unusually fussy—don't necessarily mean he's not getting enough milk)

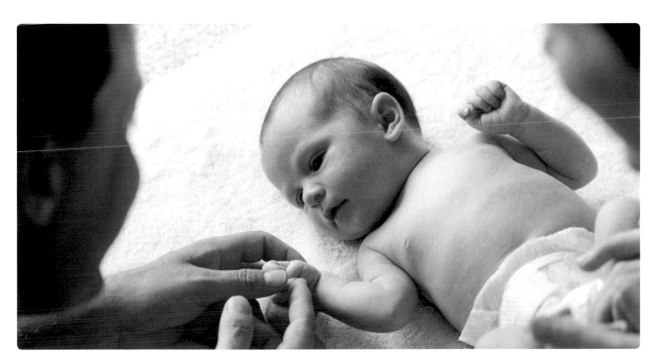

The first weeks are an important time to get to know your baby and for your baby to get to know you. Make use of this time. Soak everything in while you have this once-in-a-lifetime chance.

If you ever have questions about the amount of milk your baby is taking in, please ask someone for help. Your local lactation professional will be happy to help you make that assessment, and can refer you to your pediatrician if medical support is needed. It is also better to ask for help early on than to wait until a minor problem becomes a bigger issue.

LEARN HOW TO TELL YOUR BABY IS WELL NOURISHED

We all want what is best for our babies. In the early days, a newborn's only real job is to grow. To grow, your newborn baby attaches to you both emotionally and physically. Through the act of breastfeeding, your baby grows, gaining weight and length.

In the preceding section, you learned ways to recognize whether your baby is getting enough milk in the early days of breastfeeding. But how do you tell whether your baby is well nourished as time goes on? It is not practical or desirable to weigh or measure your baby every day; fortunately, you can tell whether your baby is growing in other ways.

CONFIDENCE CUE

When it comes to breastfeeding, expect to get conflicting information from health professionals. Many are not trained in breastfeeding specifically and have only anecdotal information that doesn't necessarily translate into real life at home—meaning they don't really know whether it works or not. Be leery of advice that doesn't feel right or sounds at odds with what you know. Find a trusted source, your lactation professional, a breastfeeding-knowledgeable physician, or friend, to corroborate that information. Most of all, trust yourself as a mother.

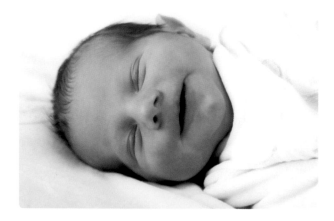

There are many things that indicate that your baby is well-fed. You should observe periods of alertness as well as peaceful sleep.

What a Well-Nourished Baby Looks Like

A baby who is getting enough breast milk is easy to spot in most cases. You will notice periods of activity and alertness, mixed with periods of restful sleep. Now, that sleep might not be as lengthy or as often as you would like, but that is normal.

Your baby's nursing pattern might give you more of a clue than anything else. Watch your baby nurse. Do you see your baby's movements as she nurses? Watch her mouth for the open, pause, and close of the suck cycle. When your baby's mouth opens, she is creating suction and drawing the milk that has been massaged out of your breast. When she pauses, she is gathering that milk. When her mouth closes, it indicates the swallow portion of the cycle. Sometimes you can hear your baby swallowing, but not always.

Things That Don't Really Tell You What's Going On

The problem with trying to judge how well a baby is nursing is that we often try to use a bunch of measurements that do not really tell us much, let alone how well our baby is taking in breast milk. You cannot tell how well your baby is nursing by judging her temperament, for example. A baby who cries after feeding might need to be burped, or may have any number of issues that are not related to the amount of milk she has taken in. This is one of the biggest breastfeeding fallacies.

Also, don't use how much milk you get while pumping as a basis for judging how much milk your baby is getting. While a good breast pump typically does a good job of pumping breast milk, a pump will simply never be as effective at drawing out milk as your baby is. You also need to consider the age and style of the pump, the timing of the pumping, and other factors. How much you pump is simply not a good indication of what your baby is getting while nursing.

And just because your baby eats frequently is also not a good reason to believe she is not getting enough breast milk. Some babies simply eat frequently. Biological reasons might be causing your baby to need smaller, more frequent meals. Or perhaps your baby is signaling a growth spurt and is nursing to help you increase your breast milk supply. You might also have a baby who prefers to cluster-feed at times. So if you look at your baby's feedings patterns, you might find that she is nursing more frequently for short periods over the course of several hours, and then going for a longer stretch of time before nursing again later.

Once again, keep in mind that feeling how "full" your breasts are is definitely not a good way to assess the amount of milk you are producing. Sometimes it is easy to fall into the trap of trying to measure the amount of milk by the size or shape of your breasts after a feeding. This is to say that you might expect that a breast, right after a feeding, would be lighter due to the lowered volume of milk. This is not true. It's more that you probably got accustomed to the feeling of engorgement, and once you no longer are engorged, it might feel as though you have less milk. But really, your body is just sending milk through the breast as your baby needs it.

CHAPTER
2

WAKE A SLEEPY BABY

Although it might be hard to believe in the midst of seemingly sleepless nights with your newborn, sometimes babies really do get sleepy, and they even fall asleep. This can make nursing them until they are full a bit harder. Babies are sleepy for various reasons. After the first hour following birth, your baby might take a very serious nap. (It stands to reason, after all. Just think of how exhausted a tiny baby must be after going through all the work it takes to emerge through the birth canal.) During this deep sleep, it is really difficult to rouse your baby to nurse. You should offer the breast by being skin to skin to see whether your baby stirs.

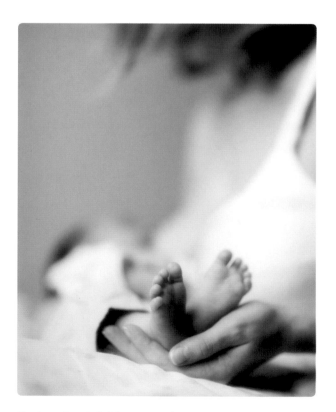

Gently moving a baby's feet is one wake to wake a sleepy baby before or during a feeding.

After this period, your baby might be sleepy for different reasons. Sometimes babies are sleepy from jaundice. Your baby might also be sleepy from pain medications that you are taking. Nursing is also hard work for tiny babies, and they can become tired from all of the sucking and swallowing they're doing. Often, babies become so relaxed while nursing that they simply doze off mid-nurse, only to wake shortly after to resume nursing once again. (These are the little ones who are sometimes jokingly referred to as the "lazy suckers"!) And babies are even occasionally sleepy because they are not getting enough breast milk. If you think you have the world's best baby because your baby sleeps all the time, chances are you need to talk to your lactation professional or pediatrician.

To wake a baby who needs to eat, you can try several tricks. One trick is to undress the baby. Being cold can often stimulate the baby into being awake. Some babies will wake up as soon as you start stripping them down.

If stripping your baby down does not work, there are plenty of other tricks to try. You can take a cool wash cloth or wipe and start to wash your baby's face or body. You might also thump on the bottoms of your baby's feet, massage his back, or stroke his cheek to wake him up. You might also use your hand to wiggle your breast slightly from side to side to stimulate your baby to resume sucking. Avoid touching the back of your baby's head. If you do, your baby will most likely release the latch as a reflex. As you get to know your baby, you will learn what wakes him up with great regularity.

Waking a baby so that he can nurse is important. Not only will it help to initiate more nursing sessions, but your baby will also be more likely to nurse well when he is awake. These tricks will come in handy during these first few weeks when being awake is a key to nursing success. If you find yourself getting sick of having to wake your sleeping baby continually, don't fret. This sleepy phase will pass. After a while, you'll find your baby has learned to multitask and can eat while falling asleep, and even while sleeping.

LEARN TO BURP A BABY

Crying after a feeding might be a sign that your baby needs better burping. The purpose of burping is to help your baby expel any air that is in her system. This air gets taken in while eating. Although breastfed babies require less burping than bottle-fed babies, because they take in less air, you will want to try to burp your baby after every feeding until you learn what your baby needs at each feeding. Some babies need lots of burping, while other babies need very little.

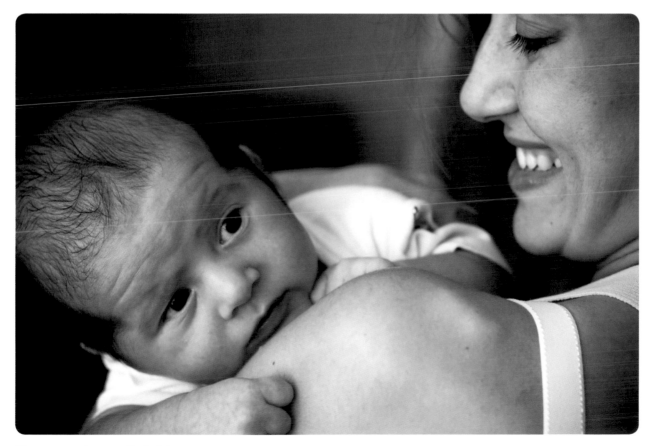

There are several ways to effectively burp a baby. Find the method that works best for your baby at the proper stage of their development.

The Best Burping Techniques

Burping your baby is an important step in assuring their comfort and contentment. If a baby is not properly burped, it can lead toirritability, sleep disturbances, or spitting up. Be patient with this essential process. It becomes easier as your baby grows stronger.

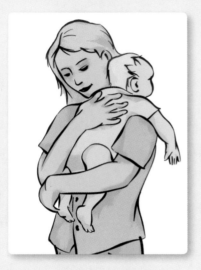

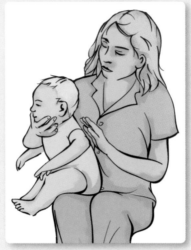

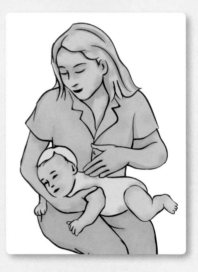

Hold your baby over your shoulder while supporting his neck. Apply gentle pressure against his abdomen by rubbing and patting his back until he expels the excess gas.

Position your baby in a seated position supporting her head by cupping her chin in your hand, depending on how much neck strength she has achieved. Her legs should be extended forward. Pat and rub her back until she is able to pass the excess gas.

Drape the baby across your lap with your legs crossed or spread so that pressure it applied against his tummy. Support the baby with one hand while you rub his back with the other until the gas is expelled.

When you think of burping a baby, the classic position that comes to mind is one in which the baby is placed over the shoulder. This can certainly be an effective way to burp a baby. This is particularly true in the early weeks when your baby does not have a lot of head and neck control. This burp hold gives you a lot more control. It's a good idea to throw a burp cloth over your shoulder, and be sure it extends down a bit toward your back. This will protect you and your clothing should your baby spit up.

Place your baby's head a bit over your right or left shoulder. With your hand on the same side, wrap your arm around your baby's bottom. Using your opposite hand pat your baby firmly between the shoulder blades in an upward motion. This will hopefully dislodge any air.

While over the shoulder might seem like the most obvious burping method, other positions are equally effective. You can also hold your baby on your lap to burp her. Place your baby in a sitting position on your lap. Place one hand under your baby's chin while you lean your baby slightly forward. Have a burp cloth in the hand that's holding your baby's chin. Use your other hand to tap gently using upward strokes on your baby's back.

A third way that is actually a bit easier with tiny babies is between your thighs. Using your thighs, gently grasp your baby at the waist. Place a burp cloth over your thigh in the direction that the baby is facing. Use one hand to hold the baby up slightly under the chin; use your other hand to gently burp the baby.

How long it takes to burp really depends on the baby. Some babies will burp as soon as they sit up, while others take a while. You can quit burping after a few minutes if nothing is coming up. You will also grow to know whether your baby takes a short or long period to burp. Some babies will outgrow the need to be burped. Other babies require burping for a while.

KNOW HOW TO END A FEEDING

Ideally, the best way to know that a feeding session with your baby has ended is that he has stopped nursing and has released your nipple from his mouth. The baby will no longer be rooting and actively trying to be fed.

Sometimes you will need to end a feeding or even simply break a latch because it is painful or feels "wrong." To do so, gently insert a clean finger just into the corner of your baby's mouth. You might

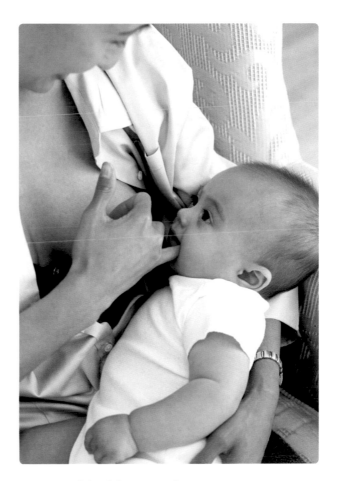

Be sure to gently break the suction with your finger when ending a feeding or your nipples will become sore very quickly.

hear the suction break, or you might not. You can then relatch your baby or do whatever you need to do. Whatever you do, do not try to pull your breast out of your baby's mouth without first breaking the latch, as this will be quite painful!

You should only infrequently need to end a feeding before your baby is done. It is important for your milk supply and your baby's weight gain and satisfaction to know that your baby is getting enough milk. Babies need both foremilk—the thinner, lower-fat milk the baby gets first—and hindmilk, the higher-fat, creamier milk that flows after foremilk. Foremilk is rich in the carbohydrate lactose, which babies need for energy and brain development, while hindmilk's fat calories are important for growth. If you end a feeding prematurely, you might find that your baby does not get adequate amounts of both foremilk and hindmilk.

DISCOVER ALTERNATIVE FEEDING METHODS IF YOUR BABY CAN'T NURSE AT FIRST

Sometimes babies cannot or do not nurse immediately after birth. The most frequent reason this can happen is that you and your baby are separated due to a medical need for you or your baby, or because of hospital scheduling. You might also have a baby who has a medical issue that makes breastfeeding more difficult, such as an oral anomaly (tongue tie, cleft palate, etc.). In rare occasions, a newborn will simply refuse to latch on. This is sometimes related to birth trauma or even vigorous sucking at birth, but sometimes there is no obvious cause.

If you have a baby who is not nursing well, you must first make sure your baby is fed. Ensure that your baby is fed your breast milk in the way that is most conducive to protecting your breastfeeding relationship. While many hospitals and lactation consultants know about these options, they might not be first on their list for a variety of reasons, but mostly because these medical aides are not thinking about the future, but simply this one feeding.

When you consider things in the context of this feeding and the future of your breastfeeding relationship, you might think about solutions differently. Your baby is at a greater risk for nipple confusion if artificial nipples have been introduced. Babies who experience nipple confusion might push the breast away or refuse to latch on. Or they might latch on and then pull away crying. This creates a frustrating nursing experience for both mother and baby.

To this end, using a simple alternative to the baby bottle and nipple can save a whole host of worries. A few different types of alternative feeding methods are available: See photos, page 65.

- **Syringe:** A syringe is a simple way to feed your baby medicine or small amounts of breast milk. You simply take a small syringe and remove the needle. You can get these at the hospital or from your lactation consultant or pediatrician. Insert the syringe into the corner of your baby's mouth gently, and slowly release the fluid.

- **Newborn cup:** Newborn cups are made from really flexible plastic. They can be rounded or they can be rectangular. They resemble

Alternative Feeding Methods

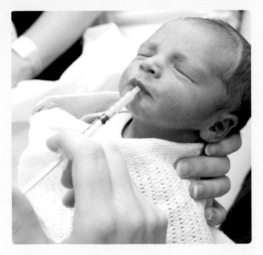

A syringe is a good, short-term solution for feeding a baby in an alternative manner.

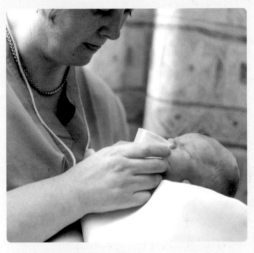

Cup feeding is a great alternative for short- and long-term feeding without using nipples.

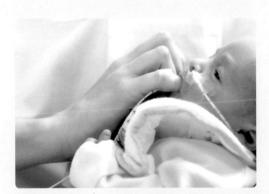

Finger feeding can be done in many ways. It also helps to teach your baby to suck and rewards your baby for doing so. This can be achieved even when baby is receiving nutrients from nasal gastric tubes and other feeding methods.

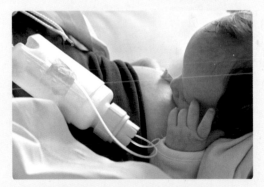

A Supplemental Nursing System (SNS) is a great way to feed your baby at the breast and yet provide more milk during the feeding. Your breast gets stimulation, which helps milk production, and baby is at the breast feeding.

a plastic cold-medicine cup, except that new-born cups hold more, are more flexible, and are designed not to spill! The most important thing to bear in mind with a cup is that you are not to pour breast milk or medication into your baby's mouth. You will simply tilt the cup until the fluid is at your baby's lip. Your baby will actually lap the breast milk up like a kitten.

TIP Protect Your Milk Supply

If your baby is having problems nursing, be sure to protect your milk supply. All forms of supplementing can have a negative effect on your breast milk supply. If your baby is having trouble nursing, you should begin pumping with a breast pump as soon as possible. Pump often at night, and more often if you are having difficulties with milk supply. (For more on pumping see chapter 9.)

- *Finger feeding:* Use a finger-feeding system if you need to feed your baby larger quantities of liquids for longer periods of time. You can make a finger-feeding system with a large syringe and a thin catheter taped to your finger with paper tape. Your baby would then nurse on your finger. The baby's suction actually pulls the milk out of the syringe and into her mouth, so this method is infant led.

- *Supplemental Nursing System (SNS):* The SNS is used to supplement a baby's feeding while stimulating the nipples and breasts to produce more milk. Such a method might be a first step back toward breastfeeding for some babies. Mother will wear a small collection bag on a necklace that hangs between her breasts. As with finger feeding, a small catheter is taped to the nipple. As the baby nurses at the breast, the breast is stimulated but the milk comes from both the breast and the container. A similar product is available, called the Lact-Aid Nursing Trainer.

How to Choose a Supplemental Feeder

The supplemental-feeder system you choose will depend on many factors. First, consider why your baby needs to be fed away from the breast. For how long will you need to use this solution—just a few feedings, or a lengthier amount of time? Is your baby getting medication or just breast milk through the feeder?

Breastfeeding Affirmation

I am patient with myself and my baby as we learn about each other.

For example, a syringe is a great way to give a baby a bit of medication. The syringe can then be tossed fairly easily and you do not need to worry about cleaning it. However, it would take a long time to feed a baby a substantial amount of breast milk via a syringe. So as a long-term feeding solution, this might not be the right choice for your family.

Self-Care Tips

It can be easy to overdo it after having a baby. Your body must heal from giving birth, even if you had an easy birth. Your mind and emotions are still swirling from the pregnancy, the birth, and now a new baby. Doing too much or ignoring your body can lead you to have physical manifestations of problems, such as increased bleeding and infection. Taking small steps toward caring for yourself will go a long way. Here are some things to consider:

- Fit in a shower every day.
- Get dressed every day.
- Find time for a postpartum massage in the first month, even for thirty minutes.
- Buy a new outfit.
- Get a pedicure or manicure.
- Get out of the house once a week.

CHAPTER
2

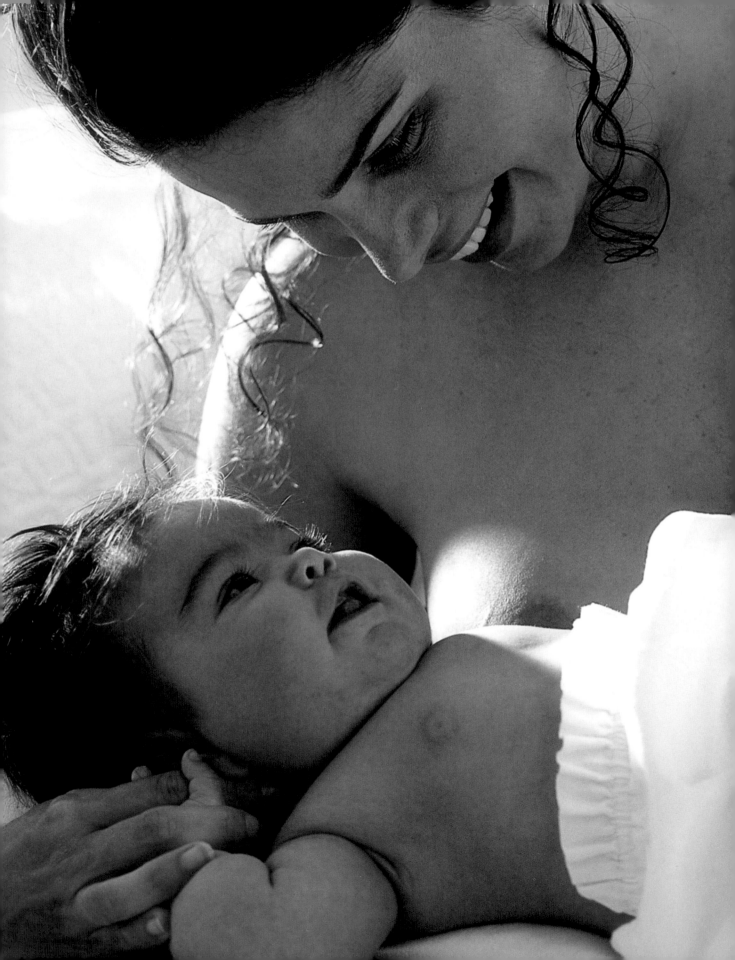

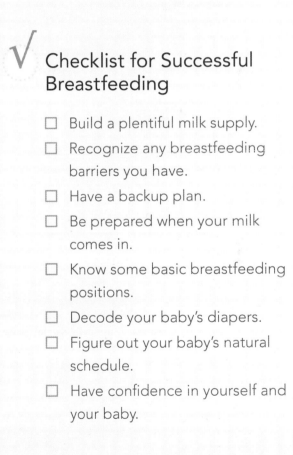

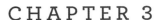
Get Your Breastfeeding Relationship Going

√ Checklist for Successful Breastfeeding

- ☐ Build a plentiful milk supply.
- ☐ Recognize any breastfeeding barriers you have.
- ☐ Have a backup plan.
- ☐ Be prepared when your milk comes in.
- ☐ Know some basic breastfeeding positions.
- ☐ Decode your baby's diapers.
- ☐ Figure out your baby's natural schedule.
- ☐ Have confidence in yourself and your baby.

The first days and weeks with your baby are so important as you establish your breastfeeding relationship. Start off on the right foot now, and you will experience many benefits later on. Above all, keep your baby close to you, breastfeed often, follow your baby's lead, and you'll build a plentiful milk supply. Don't get discouraged if you hit some obstacles in the early days of breastfeeding—pay attention to difficulties and address them early on, and soon enough you'll be breastfeeding like a pro.

BUILD A PLENTIFUL MILK SUPPLY

Breastfeeding your baby can be a beautiful thing that is part physical sustenance and part emotional nurturing. While lovely feelings and emotions go along with nurturing your baby in such a special way, it is essentially about helping your baby to grow by providing him with breast milk. Your supply of breast milk is key to your baby's growth. Building a plentiful milk supply will help you and your baby get your breastfeeding relationship off to the right start and ensure that you will be successful.

Breastfeed Early

It cannot be stressed enough that early stimulation of the breast is the best way to build your milk supply. This is true for all mothers. Your hormones are primed right after birth to help you create the best milk supply possible. This is not to say that if you stumble at first your breastfeeding possibilities are gone. But to have the optimal chance, it is best to get started early.

The early feedings might be short and sweet. You might find that initially, breastfeeding feels weird or awkward because this is unfamiliar territory for both of you. But you and your baby will soon get the hang of breastfeeding.

Breastfeed Often

Breastfeeding is a strictly demand-and-supply proposition. Put simply, your baby demands your breast milk and your body supplies it. The more times your baby nurses (demands breast milk) the more available and abundant your milk (supply) will be for him.

This delicate process is true throughout the course of your nursing span. Your breasts will alter how much milk they make as your baby goes in and out of growth spurts, producing more milk as he needs it. As your baby begins to add solids, your body will slowly decrease the amount of milk it produces.

It is remarkable how well your body can adjust in terms of milk supply once you and your baby have established your nursing relationship. Over time, your body will become more adept at producing milk and responding to your baby's needs on cue. Eventually, your supply can easily vary on an even daily basis, producing more or less milk as needed, according to your baby's hunger levels at the moment.

So if you find yourself thinking that you need more breast milk, there is always a cure, and it's always the same, no matter how long you've been breastfeeding. It is a simple one: Breastfeed more often. Sometimes you might need to get really insistent with this, meaning that you need to make the time to really do it and get the support of those around you. You might even need to take the twenty-four-hour cure: Stay in bed all day, with no one but your baby! Let others wait on you. This is a great way to reboot your milk supply, as well as give your body a break to heal from issues such as blocked ducts or mastitis.

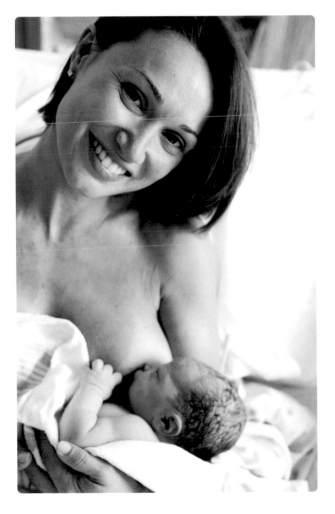

The Forty-Eight-Hour Cure

When faced with nearly any breastfeeding problem, but specifically when it comes to low milk supply, you can try the forty-eight-hour cure, which is an extended version of the 24-hour cure, which is used for minor problems. In short, you should basically do nothing but rest and work on nursing your baby. Get in bed, watch television, read a book, and nurse your baby. Have someone bring you food, and get up only for bathroom breaks and perhaps to take a quick shower. (Or better yet, take a bath with your baby.) This closeness will help you to ensure that you are nursing whenever your baby needs milk. Within forty-eight hours, your milk supply should show signs of being on the mend. Although this may be difficult for some families, this is the fastest, easiest, and least expensive way to increase your milk supply. It is worth finding friends to help you accomplish this or even hiring a babysitter for older children if needed.

Sometimes you just need a quick break from everything else you're doing. Going to bed with your baby and doing nothing but nursing and relaxing for a few days can be very helpful in refocusing on your priorities.

CHAPTER
3

RECOGNIZE ANY BREASTFEEDING BARRIERS YOU HAVE

In some instances, you will be able to predict problems you might have with breastfeeding before you give birth. In others, unexpected circumstances might catch you off guard when your baby is born. Either way, you can deal with these issues by being aware of and proactive about what is happening. Assess these situations as soon as you recognize them, and then take steps to protect and strengthen your ability to successfully breastfeed.

Pre-existing Conditions

You might have a propensity for breastfeeding problems if you have experienced:

- Surgery on your breasts, such as a breast reduction (see pages 180)
- Certain autoimmune disorders (e.g., hypothyroidism)
- Polycystic ovarian syndrome (PCOS)
- Lack of glandular tissue in the breasts

If you have experienced any of these situations in your life, you will want to talk to your practitioner before you have your baby. You should ask about any signs and symptoms you should look for after the birth of your baby. You might also want to start working with your lactation professional before you give birth. While not all women who have experienced the preceding issues will have difficulties with breastfeeding, it is possible. Knowing ahead of time can help you to prevent major problems by being aware of potential issues.

Predict Potential Complications

There are also birth factors that could indicate your baby might have issues with breastfeeding. These include any of the following:

- Being born prior to thirty-seven weeks of gestation
- Being born after an induction
- Having a physical defect of the oral cavity (cleft lip, cleft palate, tongue tie)
- Being born by cesarean
- Being born after a medicated labor

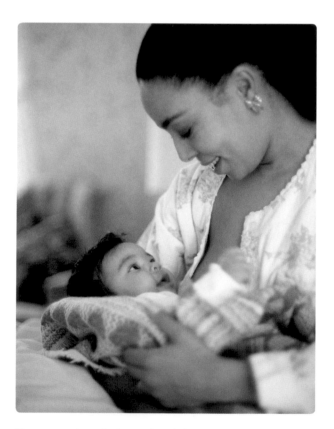

Knowing your breastfeeding goals and identifying barriers can help you become successful at nursing.

Many of the things on this list affect how your baby sucks. Sometimes it's related to your baby's maturity. For example, even slight prematurity can cause breastfeeding issues. This can happen even after thirty-seven weeks, particularly after an induction or scheduled cesarean. Sometimes you are dealing with medications that weaken your baby's reflexes or responses. Some of these signs are so slight that you might not notice your baby is having trouble. These are called subtle effects. Babies born without labor or by cesarean section after labor might also have the disadvantage of more fluid in their lungs.

Other things can happen at birth that will also impact your baby's breastfeeding ability. Vigorous suctioning is one that can often leave your little one with a very sore mouth. This might make your baby have no desire to suck on anything.

HAVE A BACKUP PLAN

Sometimes circumstances could prevent you from nursing early or often. This might be illness in you or the baby. It might also be breastfeeding challenges. Whatever the reason for the lack of breast stimulation, have a backup plan.

Typically, your backup plan will include a breast pump. If you and your baby are separated, get a breast pump and pump! Ideally, you should be able to double-pump. You should stimulate each side for ten to fifteen minutes. Pump every two to three hours during the day and every three to four hours at night. This will help until you and your baby are back together.

In your first attempts at pumping, you will not get any breast milk. When you do get milk, you can save it for the baby. This is a temporary solution. (Be sure to check the section on pumping breast milk for more specifics.)

Using your breast pump can also be an effective way to increase your milk supply no matter what the age of your baby. There might be times when expressing your milk, either by a pump or hand expression, is helpful.

Also remember to help yourself by giving your baby the expressed breast milk in the most productive manner. For some babies, that means finger-feeding them a bit of food to satisfy their hunger, and then still letting them try to nurse; then, if need be, finishing the feeding with a bit more of the expressed milk. Other babies are content to work on nursing without any initial finger-feeding, and instead finishing their feeding with expressed milk.

Avoiding artificial nipples in your baby's early days or whenever you are having breastfeeding challenges can be a good idea. Since nipple confusion is something that you can't really predict, do what you can to err on the side of caution and save yourself from adding any extra problems to the mix.

BE PREPARED WHEN YOUR MILK COMES IN

In the early days after birth, your baby is snacking on colostrum. As mentioned previously, this golden, premilk substance is extremely rich in antibodies, and it also helps your baby to flush the meconium from her system. But eventually, your breast milk will come in.

Most women will see their breast milk come in between two and four days after giving birth. This can be delayed for a variety of reasons, including if you have had a cesarean birth. This is good to know so that you can be patient and not expect the same results as you would if you had given birth vaginally. After a C-section, you can expect your milk to take about a week to come in fully.

If you have been feeding your baby by following her cues, you are unlikely to experience engorgement or at least your engorgement will be less. Feeding your baby on demand lessens the likelihood of engorgement from too much breast milk. However, some moms might still experience some engorgement due to excess fluids in labor, hormones, and so forth. Engorgement is painful for most mothers. Your breasts might become very large, hard, and sore. This can also make it difficult to get your baby to latch on.

If you experience engorgement, there are a few things you can try to help resolve the problem. First, help your baby to have an easier time latching. Try to hand-express just enough milk so that your nipple is not rigid. This will help your baby to nurse, which will in turn make you more comfortable.

You can also use some cold compresses in between feedings. Or try wearing cabbage leaves in your bra for a few minutes to help reduce the swelling from engorgement. (Just be sure not to overdo it with the cabbage leaves, because they can cause your milk supply to dry up.) A good nursing bra can also be helpful.

You should avoid using a breast pump, because that will only signal to your body to make more breast milk. Other things to avoid include hot compresses and breast stimulation of any kind (other than your feedings). This includes shower sprays.

Typically, after a few hours to a few days, your breasts will begin to feel better in general. At first it will only be after a feeding. But as your body figures everything out, you will find that you are not over-producing milk to the point of engorgement.

KNOW SOME BASIC BREASTFEEDING POSITIONS

Breastfeeding positions are a starting point to help you as you get used to nursing your baby. They are designed to help you and your baby get into a reasonable position to nurse so that you are comfortable and your baby can get a good latch. They will hopefully help you to prevent pain and get breastfeeding off to a good start. Once you and your baby have a breastfeeding relationship established and the latch comes naturally, you will, for the most part, stop thinking about breastfeeding in terms of which position to use. You might choose a position for a specific reason, but not typically at every feeding. In the meantime, here are some specific breastfeeding positions to try until you and your baby's relationship reaches that point.

Cradle Hold

The cradle hold is the position that most people imagine when they think of breastfeeding. In a seated position, in a chair or bed, mother has the baby's head in the crook of her right arm, with the baby facing her right breast. The left hand is used to express breast milk if needed, to support the right arm, or to help mother remain comfortable with her cup of water, her book, or the television remote.

This position has some advantages in that it is recognizable. This fact can be a comfort to some mothers. It also allows you to see your baby and your breast fairly well. And having a hand free is an added bonus.

Cross-Cradle Hold

The cross-cradle hold is a different take on the traditional cradle hold. In fact, unless you were paying really close attention, you might not notice the subtle but important difference. In the cross cradle, the baby's head is at the mother's right breast, but the baby's body is supported by the mother's left arm. Her left hand is at the base of the baby's neck, supporting it and helping to direct the baby gently. The mother's right hand is then free to help with breastfeeding or with whatever else she would like.

Many moms feel more comfortable using this hold because the use of the other hand is helpful in getting baby to latch. Since your baby's head is not resting on the crook of your right arm, your baby has a bit more mobility, which helps with the latch.

CHAPTER
3

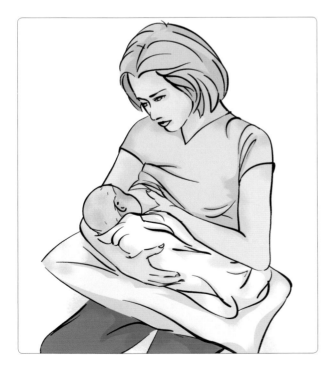

Cradle Hold

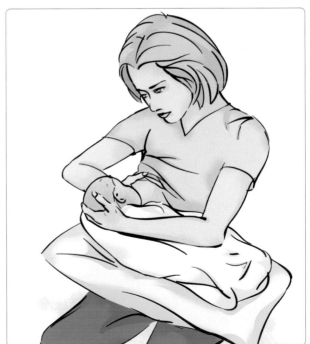

Cross-Cradle Hold

Football Hold

The football hold is named for the position of the baby, under the arm. The baby is placed face up, under the mother's left arm, with the baby's bottom up against the back of a couch or bed. If that is too deep, a pillow is placed between the baby and whatever the mother is leaning against. If the baby is long, the mother might want to bend the baby's legs at the hips. The baby's legs would go up along the mother's back toward her armpit. The baby's head would then rest in the mother's left hand, while she uses her right hand to support her breast.

If you choose this position, you can use your left hand to adjust the depth at which your baby is sitting back next to you. It helps if you rest your baby against your forearm, but this is not neces-sary. You might also need to brace your arm and the baby's weight with something like a pillow under the baby. This prevents you from leaning into your baby. Leaning into a baby can cause back pain, neck pain, and soreness.

The football hold is often recommended after a cesarean birth. This is because your baby won't be lying across your lower abdomen, where your incision is located. That being said, if this position does not appeal to you, you do not have to try it. Just know that it is one of many positions available to you and your baby.

Saddle Hold

In this position, the baby sits facing his mother, straddling her leg, like a person sits in a saddle. The

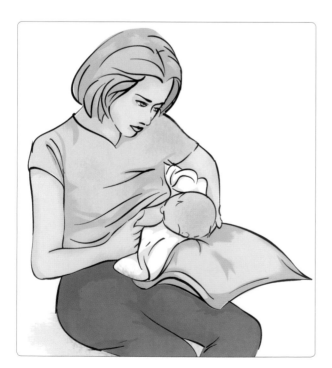

Football Hold

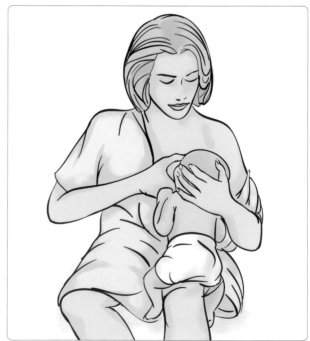

Saddle Hold

baby sits straight up and nurses on the breast at the same side he is facing. Mother can support the baby with either hand, using the remaining hand to support her breast, if needed.

The saddle hold is usually best for older babies, though sometimes a saddle or straddle hold is best for a younger or smaller baby. If your baby suffers with reflux or has other oral difficulties, this might be a good hold to try. The younger the baby, the more support you will need to give to achieve the optimal saddle hold position.

Side Lying

To use this position, the mother lies down on either side of her body. If she is lying on her right side, she can either use her right arm (the one on the bottom) to prop her head up to watch, or she can extend it above her head as she lies down to rest. The baby, also on his side, is placed facing the mother's breast. Her left hand is available to make any adjustments to her breast or the latch as needed.

Some women with larger breasts are able to nurse from both breasts while lying on one side. This can even be accomplished without disturbing the baby. You might need to turn slightly more toward your abdomen to nurse from the top breast, although this is not recommended during sleeping feedings.

This position is great for nursing at night or during naps, as it helps new moms to get much-needed rest! It is also helpful for mothers who have had cesarean births, if their incision is aggravated by nursing. It can also be useful if you have large breasts.

Semirecumbent

This position is easy. The mother simply props a couple of pillows under her head and upper back and reclines backward. The baby is placed heart to heart and is allowed to decide which side to choose and how to nurse. Of course, the mother can guide the baby if necessary. But this will allow the baby to lead when it comes to latch, helping only when needed.

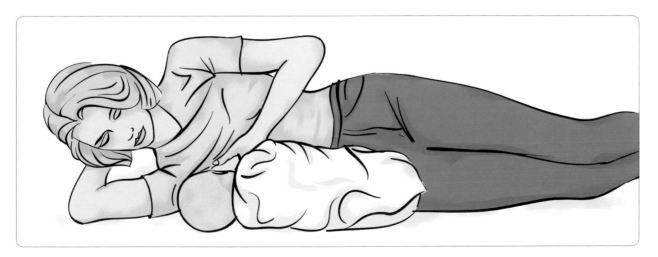

Side-Lying Hold

The semirecumbent position is great for babies who are small, for mothers who have larger breasts that seem to overwhelm babies, for babies who are having latch difficulties, or when forceful letdown or overactive milk-ejection reflex is present.

Breastfeeding positions are as unique as you and your baby are unique. Every breastfeeding duo has a certain nursing position that works for them. The suggestions that breastfeeding professionals and other mothers might give you are great ways to get started. Just remember that as you and your baby learn to nurse, feel free to alter the positions and do what feels right for you both.

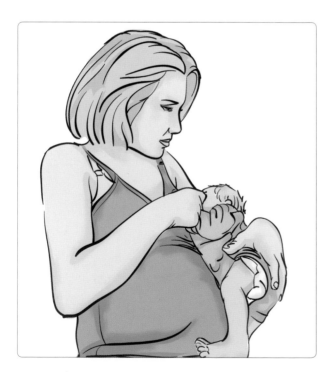

Semirecumbent

Pillows or No Pillows?

Breastfeeding pillows are all the rage these days. The goal of a breastfeeding pillow is to help you to nurse more comfortably. This means you would not lean in any one direction to reach your baby, thus preventing soreness. A breastfeeding pillow is often intended to help support your baby to encourage a good latch.

Plenty of breastfeeding pillows are available. Some have specialty tricks or attachments that are supposed to make them function better than other pillows. The truth is that any pillow can be effective, even the pillows from your couch.

Before you spend money on a breastfeeding-specific pillow, wait to see what you prefer after your baby is born. You might find that you do not need a breastfeeding pillow. Or you might find that you do need one, but that a specific one is best for your needs.

Do be careful when purchasing a breastfeeding pillow. Most are good for only one thing: help with nursing. When you start looking at pillows that claim to do it all, be worried. Do not waste your money on a pillow that you do not need, and do not risk your breastfeeding relationship on a pillow that claims to do too much. While a pillow that is designed to help your baby learn to sit up later or to use as a prop now might be nice, it is certainly not helpful for most mothers when breastfeeding.

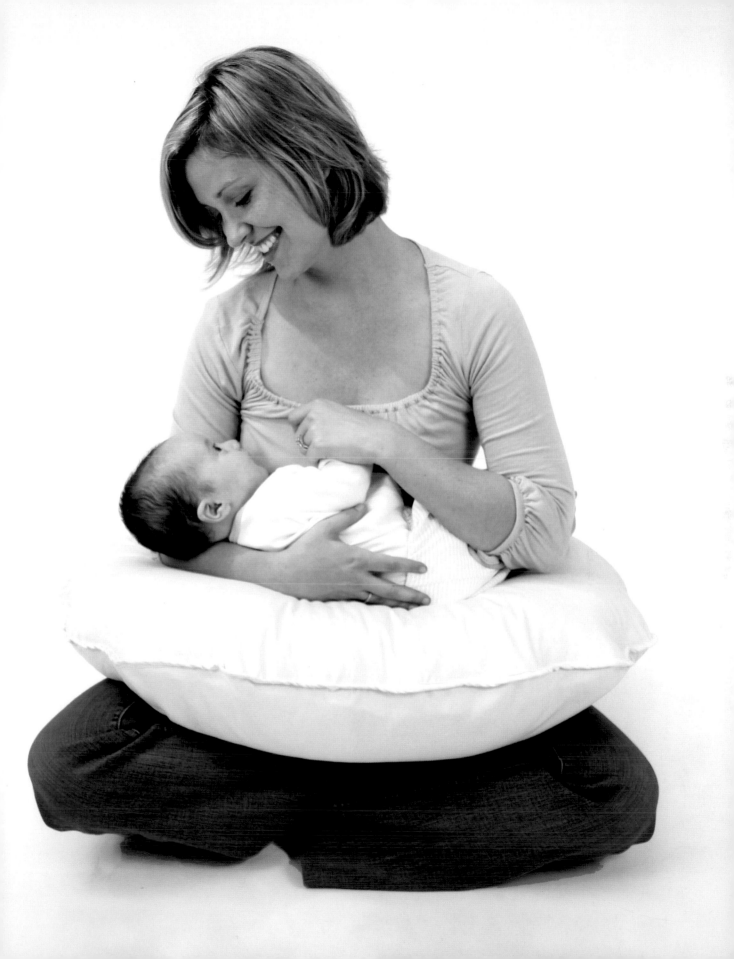

Use "Baby Wearing" to Your Advantage

The first days and weeks with your baby are so important as you establish your breastfeeding relationship. Start off on the right foot now, and you will experience many benefits later on. Above all, keep your baby close to you, breastfeed often, follow your baby's lead, and you'll build a plentiful milk supply. Don't get discouraged if you hit some obstacles in the early days of breastfeeding—pay attention to difficulties and address them early on, and soon enough you'll be breastfeeding like a pro.

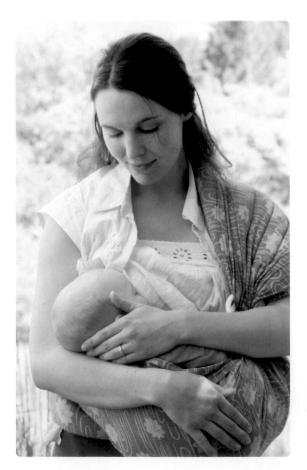

Breastfeeding in the sling

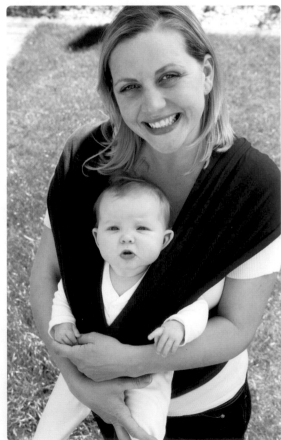

Wrap-style sling

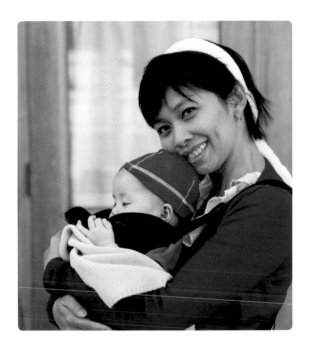

Baby Björn-style

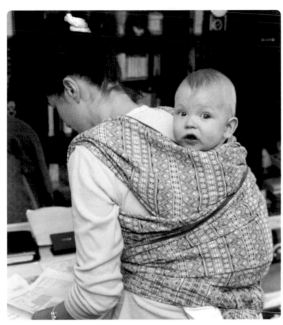

Wrap-style sling alternative

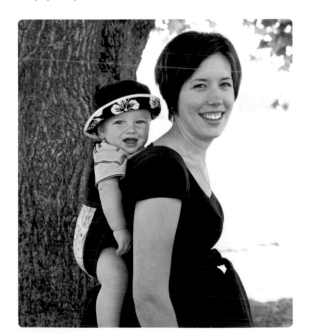

Mei-Tai Style

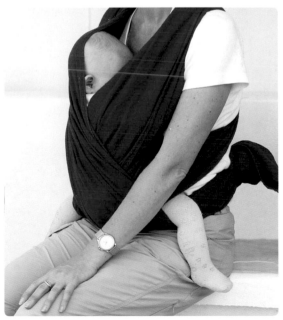

Wrap-style sling alternative

WOMEN'S WISDOM:

You know where to go for help and you know when to ask for breastfeeding support. Asking someone to watch you breastfeed can make you feel a bit more confident if you're concerned. So, do not hesitate to ask a knowledgeable friend or lactation professional to watch you latch or nurse your baby. This can help you to gain confidence in your ability to nurse your baby, but it can also help you to figure out some minor adjustments that might make your life easier. You can do this even if you are not experiencing problems. Many moms try this in the hospital with the lactation consultant on staff, just to be sure they've got things right.

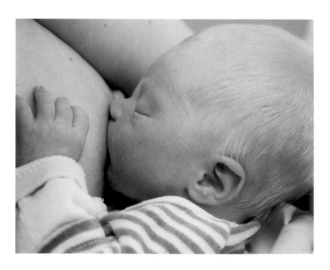

When you wear your baby, you are close. This means you are aware of the subtle changes your baby goes through. You are much less likely to miss the hunger cues of a baby who is with you constantly. Being more attuned to your baby's needs can be a big benefit when it comes to many aspects of parenting, from breastfeeding to discipline.

Not only will you be more attuned to your baby and her needs, but you will also experience other benefits of baby wearing. Babies whose parents wear them tend to cry much less often and tend to be more likely to feel calm and content. This can help everyone experience a smoother transition together as a new family. The days of holding your baby all the time pass so quickly. Before you know it, your newborn will be a squirming, crawling infant, and then an on-the-go toddler. Try to enjoy these days of closeness while you have them!

For new parents, it can be difficult at times to blend tending to baby and managing day-to-day necessities. After all, the constant requirements of daily life, such as cooking and cleaning, do not go away. Mothers are always in a rush and seem to keep moving from one task to the next.

A sling or baby carrier can help you to move more seamlessly through the day, mixing your new role as a parent with the hectic demands of life more successfully. Instead of putting your baby down while you do housework, fold laundry, or wash dishes, pop her in the baby carrier, though use with caution when cooking. Even if you're just going for a walk, skip the stroller and put your baby in a sling.

This added time in your arms is valuable. Baby wearing is also a great way for working parents to reconnect with their babies when they get home.

That being said, not all baby carriers are made equally. Some baby carriers, such as slings and pouches, are designed so that you can nurse your baby while you wear them. These carriers also allow your baby to assume various positions.

You'll have more mobility when you nurse your baby in a baby carrier. Carriers also give you some modesty while nursing. And there's an added bonus to using a baby carrier: It prevents strangers from trying to touch and hold your baby.

Baby packs are the other major type of carrier to consider. They are designed so that your baby can face either outward or inward, but they allow your baby to be in an upright position only. These carriers can be more uncomfortable for younger babies—they work better as babies get older and have developed greater body control. It is also next to impossible to nurse your baby in a front pack.

When choosing a sling or baby carrier, here are some key things to consider:

- Will it grow with the baby?
- Can the baby sit up as well as lie down in the carrier?
- Is it possible to nurse in the carrier? Discreetly?
- Is help required to put the carrier on?
- Will it fit multiple people?
- What will it be used for? (Walking, every day, hiking, etc.)

- What are the weight and height requirements and limits?
- Does the carrier require any special inserts for newborns?

Test a variety of baby carriers to find the right one for you and your family. Borrow some of your friends' baby carriers to try them out. Even without a baby in them, you can get a better idea of whether a particular carrier feels like it will be a good fit for you and your baby. While this might put a cramp in your baby-shower registry plans, having the right carrier will be a blessing.

Once you've made up your mind, begin to use the carrier as soon as possible. Some families don't introduce a baby carrier soon enough. Your baby is ready for a baby carrier nearly immediately, assuming she can lie down in the carrier. Upright baby carriers place too much pressure on your baby's pelvis and might not be recommended.

Frequently, parents do not use baby carriers correctly, so be particularly careful about learning proper use. Most baby carriers now come with written instructions as well as videos. If you have a friend or even a salesperson who has used the carrier you've selected, be sure to ask him or her to help you, as this can be the best way for many people to learn. You might look for baby slings at local specialty shops for breastfeeding and baby care, as larger chain stores tend to have only the front packs, which are not as helpful for breastfeeding.

CHAPTER
3

If you do not have anything locally, do not despair! You can easily find something at online stores. A simple search for terms such as *baby sling, baby pouch,* and *breastfeeding carrier* will turn up many such stores. Look for a versatile carrier that will perform the tasks you need. In your search for carriers you might want to include these brands:

- The Maya Wrap
- The Moby Wrap
- The Original Baby Sling
- Mei Tai
- The Over the Shoulder Baby Holder

DECODE YOUR BABY'S DIAPERS

As your baby is nursing and growing during the first days, weeks, and months of life, remember: Watching your baby's diapers is one of the easiest ways to see how well he is doing. It is simple and easy to quantify. It is also a key area of discussion in many places, from your pediatrician's office to your parents' house, making it an easy point of reference no matter who you are talking to about your baby.

The First Few Days

During the first few days of life, major changes are going on in your baby's tiny system. Keep in mind that your baby has never been hungry or had a need to eat on his own before. This is completely new territory. In the first three or four days, you should see at least one wet diaper and one dirty diaper for every day your baby is old. This means you would have one wet and one dirty diaper on day one, two wet and two dirty diapers on day two, and so on.

The amount of stool in a dirty diaper should be roughly the size of a quarter (about 2.5 cm). In the first few days, your baby's stool will consist of meconium, a substance that has lined your baby's intestines. This thick, tarry black stool will take a few days to clear. It will turn from black, to green, and then to the yellow, seedy soft stools of a healthy, breastfed baby.

Wet diapers might be harder to judge if you are using disposable diapers. But you should look for about 3 tablespoons (45 ml) of fluid. If you are having trouble telling whether your baby is wet, use a tissue in his diaper. When it is wet you will know that your baby has urinated. You can also practice by placing three tablespoons of water in a diaper to see how it feels. Your baby's urine should be pale yellow to clear in color.

After your breast milk has come in, you will notice an increase in the number of dirty diapers. You might see upward of six to eight wet diapers per day in the first days after your milk has arrived. You will also notice at least three to four dirty diapers per day. Some babies will go to extremes on this end, having a bowel movement every time they are fed. This is also considered normal.

The First Weeks to the First Month

After the first few days, your baby's stool pattern usually stays the same for the first month or month and a half. You should expect at least three or four dirty diapers per day. Remember, to be considered truly dirty, a diaper must have about a quarter-size (2.5 cm) stool in it. Keep in mind that the stools of a breastfed baby are yellow, seedy, and very soft. Many families mistake their babies' stools for diarrhea when they are actually quite normal.

Look for six to eight wet diapers per day in the first month. It might be easier to tell whether a cloth diaper is wet than a disposable diaper. Although you might find that you must change cloth diapers more frequently, this can help to prevent diaper rash.

TIP

Urine-Indicator Diapers

There are now diapers with urine indicators being sold. Many do not work as well as you would expect. If you think your indicator isn't working, try the tissue test in your baby's diaper.

CHAPTER 3

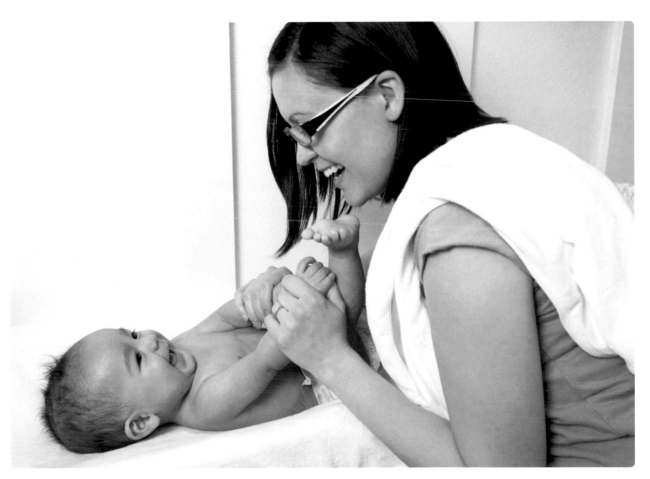

Your baby's diapers will hold clues as to how well your baby is breastfeeding.

Moving On

As your baby gets older, you can expect a drastic difference in his diapers. There is a big variance in what is considered "normal," particularly when it comes to bowel movements. You might notice that your baby goes from having a bowel movement at every feeding, or more frequently, to much less frequently. As long as your baby's stool looks normal and is not hard or painful to pass at that time, your baby is not constipated and needs no treatment.

Your baby's wet diapers should remain about the same. As your baby's bladder capacity increases with age, however, you might find that he can hold his urine a bit longer. This also means that the diapers are likely to be wetter than previously.

The Bowel Habits of the Breastfed Baby

After the first three or four weeks, your baby's bowel habits might change drastically. As mentioned previously, some babies begin to have bowel movements much less frequently, perhaps every three or four days—though, even going up to two weeks without a bowel movement can be normal, in some instances. This can be concerning to parents who worry about constipation and whether baby is getting enough to eat.

You will be able to tell if your baby is having a problem. Is your baby eating well? How often does he have wet diapers during the day? When your baby does have a bowel movement is it a normal breastfed bowel movement? If you answer yes to these questions, your baby is not suffering from constipation.

FIGURE OUT YOUR BABY'S NATURAL SCHEDULE

Parents spend a lot of time thinking about their baby's schedule. It is fairly normal in this day and age of calendars, clocks, and electronic tracking devices. The truth of the matter is that your baby doesn't know how to read a calendar and can't work a digital assistant yet.

As we all live our lives, a natural schedule and pattern typically emerge. This is something that we all hope our babies will do fairly quickly. We also anticipate that the baby's schedule will naturally work well with our family's life.

Some families will try to force a schedule on a small baby. This, particularly when it comes to breastfeeding, can be very detrimental. Strict feedings and guidelines for nursing can lead to many problems. Babies whose parents put them on strict feeding schedules in the early months (and sometimes even later) can experience growth restriction, dehydration, and other issues, including malnutrition.

The good news is that babies have their own rhythm. It might take some patience, but if you let it, a pattern will emerge. This internal rhythm or schedule will also be much easier to manage than any that you try to put on your baby.

Once your baby has established a pattern, there are ways to tweak it to be more family friendly. This means that if your baby is used to napping at two o'clock in the afternoon and you really need that nap time to start a bit earlier, you can help to mold that schedule a bit. But the flexibility is beginning with the baby's schedule, not yours. Unfortunately, babies are not convenient. But they are much easier to be around when we listen to their needs.

HAVE CONFIDENCE IN YOURSELF AND YOUR BABY

Too often, new mothers—even those who are experienced—get wrapped up in how much milk they are making for their babies. With baby bottles and other food products, we know exactly how much goes in. The amount is quantifiable. Breast milk is different. It is, in a way, a leap of faith.

Try not to fixate on all of those extraneous things. Remember, your proof is in the baby. If your baby is happy, has wet and dirty diapers on a basically normal schedule, and is healthy, you are producing the perfect amount of breast milk for your baby.

And don't forget that second easy trap that mothers sometimes fall into when it comes to breastfeeding: measurements. Measurements of

CONFIDENCE CUE

Let's face it: Worrying about your baby is normal. At first, it might seem perplexing to you as you learn your baby's signals, but your baby is giving you the answers you need. When in doubt, check it out! Check the diapers. How many diapers are you seeing each day? How many are wet? How many are dirty? Check your baby. Is he happy? Is your baby awake and alert sometimes? Does he have some restful periods? (Even if you think they are too short and not frequent enough.) Remember, charts are about averages, so you should ignore the charts whenever possible. You know your baby, and his particulars are what count.

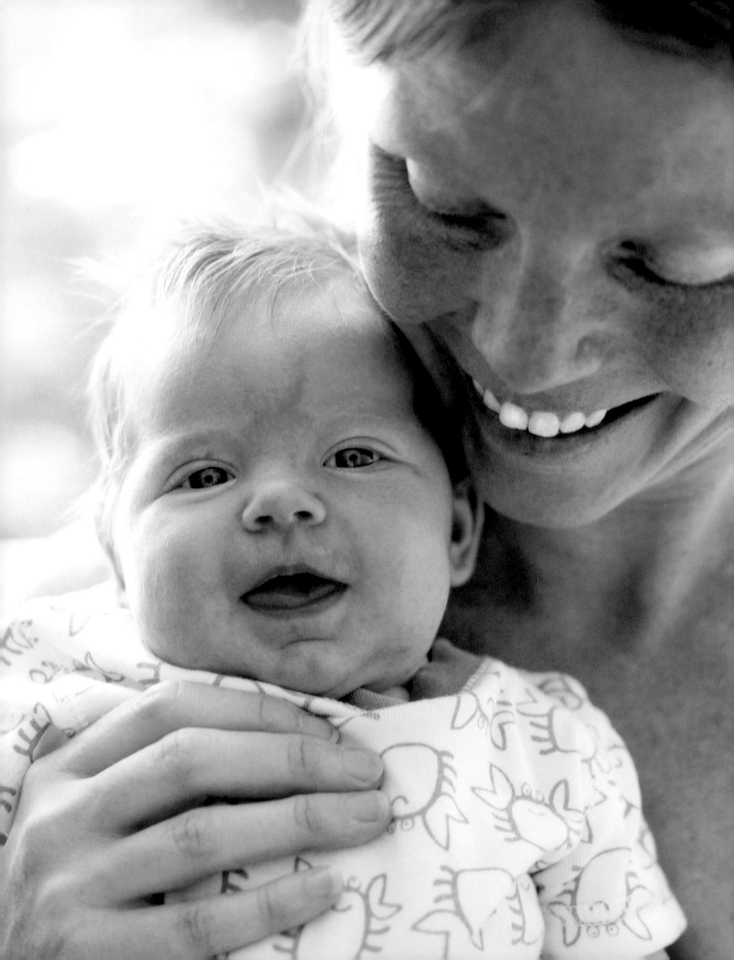

time, to be exact. Do you watch the clock when your baby is nursing? Do you watch the clock between feedings? Do you wonder how much breast milk is going in? This thought process can take you down a slippery slope.

If you find yourself concerned, double-check your list of ways to see whether your baby is getting his needs met. Also, don't underestimate how much more confident you'll feel if you tap into a solid support system—read chapter 4 for advice on how to do this! Call your lactation professional for a pep talk. Consider going to a support group meeting. You'll quickly learn that you're not alone and that other mothers feel the same way too. For many newly breastfeeding mothers, it is sometimes easy to feel overwhelmed by the inability to quantify and measure their babies' milk intake. After all, that's what happens when we are conditioned to measure everything from minutes to serving sizes. Just remember that the number of ounces, minutes nursed, and hours between feedings are not what will ultimately tell you whether your baby is thriving. Be observant and follow your instincts: You and your body know your baby best.

If your baby is gaining weight and content you are succeeding. Have confidence in yourself and in your baby. You are a good team.

Breastfeeding Affirmation

I am a good mother to my breastfed baby.

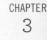

Self-Care Tips

It can be easy to lose yourself in a newborn. Remember that you need care too. Some mothers find they feel more overwhelmed a month into having a baby than they did at the beginning, right after birth. Be sure to ask for help if you need it. Here are some things others can help you with:

- Doing laundry
- Bringing a meal over
- Running errands
- Taking an older child out
- Holding the baby while you shower or sleep for thirty minutes
- Loading the dishwasher
- Writing thank-you notes that you dictate
- Lending an ear or a shoulder
- Doing whatever else you find the most helpful

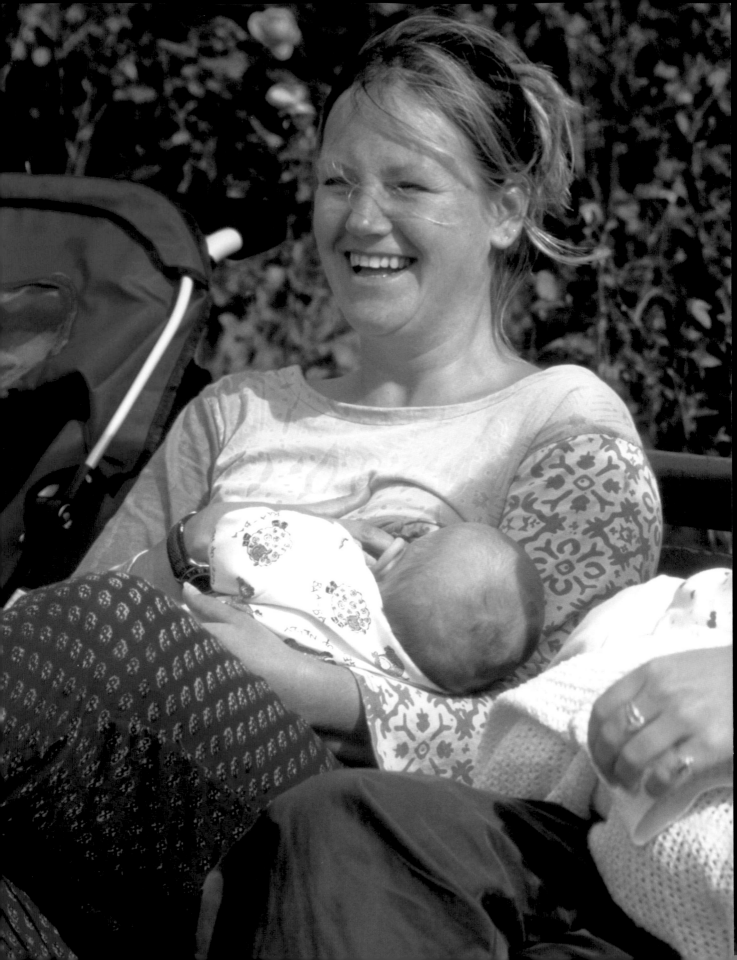

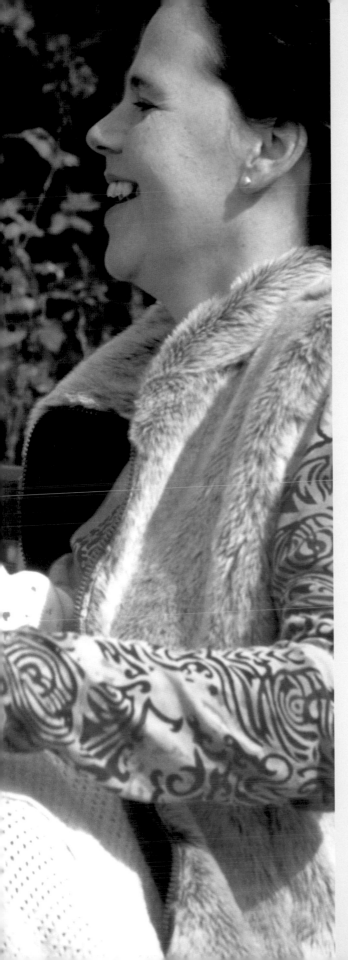

Ask For and Get Support When You Need It

✓ Checklist for Successful Breastfeeding

- ☐ Identify your breastfeeding support system.
- ☐ Know where to go if you need help with breastfeeding.
- ☐ Ask for help during the first few days.
- ☐ Find answers to your breastfeeding questions.
- ☐ Talk to other breastfeeding mothers.
- ☐ Attend a breastfeeding support group.

A new mother will need support for breastfeeding in many forms. She will need a cheerleader—someone to tell her what a great job she is doing, even when it is difficult. She will need a teacher—someone to show her how to breastfeed and how to make breastfeeding fit into her life. She will need a confidante—someone to talk to when breastfeeding is difficult or perplexing. Sometimes these people might be in her family or circle of friends. Other times a new mom will have to expand her existing network to find all of the support she needs.

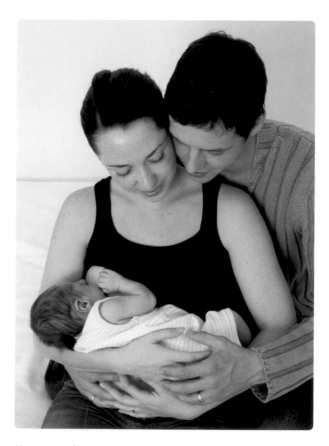

Having a good support system is one of the keys to a successful breastfeeding relationship.

IDENTIFY YOUR BREASTFEEDING SUPPORT SYSTEM

Breastfeeding takes support. Now, hopefully, we all think we have a lot of support already in our lives. Think of those people you know you can count on for support, and be ready to rally them when needed. You might also need to cultivate support from new individuals you seek out as you begin your breastfeeding journey.

Husband or Partner

One of the most important people to have support from for breastfeeding will be your husband or partner. Although breastfeeding is natural, it can take both you and your baby some time getting used to it. Given the fact that we are typically not as familiar with breastfeeding as previous generations have been, we have lost the art of support as well.

To be supportive, husbands and partners have to understand what a mother's breastfeeding goals are for her baby. They must also try to know and understand the whys behind her goals. So if, for example, a woman's goal is to breastfeed exclusively for six months, it would be helpful to know if that is based on the American Academy of Pediatrics (AAP) statement of belief about breastfeeding or if it is her personal goal.

Sometimes breastfeeding goals aren't based on just one thing. They can have a lot of complex motivations behind them. It can also be hard for women to articulate their goals for breastfeeding. Being open to talking about it is very important.

For husbands and partners, the best way to get to know this information is to have conversations. These can start during pregnancy and continue. For example, as you learn to nurse, you might find that your breastfeeding goals change. Or perhaps the reasons behind your pursuit of breastfeeding have changed the longer you breastfeed.

If your partner has issues with breastfeeding or your specific situation, you will need to have a calm discussion with him about that. Together you will hopefully come to an agreement. Be mindful of what your husband or partner might be feeling: Perhaps he is feeling left out of feeding time or is jealous of your closeness with the baby. There are ways to help alleviate these feelings without compromising breastfeeding.

Dealing with the issues head-on is important. If you do not have these discussions, you might find that your partner is doing things that undermine his ability to support you, either knowingly or unknowingly.

Family Physician or Pediatrician

Perhaps when you asked your baby's doctor his or her beliefs about breastfeeding you heard the magical phrase, "Breastfeeding is best!" This is great, but it does not really tell you how your baby's doctor feels about breastfeeding, nor does it tell you how much support you will get from him or her.

When you walked into the pediatrician's office did you take a good look around? Did you find subtle formula advertisements? Look for small things

such as pen holders or key rings that announce a specific brand. You might also be given a welcome bag that is sponsored by a formula company. This can be a sign that your physician is not as committed to your decision to breastfeed as you would like.

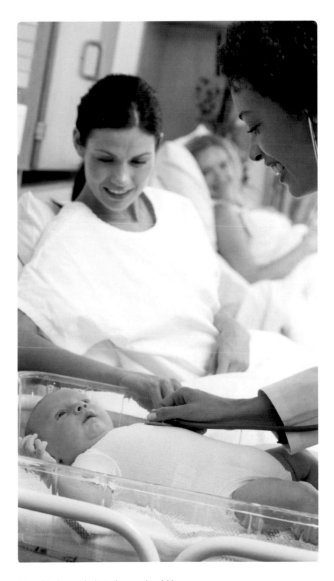

From birth your baby's doctor should be on board to help you achieve success when you breastfeed.

Be sure to have a frank discussion up front with your doctor about their breastfeeding philosophy. Hopefully, you will see signs or be given information that pertains to breastfeeding, such as a schedule of classes offered by your pediatrician or local breastfeeding support groups, information on breast pump rentals, and so on.

You can begin by asking your baby's doctor a series of questions about how he or she will be supportive of breastfeeding. This might include questions such as the following:

- What kind of training do you have in breastfeeding beyond what you received in medical school?
- Do you routinely update your breastfeeding education? Who sponsors the education that you have?
- Do you have a copy of Hale's *Medications and Mother's Milk* should I need to take medications while nursing?
- Does anyone on your staff hold an International Board Certified Lactation Consultant (IBCLC) or Certified Lactation Counselor (CLC) credential?
- Does your office offer specific lactation support?
- Do breastfed babies have a different schedule of appointments?
- What is your first step if I come to you with breastfeeding problems?
- Do you have a lactation support person to whom you routinely refer patients?

- Do you use breastfed infant growth charts from the Centers for Disease Control and Prevention (CDC)?
- When would you recommend supplementation?
- What percentage of your patients breastfeed their babies?
- When do you recommend weaning?
- How can you best help me succeed in my plans to nurse my baby?
- Have you or your partner ever breastfed?

CONFIDENCE CUE

Plenty of people will pipe in and give you advice as soon as you have your baby. You don't even have to ask for it much of the time; it's just given freely. Some of the advice might actually be good advice that makes a difference in your life. Other advice might not be practical, workable, or your style. Remember to take the advice you need and leave the rest at the door. Some of it will apply perfectly to your situation, and some of it won't help you at all.

While these might not be the only questions you have for your baby's doctor, you will really need to understand where your baby's doctor is coming from when it comes to breastfeeding to ensure that you are getting the support you need.

If you choose a physician who is not as supportive of breastfeeding as you would need or like, there are other ways to supplement the support your baby's doctor isn't giving you. Perhaps you have a situation in which the physician does not have all of the knowledge or training that you would like, but has the desire to learn. If you have the time or inclination, you could help your baby's doctor gather more knowledge. Here are some ways that you can help your baby's doctor become more breastfeeding knowledgeable and friendly:

- Give the doctor handouts on when local breastfeeding support groups meet for his or her other patients.

- Let the doctor know of breastfeeding training opportunities in your area.

- Give the doctor feedback on various support group meetings.

- Tell the doctor about your experiences with various lactation consultants, hospitals, and so forth.

- Share your pump rental experiences with your doctor.

Having a relative who has previously breastfed or is supportive is an amazing source of support. It can really make the difference.

Grandparents

Unfortunately, breastfeeding misinformation is typically an issue with grandparents. They want to help and they want to be supportive. But they often feel like they do not know enough to be helpful or that they do not have the tools or knowledge to help you.

Be specific with them. Tell them what your breastfeeding goals are for your baby. Explain to them why breastfeeding matters to your family. Talk to them about the benefits of breastfeeding. Your feedback will hopefully help them to see how important breastfeeding is for your family. You can also try the following:

- Offer to take them to a support group meeting for breastfeeding education.

- Lend them a book on breastfeeding.

- Lend them a DVD on breastfeeding.

- Give them specific things they can do to help with the baby that are not feeding related.

- Let them know that breastfeeding will not mean they cannot be a part of your baby's life.

CHAPTER
4

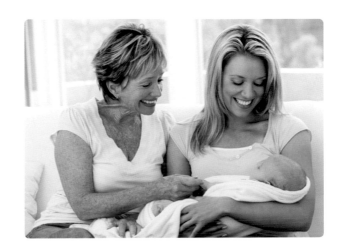

In some cases, doing these things may not solve the problem. Ongoing issues with grandparents can be very painful. You might not feel like you are being heard or validated, and they probably are not feeling great about the situation either. If this happens, let them know that you are sticking to your beliefs and goals. Explain that perhaps the discussion of infant feeding is off the table.

Friends

Your friends will hopefully be the most helpful allies you have in breastfeeding. Even if they have not personally breastfed, they might go above and beyond the call of friendly duty to ensure that you are well supported. If your friends have breastfeeding experience, you can glean a lot of really good information and support structures from them to help you in your journey.

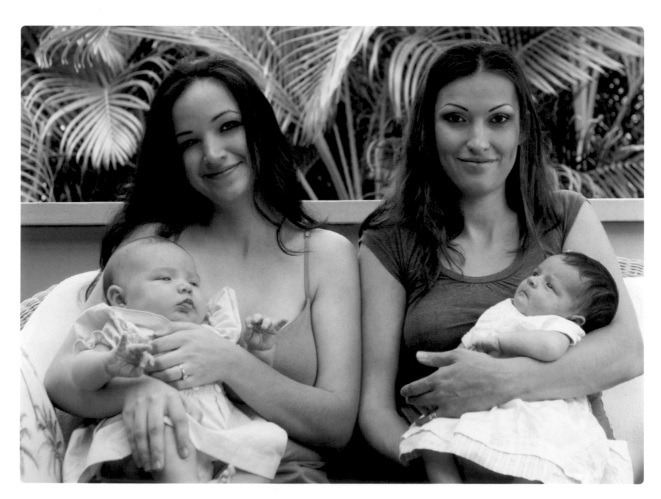

Having friends who are breastfeeding at the same time is wonderful. To be able to discuss the small, everyday questions with a girlfriend is important.

If no one in your existing circle of friends has breastfeeding experience, that's all the more reason to get out and make new friends through breast-feeding support groups and new-mom groups. Networking with other new moms in this way will help you to extend your social network to include other families who share similar parenting styles and have similar goals.

KNOW WHERE TO GO IF YOU NEED HELP WITH BREASTFEEDING

Having some support for breastfeeding is key, even if it's just calling in your husband or partner to help massage the baby's back to keep her awake and keep you company during a nighttime feeding, or turning to a group of your girlfriends who have successfully nursed for advice. Sometimes, however, you might need more than just moral support or advice from other mothers. In those cases, knowing where to go for that help is critical to getting a rapid response.

Who Is a Lactation Professional?

A lactation professional can look very different, depending on whom you ask. Some would consider only lactation consultants to fall into this category. But many more types of lactation professionals exist, each with a role to play.

Many families view a lactation professional as someone whom they can call on when there is a breastfeeding problem. While certainly that is one reason to call in a lactation professional, there are others as well. Even if you don't have any problems, it's still a good idea to see a lactation professional to ensure that everything is going well. This can help to increase your confidence in your ability to breastfeed.

It is a good idea to build a relationship with a lactation professional. The more she knows you and your baby, the better she can help you. Being able to meet her when you are not in the middle of a breast-feeding challenge or crisis is always easier.

IBCLC

The International Board Certified Lactation Consultant (IBCLC) designation is considered the gold standard in breastfeeding education and support. You will find these lactation consultants in most hospitals and lactation practices.

There are also certified lactation counselors (CL) who are trained in lactation support. They have some experience and might be using this as a step toward their IBCLC exam. Or they might need this certification for their job in a hospital or birth center.

La Leche League Leaders

La Leche League leaders have gone through intensive training to be able to support women in their breastfeeding experience, no matter what their goals are. These women are typically your first line of help in the outside world. You will find them at La Leche League meetings, online, and via phone counseling in some areas. This is a free service, though membership in La Leche League International is encouraged but not necessary.

There are also breastfeeding counselors and breastfeeding educators. These terms are vaguer, and they might mean that the person has lots of formal training or no formal training. Ask if you are unsure of the meaning.

Physicians

Your baby's physician—whether he or she is your family physician or a pediatrician—is usually not a lactation professional. His or her knowledge of breastfeeding is typically extremely limited. Of course, this can depend on when and where the physician went to medical school and had his or her training. A physician who has gone on to earn an IBCLC credential or is a member of the American Academy of Breastfeeding Medicine (AABM) takes breastfeeding seriously.

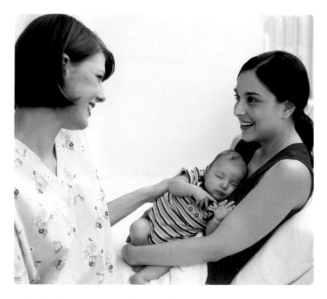

A family physician is typically limited in their knowledge of breastfeeding. Find a lactation professional for the reassuring advice you need.

Where to Find Lactation Professionals

Now that you can tell the real lactation professionals from the phonies, you need to know where to find your support. The truth is that there are many places in which you might find lactation support professionals. Where you look might depend on when you need help, what type of help you need, and what your insurance or pay structure looks like.

Group Support Meetings

Group support meetings are usually free and open to the public. They include local La Leche League meetings and similar meetings. Sometimes private lactation consultants or counselors run these meetings if they are looking to increase their skill level by gaining hours working with breastfeeding women. For some it is even a version of public service. You might also find that local birth networks offer support meetings or even educational meetings at various times. Some physicians' offices also offer support groups or classes for breastfeeding, including pediatricians, family doctors, and midwives.

Take advantage of these groups. The nice thing is that you get the attention of the lactation professional. But you also get advice from other mothers who have been there and done that. In addition, it is helpful to be near people who believe as you do about breastfeeding.

You can find these meetings by asking around. Talk to your childbirth educator, breastfeeding class instructor, or other lactation professionals you know, and look online for breastfeeding support meetings.

Not every group will be a good match; try a couple before figuring out which works best for you and your breastfeeding philosophy.

Mothers' Groups

These are not breastfeeding-specific groups, most of the time. But whenever you have a group of mothers around, you are likely to have a good idea of the knowledge base that they have. Simply start by asking around and comparing notes. If you hear the name of a group come up over and over, you know it has to be good.

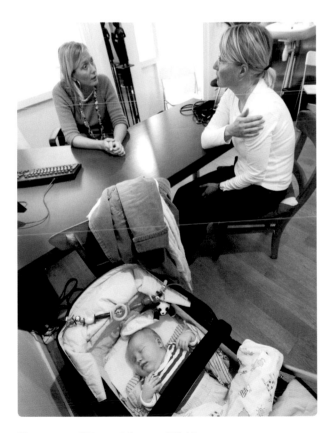

The majority of Women, Infants, and Children offices are available to help with lactation support in addition to supplemental nutrition for mothers.

WIC (Women, Infants, and Children) Office

This government program for women, infants, and children has a great system of peer breastfeeding counselors. Here you can talk to someone who has training and experience with breastfeeding. They can help guide you through breastfeeding issues and help you seek additional support should you encounter any pitfalls. This program is free to qualifying mothers.

Doctor's Office

Some family practice physicians, pediatricians, and obstetricians or midwives have a lactation professional on staff. This typically means your insurance will be billed for their time. This might or might not save you money. As with anything, the advice you get might vary. You might or might not get along, but you are always free to seek support from other places.

Lactation Consultant Practice

A few lactation consultants have their own practices. They might be located in office buildings or run their clinics from home or in your home. This can be really popular, because getting out with a new baby is difficult for some families. You might also find that they rent breast pumps. They may even provide a delivery service or in-home consultations.

CHAPTER
4

TIP

Weight Checks

Many of these providers offer free baby weight checks. That can really ease your mind if you are concerned about your baby's weight gain. Remember, weighing on the same scale at the same time of day is more accurate.

Breastfeeding Specialty Store

Some lactation consultants have expanded their practices or joined forces with others to make lactation services available at a store-type setting. So in addition to professional services, you might also be able to purchase or rent breast pumps. They might also sell nursing bras, breastfeeding clothes, pillows, and some baby-related items.

Internet or Phone

It is really difficult to do, but some lactation services are offered over the phone or the Internet. This is your best option if there is nothing in your area. However, these services should never be your first option, because there are severe limitations when a professional is not able to see the mother and baby. Even if you were passing photos back and forth, it is still not the same as watching a baby-and-mother nursing pair in person.

ASK FOR HELP DURING THE FIRST FEW DAYS

Those first few days with your baby should be fairly calm and peaceful. Unfortunately, it does not always work that way. Between the lack of sleep and the learning curve that the entire family is adjusting to, you might find that life feels fairly out of whack, even if the only change is a small bundle of joy.

Self-Care Tips

Stress is not your friend. This is true in motherhood, breastfeeding, and life in general. Some mothers can tell that stress can alter their milk supply, while others don't notice. The thing is that stress is not fun to live with, even if it doesn't bother your milk supply. Have a stress game plan. Try guided relaxation while you are nursing. This can help you to increase the benefits of prolactin and other hormones while nursing. You can also simply try counting objects or numbers to clear your mind. When you're not nursing consider a massage, a night out alone, or even a date night.

Get the Help You Need from Friends and Family

Superwoman syndrome is something that many new mothers suffer from at some point in the postpartum period. It is not uncommon to believe that you can handle your baby and everything else life throws you. What you might not realize is just how much having a baby takes out of you. This is true even when your life is not complicated and even if your birth was straightforward. Don't feel as if you need to do everything!

Getting help with your life in the first few days is really important. Knowing that you do not need to worry about food, the house, or even your pets can take a load off your mind. Truly the best thing you can do for breastfeeding success is to spend as much time as you can with your baby, even when you are not engaged in a feeding activity.

Getting help is a blessing, not a burden on those around you. You can be sure that your friends and family are more than willing to help. The problem is that many women forget or fail to ask for fear that someone will say "no" or that they will look as though they can't handle new motherhood. Instead, try to think of it in terms of letting someone feel great for being able to help you.

If you have trouble asking for help, consider this before you have the baby. It might actually work out better for you to have a list of things people can help you with. You might have a list of people to call who have offered dinner or other services such as running errands. You could have another friend agree to coordinate your list, if it helped to have someone else think about it for you.

The list also serves another purpose. It will help you to identify what your needs are, and therefore get in touch with what will be important for you. And if you have a list of your needs already written down, you can use that when people call to offer support. Then, when friends ask, "Do you need anything?" you simply give them a few of the options on a list.

When and How to Ask for Help

If you are able to plan ahead for help, that can be a large weight lifted off your shoulders. Start by thinking about what needs to be done during the period right after having your baby. Does someone need to help you with your home or your pets? Perhaps you have other children that need assistance.

Once you are home with your new baby and settling in, you might have different needs. Some of these needs can be anticipated. One of the biggest areas where you can preplan is help with meals. If you are a member of a social or religious group, they might automatically bring meals for a set amount of time. Even one or two meals can be very helpful.

If you have older children, you know you will need help with them. Even having someone to come to play with them or take them for a walk can be helpful. If they are old enough to already have friends, preplanning a few play dates can take a load off as well.

CHAPTER
4

If you can't preplan for help, try to have a list of people whom you can call for spontaneous help. This might be a family member, a dear friend, or a postpartum doula. We all need someone we can call on to go to the grocery store for toilet paper or to pick up a prescription without a lot of notice.

What Type of Help Should You Ask For?

In short, anything you can get help with you should get help with in your life at this point. Just because you have seen other women try to do everything or you think that is what is expected of you is no good reason to go it alone. Right now, your focus should be on recovering from giving birth physically and emotionally, as well as getting breastfeeding off to a good start. Throwing life in on top of that will cause you to have trouble on nearly all fronts.

Help with your home is a good place to start. See if you can find someone to help you keep the laundry going and the sink empty. If you can find a friend or two to help organize your friends and co-workers who offer help, you will be even better aligned to help yourself. Some of the following are things you could ask for help with:

- Cooking/meals
- Laundry
- Grocery shopping
- Picking up dry cleaning
- Dropping off library books
- Shuttling you to the pediatrician's office

Get Help and It Will Be Easier to Establish a Good Breastfeeding Relationship

Perhaps you are wondering, "Why all this talk about postpartum help, and what is it doing in a book about breastfeeding?" Well, the honest answer is, the more time you have to sit and get to know your baby and nurse, the better off your breastfeeding relationship will be and the easier nursing will become. This, in turn, will help you build an amazing milk supply for your baby. Plus, you and your family will benefit if you are not stretched too thin, trying to tend to your baby's needs while also doing everything else at home all by yourself. Never underestimate the power of some simple help.

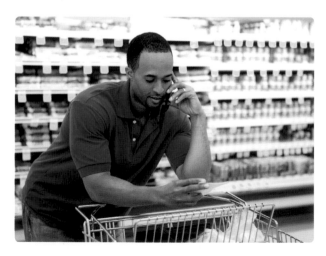

Let dad help when he can. Taking mundane tasks off your work list will be helpful.

Consider Professional Support for the Postpartum Period

Sometimes you need to call in the professionals: postpartum doulas. A postpartum doula can help you to ease your family into life with a new little one. Typically, you can have a postpartum doula come to help for varying amounts of time for the first few weeks or months of your baby's life.

A postpartum doula is trained in breastfeeding support, care of the new family, warning signs for postpartum depression, and much more. She can help you with some light housekeeping, such as doing laundry and preparing meals. A postpartum doula is also able to help you run errands or sneak in a shower. They are particularly helpful if you have more than one child, because they can help with your older child or hold the baby while you play with an older sibling.

Typically, you will meet with your postpartum doula and go over what her services and fees would be according to your needs. You will talk about what you want and need and how she can best help you. This meeting helps to ensure that everyone is on the same page.

Postpartum doulas' prices vary depending on where you live. Many offer gift certificates, so if someone asks what sort of baby gift you'd like you can always say you'd love a gift of postpartum care. Sometimes you can pay for a postpartum doula with your flexible spending account (FSA), though rules vary and you will need to talk to your company's human resources department.

TIP

Postpartum Doulas

A postpartum doula is a trained expert, usually a woman, who will come into your home and help you with the basics of running things. This can involve doing light chores, such as laundry and dishes, preparing hot meals, helping with older children, and even giving breastfeeding support and counsel. Services vary based on individuals, but start interviewing before you have a baby for the best availability.

Postpartum doulas are great for nearly every mother and family. But they can be extremely helpful if you are new to the area or if you do not have a large support base for whatever reason. They are particularly helpful to parents of multiples.

FIND ANSWERS TO YOUR BREASTFEEDING QUESTIONS

In the first weeks, you might wonder if you will get the hang of breastfeeding. You might or might not have run into multiple answers to a single question about breastfeeding at your hospital or birth center. You might be in pain, either from the birth or from

CHAPTER
4

breastfeeding. If you have any pain or unanswered questions about breastfeeding, it is always important to get help early and often.

By delaying help you can actually make your breastfeeding problem bigger than it has to be. Early intervention by a trained professional can make a huge difference in your breastfeeding relationship. Be sure to call someone as soon as you think you might have a question or problem. Call a lactation professional if:

- You experience pain when nursing.
- You have sore nipples.
- Your nipples are cracked or bleeding.
- Your baby is nursing all the time.
- Your baby's sleepy or hard to rouse for feedings.
- You're concerned about your baby's milk intake.
- You are considering supplementing.
- You are experiencing engorgement.

Lactation professionals can help to answer many of your questions. They can also help you deal with many of the problems that come up with your baby. It is not uncommon to have questions and concerns in the first few weeks of nursing, even if you have successfully breastfed another baby before this baby.

When to Call Your Doctor

There might also be times when you would want to call your baby's doctor. You would want to do this when your baby:

- Is yellowish in color
- Is not feeding at all
- Has no urinary output

A good interdisciplinary team might be needed. Your doctor and your lactation professional should work together to help you find the solution to your breastfeeding challenges. In the meantime, as you are working to smooth out your breastfeeding situation, you might have to use your home support system to give you more time with the baby. You'll need your professional team to help manage the issues, but you'll also need the home support to get everything else done so that you have time to focus on the baby.

While this multifaceted approach is ideal, it does not frequently happen. Many pediatricians and family doctors simply do not have the amount of training in breastfeeding that is required to be of as much assistance as your local lactation professional. A wise doctor recognizes this and has a personal lactation professional either on staff or readily available. Do not be surprised if you need to make this communication happen by requesting it and helping to foster the relationship.

The early days of breastfeeding can be challenging. Many mothers say that after the first few weeks, breastfeeding seems so easy and that they

TIP

Address Problems Promptly

Breastfeeding problems start small but can quickly become bigger. Get help early on to prevent further problems.

are totally surprised based solely on what the first weeks were like. The more prepared you are the fewer challenges you will have in general. While you can't prepare for every issue, having a good team ready to assist you and your baby will put you ahead of the game.

TALK TO OTHER BREASTFEEDING MOTHERS

Since you know that support is key, you might want to find someone who has actually breastfed to count on among your support group. This means you will need to find friends, siblings, relatives, or new people in your life who have already been down the breastfeeding road or who are on the road and slightly ahead of you.

It is so important to talk to someone who has already been where you are, because it can be really hard to understand all of the emotions and physical issues that breastfeeding can bring up. How can you explain to people what engorgement means if they have never breastfed an infant? Sure, these people can say they understand, but do they really?

Finding other mothers should not be difficult. First, start with people you know. Do you have any sisters or sisters-in-law who breastfed? What about cousins? They might be the perfect source for helpful hints, life experience, or even just for someone to talk to about breastfeeding.

Also check to see whether your friends have breastfed. Their support will be helpful going forward with your breastfeeding goals as well. They can help you with the day-to-day issues of

WOMEN'S WISDOM:

Breastfeeding support groups are an important part of nursing and mothering. They help you to feel like you have others who are in the same boat. Sometimes you might find yourself not feeling supported. Feeling supported is the key to your support groups. If you feel you don't click with a particular group, find a new one. No one's feelings will get hurt—it's more important to have your needs met. Try to figure out what your current support group is lacking before switching to a new one so that you can make adjustments to your thinking and criteria before you select a new group. Sometimes you also just have to dive in to the group to see whether it's a good fit.

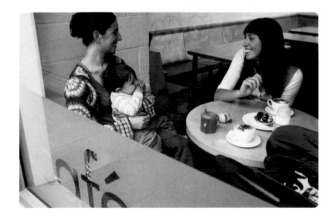

Sometimes just talking to others moms about everyday breastfeeding topics is helpful and comforting.

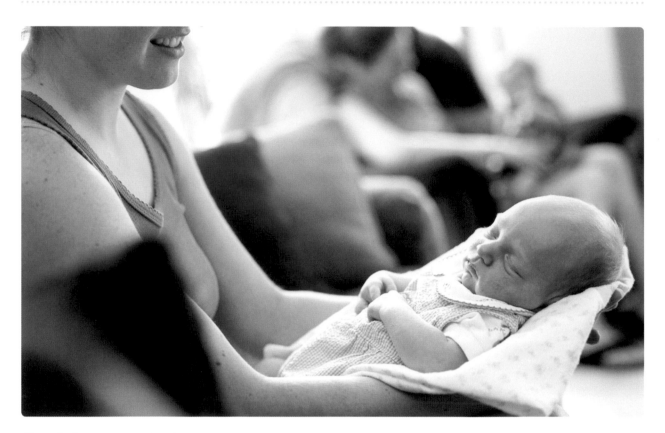

A breastfeeding support group is a place to get reassurance and offer comfort to other mothers in return. It can also branch into future friendships for you and your baby.

TIP Ways to Find Breastfeeding Moms Groups

To find a breastfeeding moms group in your area ask your OB or midwife, hospital staff, childbirth instructor, lactation consultant, or other professional. Also check out the La Leche League's Web site to connect with your local groups, at www.llli.org.

breastfeeding, particularly with breastfeeding in public. They are also likely to be sympathetic during late-night phone calls!

Since these women are all likely to be about the same age as you, it will be easier to understand where they are coming from and vice versa. That being said, do not discount information from older generations. Their perspective is likely to be beneficial as well.

If you don't find anyone in your life who already has breastfeeding experience, you can look in other places, such as mothering groups or your childbirth class. This is also a great way to extend your circle of friends to include others from new groups.

ATTEND A BREASTFEEDING SUPPORT GROUP

A support group is a place for you to go and learn about breastfeeding. It's a good idea to go while you are still pregnant to get information to help you start off breastfeeding on the right foot. Most groups will discuss the benefits of breastfeeding, how to make breastfeeding fit into your life, how to breastfeed, how to help your family support you while you breastfeed, and so on.

Once you have had your baby, these groups are still there for you. You can ask questions about breastfeeding. Typical questions might concern how your baby is doing, how to tell whether your baby is getting enough milk, and other specific issues you might be having. Some groups provide additional support outside the meeting times through phone calls and emails from leaders, as well as referring members to other area group meetings.

Breastfeeding Affirmation

I will remember to ask for help to ensure my breastfeeding success.

The nice thing about breastfeeding groups is that the educational component frequently continues beyond the basics of breastfeeding. These meetings will consist of expanding topics surrounding breastfeeding. This might include:

- When and how to start solid foods
- Sexual intimacy and breastfeeding
- Weight loss and breastfeeding
- Baby massage
- Baby-food making
- Weaning options
- Nutrition after breastfeeding

While every group is different, these are some common topics that are discussed. Some groups may have toddler meetings for the breastfed toddler and family. It is important to remember that these groups are trying to serve women with a ranges of goals when it comes to breastfeeding. La Leche League meetings often take a "salad bar" approach, encouraging members to take whatever advice they can use, and leave the rest that does not apply. Your personal philosophy should be the same.

Most women really enjoy these meetings and look forward to them. If you have found a group that you do not quite gel with do not worry. Try another group. Just as we all have different personalities, so do groups and group leaders. Simply look for a different group in your area. If there is not another group, consider starting your own!

CHAPTER
4

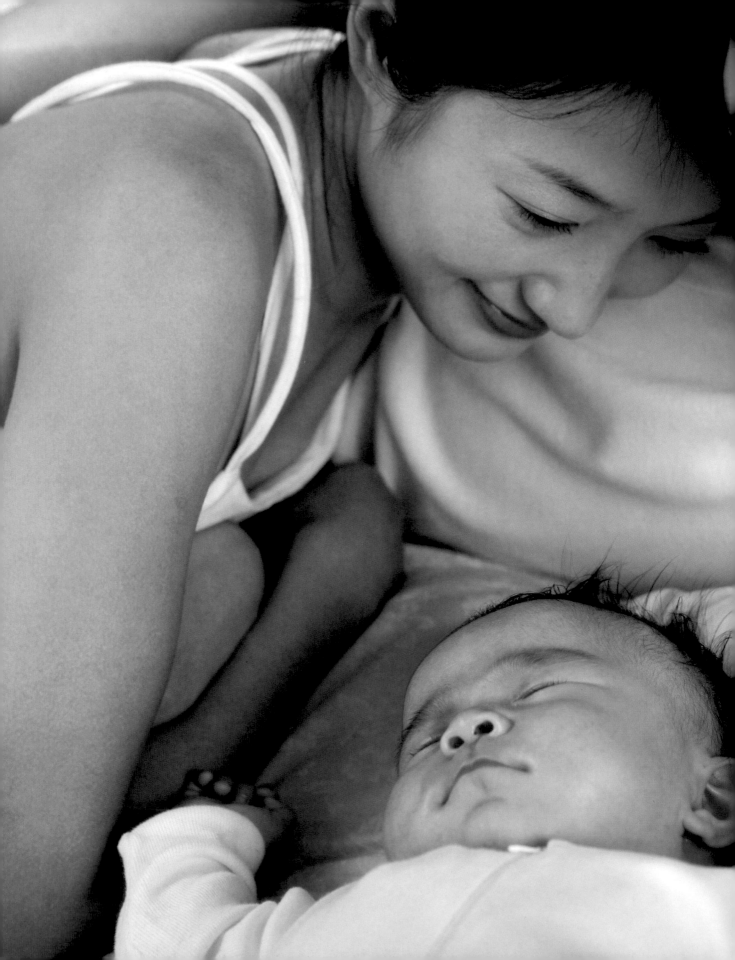

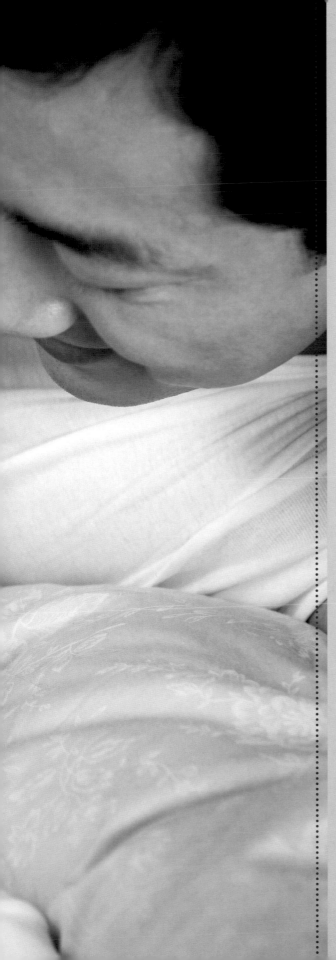

Making Minor Adjustments

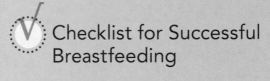

Checklist for Successful Breastfeeding

- ☐ Figure out the first rule of breast-feeding.
- ☐ Choose different breastfeeding positions.
- ☐ Find out how breastfed babies gain weight and grow.
- ☐ Deal with frequent nursing sessions.
- ☐ Learn to wake a sleepy baby.
- ☐ Handle overactive letdown.
- ☐ Deal with thrush and yeast.
- ☐ Master the art of breastfeeding at night.
- ☐ Decide whether pacifiers are right for your family.
- ☐ Deal with a nursing strike.
- ☐ Respond to comments from others.
- ☐ Prepare to breastfeed your baby with older kids around.

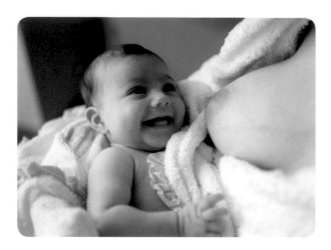

As you're breastfeeding your child, you'll soon realize that things can and likely will change at times. Your baby might favor a certain position for some time, and then suddenly one day decide that he prefers to nurse some other way. Your sleepy baby might learn to be so comfortable while nursing that you'll have to wake him up to maximize feedings. A growth spurt might bring extra nursing sessions some days, as your baby's appetite soars. Don't let these changes throw you—read on, and you'll be prepared to respond and adapt as needed, as well as become a savvier nursing mom in the process.

FIGURE OUT THE FIRST RULE OF BREASTFEEDING

It sounds simple, but it's true. The very first rule of breastfeeding is to feed the baby. This statement can mean many different things to many different people. But what you need to know about this mantra is that feeding the baby will solve many of your issues. It's also an acknowledgment that no matter what, your baby needs to eat.

Is Baby Eating Well after the First Few Weeks?

The first few weeks are unique when it comes to breastfeeding. Sometimes breastfeeding gets off to a rocky start for a variety of reasons. Once the relationship is well established, it is easier to say what you should look for regarding the patterns your baby is showing.

Recall that your baby will nurse eight to twelve times per day, at least in the beginning. During these feedings, you should watch and listen. You should notice whether your baby is sucking rhythmically. Do you see that your baby's mouth is opened wide with his lips flat against the breast? Can you hear him pause while nursing? You might even be able to hear him swallow.

In general, ask yourself how your baby is doing. Does your baby look healthy? His skin should have a good tone. His weight should be increasing at an acceptable pace.

Does you baby have periods of alert play? Is he content to interact with people during this time? Is it hard to rouse your baby? Believe it or not, the definition of a good baby, one that sleeps a lot, can often be a sign that the baby is not getting enough breast milk. Babies who wake frequently are not "bad" or "difficult" babies. When a baby wakes often it is simply a natural way of ensuring that he is eating enough to grow and be healthy. Remember, your newborn baby's stomach is so tiny—it needs to be filled frequently.

CHOOSE DIFFERENT BREASTFEEDING POSITIONS

You have already seen the basics of the major breastfeeding positions listed in chapter 3. But you have to realize that rarely does anything go by the textbook, including breastfeeding. So it's important to look at each position from a different angle to see whether you can tweak the position to make it work better for you and your family.

Sometimes necessity is the mother of invention. You simply find that you naturally alter how you nurse in a certain position. You might not even notice that you have made a minor adjustment here and there, altering the position to fit you and your baby's needs.

Finding Other Positions

You can use plenty of other positions to breastfeed your baby beyond those mentioned in chapter 3. Some you will create because they work for you and your baby, some you will see other mothers and their babies using. You will see more options for positions in this book as the chapters go along. Some might be used for a specific condition or issue, but they might also work for you and your baby even if you don't have that particular issue. The point is that you need to use what works. There is no one right way in which to position your baby for optimal feeding.

WOMEN'S WISDOM:

A good latch is key to your breastfeeding success. Once you get a good latch going, everything else will follow nicely. So what if your positions don't look exactly the same as the ones other mothers use or those that this book says work? If your baby is getting milk, you aren't in pain, everyone is happy, and the latch is good, who cares. Remember that breastfeeding is as individual as the mothers and babies who do it!

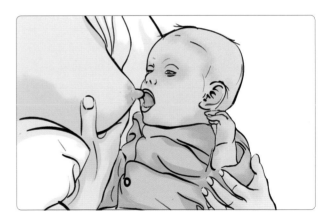

Be sure to point your nipple toward the roof of the baby's mouth. This enables your baby to take more of the areola into his mouth.

CHAPTER
5

FIND OUT HOW BREASTFED BABIES GAIN WEIGHT AND GROW

Perhaps you have heard the slogan: human milk for human babies. It is true. Breast milk is specifically designed for your baby. Your body knows exactly what your baby needs and provides it in exactly the right proportions. If your baby was born early, your body knows and alters the content of the breast milk to accommodate those needs. As your baby gets older and begins to crawl around on the floor, your breast milk responds with an increase in immunities.

What "Thriving" Really Means

Bigger is not necessarily better when it comes to your baby's weight. Babies are said to be "thriving" for a number of other reasons as well. Does your baby seem happy and is she responsive? Does she look healthy, and is her body filling out well? As she gets bigger, are you noticing growth in her cognitive development? Your breast milk is helping your baby to grow in all of these ways. As long as your baby is nursing well, wetting enough diapers, and gaining weight, it doesn't matter where she falls on the growth charts. Healthy babies grow at their own pace!

The fat and protein content of breast milk also changes. Not only does it change as your baby gets older and bigger, but it also changes throughout the course of each day. This means that the breast milk your baby gets in the morning is not the same breast milk your baby gets at night or even in the afternoon. The caloric content varies to suit your baby's needs at different times of the day.

Breastfed babies grow well. But they grow very differently from babies who are not breastfed. Be sure not to get bogged down in comparisons of your baby's growth versus any other baby's growth. Everyone grows differently.

Breastfed Babies and Growth Charts

Most parents have well-baby visits with their pediatricians. The baby's height and weight are checked at these visits. When you take your baby to the pediatrician for a weight and height check, the doctor will mark your baby's measurements down on a chart. This is known as your baby's growth chart.

At each check, your baby is assigned one percentile for height and one for weight. This lets you compare your baby's growth with national averages for children of the same age and sex. You can also begin to see a pattern emerge, called a growth curve. There is a fiftieth percentile and a curve that goes along with it. If your baby girl at, say, two months of age, is in the forty-fifth percentile, it means that 45 percent of two-month-old baby girls weigh the same as or less than your baby does and 55 percent of two-month-old baby girls weigh more than she does. It is a way to figure out how your baby compares with other babies at the same age. Know that what is more important is the curve, rather than the overall numbers.

If your pediatrician is seeing that your baby is really low on the growth charts, you both might be concerned. The first thing to do is to ensure that you and the pediatrician are using the growth charts meant for breastfed babies. The Centers for Disease Control and Prevention (CDC) put out these charts, and they are based on solely breastfed babies. The other growth charts relied more on formula-fed babies, who tend to be heavier and gain weight more quickly than breastfed babies. Obviously, a breastfed baby will look strange on this chart.

Another thing to look for when your baby prefers to hang out at the bottom of the growth chart is that curve. Is your baby growing in a curve that is appropriate for her? Has it been consistent? If the answer is yes, there is likely nothing wrong and you

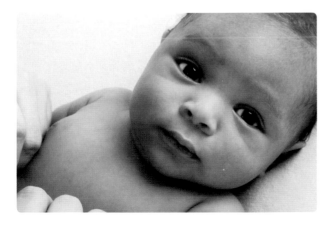

Frequent nursing can sometimes wear on you. Remember why you're doing this—a good look at your baby, thriving and happy, is the best reminder.

simply have a baby who is more on the petite side. Remember to discuss all concerns with your baby's pediatrician.

DEAL WITH FREQUENT NURSING SESSIONS

Some babies nurse more frequently than others. They might have missed the in utero class on how frequently they should be feeding. While textbooks believe that eight to twelve times per day is an adequate number of feedings, sometimes it can be more.

The most common reason for your baby to be nursing more than the average is that he is going through a growth spurt. Growth spurts occur several times in the first six weeks and then slow a bit. But they continue to occur throughout the first year. During a growth spurt, you might notice your baby nurses very frequently. This is the way nature intended for your body to get the signal that more milk is needed. Remember, your body works through a demand-and-supply tactic. Your baby is the demand, and you are the supply.

Look for ways to improve your technique to help you breastfeed more effectively. Let's say you have a baby who is gaining weight but is nursing frequently or for long periods. You might be able to reduce that time by making minor adjustments to the way the baby is latched on. Perhaps your baby could move slightly or get a deeper latch for a better milk transfer rate. If you have gotten used to nursing with the open position, try something else for a bit to see if that doesn't help to reduce the length or number of feedings.

Frequent Nursings?

If you think your baby is nursing more frequently than normal, keep a chart for three or four days. Sometimes it's the sleep deprivation talking and you find out that your baby nurses less often than you previously thought. It just feels like a lot when you are being awakened during the night! If night nursing is getting to you, try feeding your baby while lying down. (See chapter 3 for more on the side-lying position.)

Other babies simply take a long time to eat or eat frequently. This is where adjusting your expectations is best. You cannot spoil your baby by feeding him. It does not work that way. Your baby needs to eat. Breast milk is the best food, and it's perfect for him. Remember, your baby needs to nearly double his birth weight by the half-year mark. Frequent nursing may be what he needs to accomplish that goal.

If staying home to wait to feed the baby is driving you crazy, try something new. You can become a whiz at discreet feeding. Try out your new skills in a restaurant with friends. You could even consider going to see a movie, and just nurse during the movie to help keep your little one quiet. (For more tips on nursing in public, see Chapter 6.)

LEARN TO WAKE A SLEEPY BABY

"Never wake a sleeping baby!" That's what our grandmothers and mothers told us while we were growing up. That might be true of a nice, full baby who is eating well. But the problem is that sometimes you have to wake your baby to make sure she is eating enough, especially in the early weeks.

Why Would You Wake a Baby Who Is Sleeping?

You would need to wake a sleeping baby for two main reasons:

- Baby is sleeping more than she should because she is sick.
- Baby is not gaining weight very well and needs to eat more frequently.

Though the truth of the matter is that why you need to wake the baby to eat really does not matter. What matters is that you wake the baby to eat if the baby is not waking up often enough on her own. This will help you get in more feedings and make sure any issues with the baby are resolved.

Some Techniques That Work

Some babies wake up the minute someone walks into the room. Other babies are great about rousing when picked up. But then there are the babies who just sleep through anything. Sometimes this is because they are just naturally heavy sleepers and other times it's because they are not feeling well.

No matter the cause of the sleepiness, sometimes you need to wake your baby. If you are trying to wake your baby for a feeding, you have a couple of choices if simply picking her up and putting her near the breast doesn't do the trick.

Give your baby a rubdown. Sometimes rubbing your baby will encourage her to wake up. You can rub her back, even through her clothing, stimulating her to awaken. You can also give a mini massage on her arms and legs to try to get her to stir.

Have your baby sit up. Sit her bottom on your lap, and hold her in a sitting position. It usually helps to have one hand under her chin so that her head does not flop forward. You can also try to lay her back and sit her up a couple of times, hoping that the movement helps. You might even combine this with a back rub.

Consider a change. If your baby is snuggled up nice and warm, usually taking off her clothes or changing her diaper will cause her to wake up. None of us like to feel the cold air on our bodies, and babies are no different. If you don't want to remove all of her clothing, you can try simply removing any blankets or swaddling at first. If that doesn't work, move on to getting her down to her diaper.

Use a wet wash cloth. This can also be an effective arousal tool. Use the wash cloth to wipe off your baby's face. Sometimes this will wake your baby right up. But some babies need to be nearly fully stripped and washed down. Some mothers have said that full baths work really well.

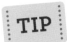

TIP

Time to Eat

It can be difficult to remember how long it has been since you last fed your baby. Keeping a small chart or even setting the oven timer to help remind you can be such a blessing if you need to remember to wake a sleepy baby.

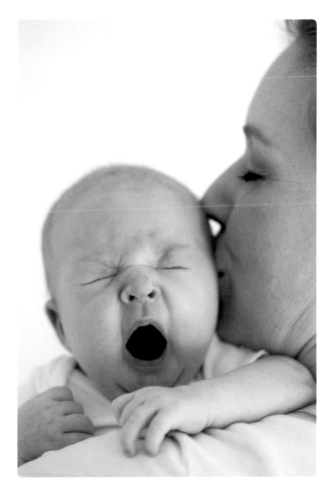

Sleepy babies might not be the best nursers. Try waking your baby up a bit before nursing if you're having troubles.

CHAPTER
5

CONFIDENCE CUE

Breastfeeding at night is the ultimate challenge. During the day, you've got books to read and other things to keep you busy. There are people to help you out. But at night, it's a different story. It's just you and the baby. Instead of dreading nighttime wakings, make the most of the quiet hours. Everything is calm. Try going skin to skin with your baby for nursing sessions, or just for snuggle time. Snuggle up, and let baby latch on. Sometimes when you're not trying very hard, that's when the breastfeeding magic happens. When all the attempts have finally worked and each one has left a small imprint, things come together. Remember, nights are good, no-pressure times, even if you're tired.

Sleeping between breasts can also be an issue for many babies. Your baby might nurse well on one side and then fall asleep before switching and finishing on the other side, only to wake up and nurse again shortly thereafter. This can be quite frustrating for moms, especially during middle-of-the-night feedings when the goal is to get everyone back to sleep! If your little one gets too relaxed and sleepy mid-nurse, know that these techniques will also be helpful in the middle of a feeding as well.

HANDLE OVERACTIVE LETDOWN

Forceful or overactive letdown can be a problem for some breastfeeding mothers and their babies. It frequently occurs with an oversupply of breast milk. You may have an overactive letdown if:

- Your baby chokes or gags while nursing.
- Your baby gulps when nursing.
- Your baby bites down with his gums as if to slow the flow of milk.
- Your baby is gassy.
- Your baby is a noisy nurser; for instance, he clicks while breastfeeding.
- Your baby spits up a lot but is still gaining weight.
- Your baby avoids breastfeeding.

If you think you are having an issue with an oversupply of breast milk or with overactive letdown, there are some tricks you can use to help make breastfeeding less stressful and make your baby happier.

To help your baby to cope with overactive letdown, you can try changing positions. Typically, a good position to nurse in is one in which your baby's throat is above the nipple. Think of this as the milk trying to flow against gravity, which can slow it down for a bit and give your baby a chance to get on top of the flow. Some of these positions include the following.

- **Side lying:** This is probably the most "normal" breastfeeding position to use with an overactive letdown. Choose a side to feed your baby from—left or right. Whichever side you choose, lay with that breast closest to the bed or floor. Your baby should be lying facing you, also on his side. This is a great position to try with a newborn baby, although sometimes it takes some practice to get the hang of it when you're a first-time mom. Stick with it—keep trying this position. Once you do figure out how to nurse while lying down, it will be a blessing!

- **Reclining cradle or cross cradle:** The way you would hold the baby for both of these

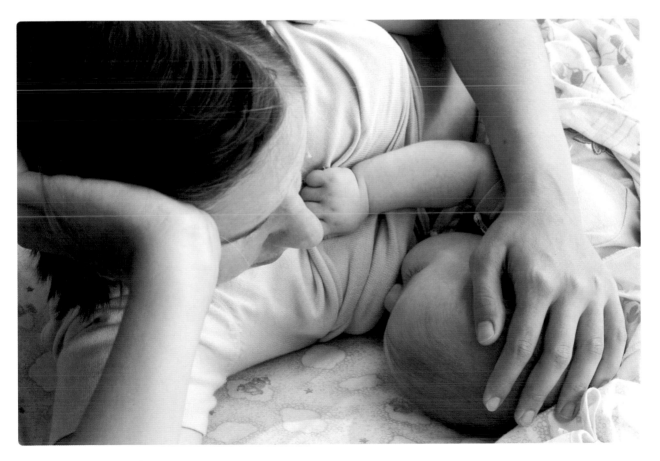

For a change in position, or when you're feeling tired, side lying is a great way to breastfeed.

positions is the same. (See page 75 for a description of the cross-cradle hold.) Your hands should also be in the same positions. What is different is that you are reclining. You can be on your bed or the couch, or even in a reclining chair. Prop yourself up slightly with pillows for comfort.

- **Baby sitting up, facing mom:** For an older or more agile baby, you can try a version of the straddle position. Here, baby sits up and leans over your lap to latch on.

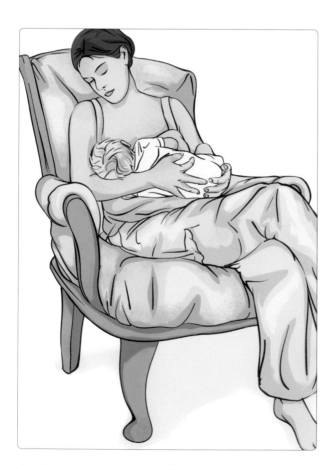

This classic nursing position is good for almost every baby. A nice, comfortable chair can make all the difference.

- **Recumbent feeding:** This position sounds and looks weird, but it is very helpful for some mothers and babies. Simply lay back until you are completely recumbent or nearly completely recumbent. Place your baby belly to belly with you, with baby's brow just above your nipple. Let your baby nurse while lying down in this manner. This might be a difficult position for a newborn with little head control, but it can work well for older babies.

Tips for Treating Overactive Supply and Letdown

Other tips and tricks can help as well, although these are more for treating the symptoms of overactive supply and letdown. For example, if you have a baby who is extremely gassy but otherwise seems fine, consider burping him more frequently. This might even mean stopping in the middle of a feeding to burp him if needed.

If your baby nurses well at the beginning of a feeding, but has trouble with letdown, you can experiment with taking him off the breast for a minute or two. As you begin to feel the milk rushing, pull him off the breast gently. You may even notice that your breast milk sprays. Once that spraying has stopped, try to put the baby back on the breast. If you have multiple letdowns of the same force, you can do this for each letdown.

Do not let your baby become extremely hungry. This might mean feeding more frequently. Less milk is available at one time when feedings occur more frequently, which may also help your body to regulate the milk supply issues. It might also mean your baby does not need to nurse as vigorously, which can keep him from becoming frustrated and agitated during feeding sessions.

Some mothers have reported success with pumping or hand-expressing a bit of milk before a feeding. The problem with this is that you are stimulating the breasts more, which means they will make more milk. This is counterproductive when you have an oversupply. If you do express some milk to make it easier for your baby to latch, be sure that it is only a very small amount—just enough to help your baby to latch more comfortably.

You might also try feeding your baby from one breast per feeding. This can mean your breast will have only one time of really forceful letdown, and the rest of the nursing session will have more moderate letdown. This probably goes against everything you have heard about needing to nurse from both breasts at every feeding. But this is not always necessary. In fact, some mothers have successfully nursed exclusively with only one breast.

Here your goal is to nurse from one breast per feeding. So if your baby nurses on the left side and then pops off but wants more milk in a minute or after burping, you should put him back on the left breast. At the next feeding, you would then offer the right breast. Some mothers even use each side in blocks of time—for example, offering the left breast from noon until three o'clock in the afternoon and the right breast from three o'clock in the afternoon until six o'clock in the evening. Play with the time frames until you figure out what works for you and your baby. Some mothers find that this can be beneficial when their baby is older. As your baby becomes a more adept nurser, an abundant supply can cut down on the length of nursing sessions.

How Long Will It Last?

You might notice an oversupply as soon as your milk comes in, but some mothers do not notice this until their babies are nearly at the one-month mark. Typically, this problem will correct itself within the first twelve weeks. Though it can be miserable for some families, other families find it only slightly annoying.

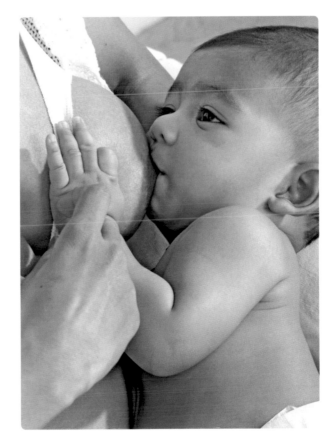

If you aren't sure about your baby's latch, ask yourself if nursing is comfortable and if your baby is gaining well. If you have achieved both, don't stress.

Whatever the case, the good news is that things will get better soon enough. Your breasts won't be spraying everywhere and your baby won't be gagging on your milk forever! Your body will learn how to regulate itself, and your baby will become a more adept nurser as he grows, making it easier for him to deal with your abundant milk supply and strong letdown.

In the meantime, however, you might want to become knowledgeable about breast pads. These cotton inserts help to prevent breast milk from leaking onto your clothing. When you have an

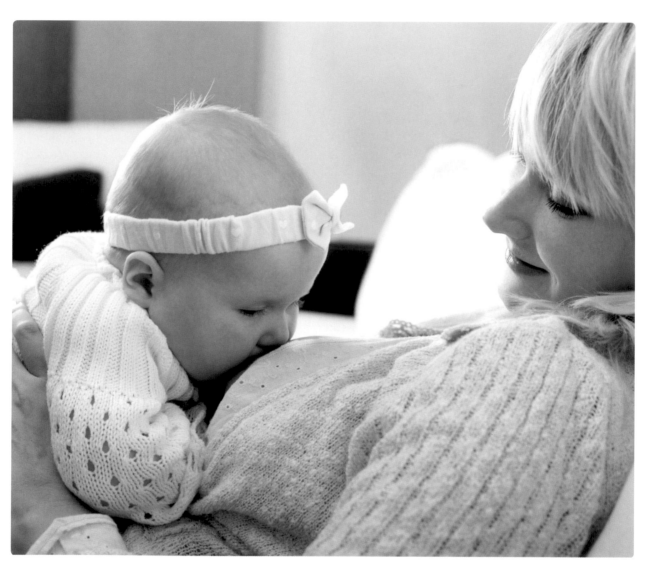

The majority of the time, babies come back to nursing fairly easily after a nursing strike.

overactive letdown or an increased supply, there's a greater chance that you'll leak. Many moms with these issues use breast pads almost every time they are in public. Be sure to pack extra pads in case you need to change them!

DEAL WITH THRUSH AND YEAST

A yeast infection is simply just an overgrowth of yeast, a fungus normally found in your body. Yeast prefers warm, dark places, such as your mouth, folds of the skin, intestinal tract, and vagina. Sometimes the body gets out of balance and is thrown off-kilter by medications or diet. In turn the yeast, which is normally present, is not kept at bay by the body's normal bacteria. This causes an overgrowth. Thrush is simply an overgrowth of yeast in the mouth.

Babies can get thrush from being exposed to yeast in the birth canal. There are also many babies who develop thrush simply due to the hormonal changes that occur after birth. If you are giving your baby antibiotics or if you are taking antibiotics, you might also be more likely to experience thrush. Some mothers and babies simply seem to be more prone to getting yeast infections than others.

Diagnosing Thrush

Typically, you can diagnose thrush in your baby without the help of your doctor or your lactation professional, though if it's your first bout of thrush it might be easier to let someone help you to make the diagnosis. You might notice white patches on the inside of your baby's cheeks. Thrush can also occasionally be on your baby's tongue. With a clean, gauze-covered finger, you can gently try to rub the white patches off. If they come off easily they are breast milk residue; if the area bleeds or the white patches do not come off easily, it is most likely thrush.

If you see some white patches at a feeding, wait for a bit and look again. If the patch is still there, your baby probably has a case of thrush. You will typically need to treat thrush for it to go away, though sometimes you can wait it out if you are not infected and it does not seem to be painful for your baby.

CHAPTER
5

The Real Deal on Nipple Shields

You might hear that using a nipple shield or other device can be helpful. A nipple shield might help to slow your milk flow for the baby. But nipple shields are a slippery slope and your baby might become dependent on them. And if you do not use them correctly you could go from an over-supply of milk to a decreased supply.

Treating Thrush

How you treat thrush will vary depending on the cause of the thrush, how your baby feels, and your outlook on medications. You have to do some simple things first before any medication is effective. These involve preventing reinfection for your baby and preventing yourself from having a yeast problem.

This means everything that goes into your baby's mouth needs to be used only once. So if your baby uses a pacifier, boil it before your baby gets it again. The same holds true for toys and anything else that goes into the mouth, including medication droppers when possible. You might even wish to cleanse your nipples after feeding. A clean, wet washcloth will do the trick.

Some practitioners will treat your baby, and perhaps you, with a medication called Nystatin. This is a prescription medication that is used topically on the spots. You might also be told to use it on your nipples. Some practitioners also use an antifungal agent known as gentian violet. If you go the gentian violet route, first coat your baby's lips with nonpetroleum jelly. This will prevent the violet color of this agent from staining the baby's skin. If for some reason you forget the nonpetroleum jelly, don't worry—the color lasts only a few days.

Yeast in Mom and Baby That Is Not Thrush

Sometimes a yeast infection occurs in the baby's diaper area. You may notice this when you are being treated for oral yeast. You might also simply notice it because your baby's diaper area is warm, dark, and moist, which is the perfect place for a yeast overgrowth.

Typically, a yeast diaper rash is going to have a raised red border. But the biggest clue will be that your usual diaper creams do not seem to help. If your baby has a diaper rash that lasts for more than two days and is not responding to traditional creams and ointments, you should talk to your pediatrician about the next steps for treatment.

There is also something known as a ductal yeast infection. This type of breast yeast infection is very painful. Many mothers say that it feels like they have shards of glass in their breasts. Again, if nursing is ever painful, you should seek help immediately. A ductal yeast infection is typically treated very successfully and quickly with Diflucan, a prescription you can get from your doctor or midwife or from your baby's pediatrician.

MASTER THE ART OF BREASTFEEDING AT NIGHT

It is really not a surprise that you will need to be awake at night to feed your baby. Every new baby will wake up to be fed at first, no matter how she is fed. The obvious reason babies wake up to eat at night is because they have small stomachs that do not hold a lot of food. But this wakefulness has recently been shown to be protective for babies as well. Since babies wake more frequently, they cannot fall into the deeper periods of sleep that can prevent them from rousing in the face of danger.

This danger can be something like hunger, but it could also be pain, fever, or something too close to their face and reducing their oxygen intake.

Once you have it in your mind that this night-time waking is protective, it is much easier to deal with it. This is not to say that you are not tired. This is not to say that it is your favorite parenting activity. But it can help put things into perspective.

Where Does Baby Sleep?

The American Academy of Pediatrics (AAP) recommends that your baby sleep in the same room as you in the first months of life. This is so that you can easily and quickly respond to your baby's nighttime needs. Parents who have their baby in the same room tend to get more sleep than those who have their baby in a separate room. You can have your baby in your room in either a crib or a small sleeping space such as a co-sleeper (which attaches to the side of your bed), bassinet, or cradle.

Some families choose to bring their baby into their bed to sleep. This is called the family bed or co-sleeping. Currently, the AAP is against co-sleeping. In my opinion, this is largely because of poorly designed studies that do not take into account safe co-sleeping practices. To co-sleep safely you must follow some specific rules:

- Do not sleep with your baby anywhere but your bed.
- Do not sleep with your baby if you or your partner has been drinking.
- Do not sleep with your baby if you or your partner has been taking pain medication.
- Do not co-sleep if you or your partner is obese.
- Be sure you have a hard mattress.
- Remove fluffy bedding and pillows.
- Place the baby in your bed so that the baby is away from heavy comforters and blankets (some families choose to turn up the heat and forego comforters, or invest in lighter weight blankets).
- Do not use sleep positioners for your baby.
- Beware of products sold to help you co-sleep, as they may not be safe.

Self-Care Tips

You will experience bumps along the breastfeeding and parenting roads. Just when you think you've got it all down, something will change and you'll be tinkering again. It's all good; you've got the skills. Anytime you feel frazzled, just remember the basics: calm mom; calm baby; quiet room; skin-to-skin contact. Add some warm water, such as a bath, and that can be helpful. Get yourself to a tranquil place, and you will help your baby to do the same.

Co-sleeping is a personal decision. But breastfeeding mothers have done so safely for years and years, as it helps tired mothers get much-needed sleep as well as fosters closeness between mother and baby, which many infants crave at night. Plus, co-sleeping mothers report being extra aware of where their baby is in the bed. They are also able to respond faster as baby wakes up, meaning they do not have to spend extra time to calm the baby before a feeding. And moms can also actually sleep through some of the nighttime feedings. If you have a baby who is waking frequently at night but you are still concerned about the safety of co-sleeping, consider whether it is a safe idea to drag yourself to the point of extreme exhaustion getting up and, perhaps, staying up, over and over again, night after night,

with a fussy, wakeful baby. In such cases, it really can be safer to follow appropriate co-sleeping guidelines so that everyone can sleep more peacefully and mom can function at her best. And contrary to what some people might say, you are not spoiling your baby by co-sleeping, responding to her needs promptly, and giving her the closeness she craves at night. This is not about where your infant sleeps, for how long, or how to get your child out of your bed. I mention bedding practices as they relate to breastfeeding. Breastfeeding mothers who co-sleep get more sleep than other mothers for a variety of reasons, including being able to respond more quickly to their babies, a lesser need for de-escalation once baby is awake (the calming from crying) as well as the ability to stay in bed to nurse. Bear in mind that many babies simply want to sleep in close proximity to their parents. Eventually, your child will learn to sleep on her own, all in due time. In the meantime, you are fostering a healthy bond that will give your child security as she grows and confidence in your willingness and ability to meet and respond to her needs.

While this is not a book about where your baby sleeps, for how long or about how to get your child out of your bed. I mention bedding practices as they relate to breastfeeding. Breastfeeding mothers who co-sleep get more sleep than other mothers for a variety of reasons, including being able to respond more quickly to their babies,

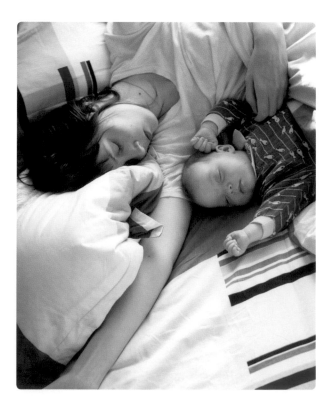

Being awake at night is rough on every parent. Moms who breastfeed and co-sleep report less sleep problems than other mothers.

a lesser need for de-escalation once baby is awake (calming from crying) as well as the ability to stay in bed to nurse.

Ways to Minimize Time Out of Bed

One of the best pieces of advice when it comes to nighttime wakings is to minimize the number of feedings by making sure your baby fuels up fully. Also try to minimize the amount of time you are up with your baby. To that end, responding quickly is key. The sooner you respond to your baby's stirrings, the calmer your baby will be. This translates into a faster feeding, which gets you back to bed sooner.

You should also try to minimize distractions and interaction at night. So, if your baby is awake and needs to be changed and to eat, do so quickly and quietly. Avoid turning on lots of lights. Do not spend a long time conversing with your baby. Sim-

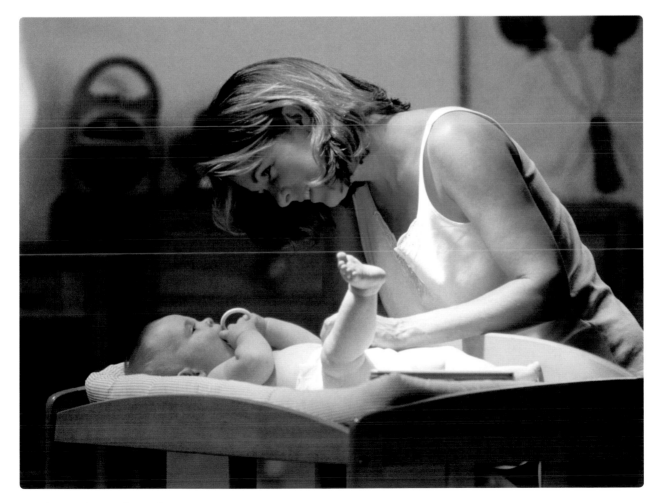

Try to be quiet during nighttime diaper changes to maintain a sense of calm.

ply and quietly change the diaper with low lights. Keep all forms of stimulation to a minimum. This will let your baby know that nighttime is not playtime. It will also hopefully prevent your baby from waking up completely, meaning she will fall back to sleep more easily.

Ways to Minimize Nighttime Feedings

Once your baby is a few weeks old, you will notice a pattern emerging. This will tell you where to start with nighttime feedings. The first thing to try is to have a consistent bedtime routine, no matter what time bedtime is for your baby. A bath, a book, easing into a gentler time of day: These are all things that signal bedtime. Your own bedtime routine can be a collection of whichever elements work for your family at bedtime.

If you go to sleep after your baby, consider sneaking your baby an extra meal just before you go to bed. Depending on when your baby last ate, this could be a top-off or a full meal. This will usually buy you a larger chunk of sleep time. This chunk might be three to five hours in length, depending on your baby. That will even possibly leave you with only one nighttime feeding, at least theoretically, by the time your baby is a few weeks or months old.

The next feeding will typically occur in the early morning. Now, this may not be when you want to wake up. In fact, you might feed your baby and then both of you may go back to sleep for a few more hours, which is your call.

Some babies want to graze all night long. They are getting comfort and nutrition from these night-time nursings. Sleeping with your baby is a quick and easy way to accommodate the nighttime feeding sessions that seem to go on for hours and interfere with your sleep schedule. Many moms note that they are able to sleep through most nighttime feedings when their baby is sleeping with them.

Your baby's doctor is unlikely to help you figure out the safest way to co-sleep. This is because the professional organizations do not recommend that your baby sleep in your bed, only in your room. Yet most practitioners know most parents are sleeping with their babies, at least in part. You may even have friends who are co-sleeping in some manner. While they can share personal experiences, you should look to the safe co-sleeping guidelines on page 123.

It is a widely known fact that parents who sleep with their babies sleep more. More sleep is something that parents can be on board with. Figure out how you can incorporate nighttime closeness with better feedings and more sleep for your family.

Sleep More during the Day

Sometimes nighttime sleep situations are not yet ready to be solved. This means you will spend a lot of time trying to make up for lost sleep. Being sleep-deprived might be what everyone says is normal, but it can also feel horrible and it can be dangerous.

Getting some extra sleep during the day can be very helpful. Not only will you feel more rested, but it will also enable you to have a clearer idea of what you need to succeed with your parenting and breastfeeding journey. So if a nap is what it takes to help you feel better, why not nap?

Seriously, everyone says to sleep when the baby sleeps, but we often listen to that little voice in our heads that says, "Just one load of laundry, and then I'll sleep. . ." That one load of laundry then becomes a cycle of dishes, and so on and so forth, until your baby wakes up. And then you do not get a nap! Even trying to lie down for a few minutes during the day, or co-sleeping during naptime, will go a long way. You can multitask—nurse and sleep!

DECIDE WHETHER PACIFIERS ARE RIGHT FOR YOUR FAMILY

Dummy. Binky. Paci. No matter what you call it, this artificial nipple causes a lot of debate in households around the world. Some people believe it is cruel to refuse to give a baby a pacifier and others think pacifiers are downright evil. The truth is that the pacifier is probably much more neutral than that. It mostly depends on how you use it.

How Babies Calm Themselves

A discussion of how babies calm is in order before you can decide about pacifier use. Babies are born with a need to suck. The reason babies need to suck is to stay alive, as this is how they get milk. However, two distinct types of sucking have been identified: the nutritive and the non-nutritive sucks. Both types of sucking will calm your baby.

The Benefits and Risks of Pacifiers

A pacifier allows your baby to suck, although your baby is getting no nutrition. This also means your baby is not suckling at your breast, which in turn means your milk supply is being diminished, even if that was not the intention.

Some mothers have vibrant milk supplies and a few minutes of a pacifier does not bother anything. This is not true for all mothers. Some mothers will lose their supply very easily.

Making the Decision

There is not a right answer when it comes to pacifiers. The truth of the matter is that only you can decide whether using a pacifier is worth the risks. The benefits might be obvious.

You can also try to delay using a pacifier. Once breastfeeding is well established and your milk supply is good, the risk might be lower. Discuss your options with your family, your friends, and your pediatrician.

CHAPTER
5

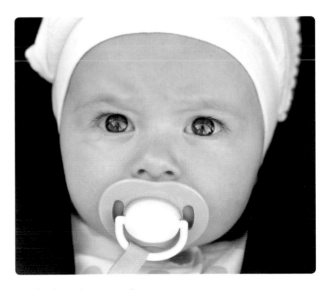

Pacifiers have their pros and cons.

DEAL WITH A NURSING STRIKE

All babies and mothers have their good days and bad days. There are days when breastfeeding or even being close is not what babies want to do. This can be frustrating for you as a mother trying to get your baby to nurse.

What Is a Nursing Strike?

A nursing strike is simply when your baby refuses to breastfeed. This can occur for a single feeding or for more feedings, up to several days. Nursing strikes can be very disconcerting for mothers. It is usually not as disconcerting for babies.

When Do Nursing Strikes Occur?

You usually will not see a nursing strike in a baby who is less than six months old. If you do, it is usually short lived. These nursing strikes are generally due to sore gums or other physical ailments that are causing your baby pain. Remember that skipping a feeding is not harmful to your baby typically.

If you are experiencing a nursing strike, there are many reasons why it might be happening. A few of those reasons include:

- Teething pain
- Ear infection
- Stuffy nose from allergies or a cold
- Changes in routine
- A lengthy separation from mom
- Distractions (talking, television, other people)
- Change in laundry detergent, perfume, bath soap
- Change in milk supply
- An inflexible feeding schedule
- "Sleep training," or letting a baby cry it out
- Travel away from home

Be sure to look for minor issues such as these before jumping to other conclusions. Sometimes the reason is simple to spot. And going back to the old laundry soap is much easier than having a baby who refuses the breast!

What Strategies Should I Use for a Nursing Strike?

When your baby is not nursing at all you will want to try a multipronged approach. First, it is imperative that you feed your baby. In an older baby who is eating solids, this is not as much of a concern. But if you are seeing a nursing strike in a baby who is not eating solids, you should do what you can to see to it that your baby is eating.

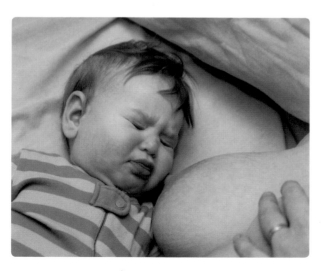

Don't take nursing strikes personally. They often end quickly.

This step is in line with another approach, which is to ensure that you are maintaining your breast milk supply. This can mean pumping your milk to make sure your supply stays up. You can use this breast milk to feed your baby from a cup, an alternative feeder, or even a baby bottle. (Which one you choose should depend on your baby's age and nursing history.) Pumping will also help you to stay comfortable and avoid engorgement, as well as avoid plugged ducts and mastitis. (For more information, see page 177.)

Do what you can to get your baby back to the breast. One of the easiest things to try is to encourage your baby to nurse when he is asleep or extremely drowsy. Sometimes this is the easiest way to get a baby to nurse again. If this does not work, you can try other approaches as well.

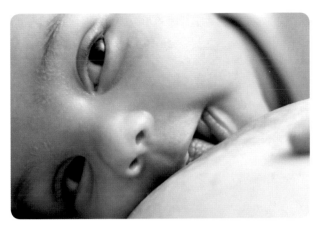

In the majority of instances, babies come back to the breast after a nursing strike.

Nursing Strike Doesn't Equal Weaning

A nursing strike is a brief period of time during which your baby does not nurse. Babies go through nursing strikes for a variety of reasons, but they almost always return to the breast soon enough. A nursing strike does *not* mean your baby is weaning. Simply ride it out and express milk to stay comfortable and maintain your milk supply.

Make sure you are available for your baby. This means both physically available to nurse when your baby is ready to nurse as well as literally able to produce your breasts quickly. Being available includes your clothes. This might be the time to wear a convenient nursing shirt and bra. This will make breastfeeding easier, and it will provide your baby with a near instantaneous result.

Staying close to home for a few days can also be helpful, though not necessary. This can be done over the course of a long weekend. Simply stay in bed with your baby and have some down time. This is often called the forty-eight-hour cure.

If that is not possible, simply be available for your baby as much as possible. Also try carrying your baby in a sling. This can help you to go about your life while keeping your baby closer.

Also try various nursing positions. Perhaps your baby isn't nursing as well as normal because of some pain that you cannot find. It could be the place where he got a recent shot or even a bruise

CHAPTER
5

from an attempt to walk. Whatever the cause, it might hurt for your baby to nurse in your normal nursing position.

Some mothers also find that walking or rocking is helpful. The motion might distract a baby who is reluctant to nurse. You can also try the opposite and go for a calm, quiet, and still environment to see if that helps.

Monitoring your baby for adequate intake is something to help keep your sanity. Checking for five to six really wet diapers per day will ensure that your baby is getting enough to eat. You should not starve a baby so that he "gets over" a nursing strike. This will only cause more problems.

The good news is that while nursing strikes can be physically and emotionally exhausting for you and your baby, they are frequently short lived. Nevertheless, the few days to more than a week that a nursing strike lasts can seem really long. You might never figure out what caused the strike. But remind yourself that this is not weaning, which babies almost never do abruptly or before a year and a half or two years of age. When in doubt about a nursing strike, seek feedback and advice from those around you who are supportive of breastfeeding.

RESPOND TO COMMENTS FROM OTHERS

As you are making your way in your breastfeeding relationship, you may notice that many people have opinions about what you are doing or how you are doing it. However, as you and your partner agree on what is going on in breastfeeding and parenting,

and your decisions are right for your baby, you are fine. You also need to know that presenting a solidified front is a benefit when relatives or friends try to divide you.

Breastfeeding is a topic that will draw people to talk. Others will always have advice for you, no matter how your breastfeeding is going. If your breastfeeding is running into trouble, they will have sixteen ways to make it all better! If your breastfeeding is going well, they will tell you what you can do to wean your baby. All of this unwanted advice is a wild ride.

The bottom line is that people will probably say some things that you disagree with, and you will need to respond. Have a few handy retorts ready as well as some solid facts, and you will be prepared. For example, if someone tells you that breastfeeding is of benefit in only the first weeks and suggests that you wean your baby now that you are going back to work, you can give him or her the facts: Breastfeeding is always nutritionally beneficial.

Another technique is to tell such people what the breastfeeding experts say. If you're running into some breastfeeding snags, for instance, you might hear that you could always supplement. But what you really want and need is to have some help with breastfeeding. So you could explain that your lactation professional has advised you to do "x, y, or z" to help you maintain your milk supply.

If your mother-in-law is offering her home remedies for a low milk supply, you know she is trying to be nice, even if it is annoying you to death. You can share with her some of the tips you have been using from various sources. This will allow her to participate, even without you having to follow her suggestions.

Sometimes people just butt in and offer unsolicited advice. If they do not understand the benefits that breastfeeding brings to mother, baby, the family, and society, you probably will not be able to enlighten them. Simply ignore them. Many mothers find that this is the way to go, but sometimes it's not possible to ignore their comments. In such cases, tell them their comments are annoying you, and perhaps they will stop.

PREPARE TO BREASTFEED YOUR BABY WITH OLDER KIDS AROUND

Nursing your baby with a toddler or an older child running around can be a fun experience. Sometimes the cute things your older child asks or says just blow you away. Other times you are harried and wish you were alone a bit more with the baby. Whatever the case, it can be a challenge to juggle older kids when you have a new infant. Nevertheless, there are ways to cope confidently with these issues.

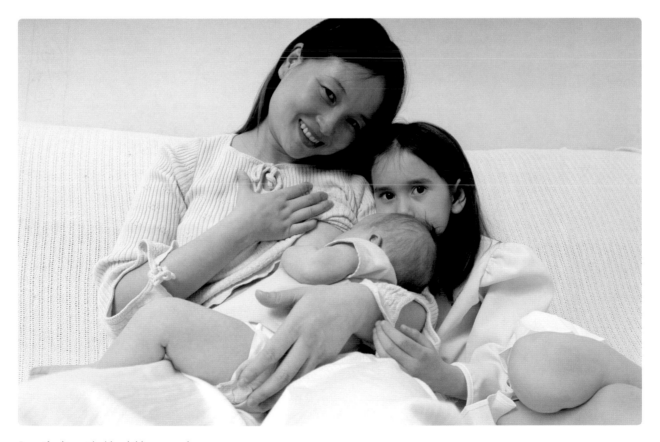

Breastfeeding with older children around can be both challenging and rewarding.

CHAPTER
5

Touched Out

Many new mothers who have more than one child experience the feeling of being "touched out" from time to time. For instance, after nursing your newborn, you are likely to want to be left alone, when your older child really just wants some hugs and cuddle time. This is when it gets tough.

This touched-out feeling is normal. Sometimes expressing to your older child that you need a break is enough to get some needed space. Some mothers choose to explain it in terms of needing a time out. However you choose to, try to be patient in explaining your feelings to your older child, and make sure you re-engage with your older child as soon as you feel like you've had a bit of a break.

Entertaining Your Other Children While Breastfeeding

While you are breastfeeding your baby, it's a safe bet that your other children will also want attention at times. It would be great if you always had someone else with you to pinch hit, but that simply is not realistic for most families. There are many moments when mom is the only game in town. For those times when you feel as though you can't split yourself into enough pieces to attend to everyone, here are some tricks of the trade.

One is a goodie box. This special box of really fun, really special, and really quiet toys should be something you bring out only when you are nursing. This helps your older child enjoy something special while you get a bit of a break. These toys can be puzzles, felt boards, bubbles, coloring books—anything that is quiet and self-contained.

You can also choose to use breastfeeding as reading time. After you have your baby latched on, pick up a book and read to your child. Snuggle up close to your older child on the opposite side, and he or she will sit right down and listen. Your older child will come to enjoy this special quiet time that goes along with breastfeeding.

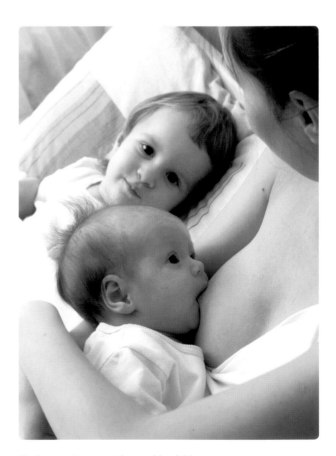

Find ways to interact with your older child while you are nursing. Telling stories or singing songs reminds them that they are still special.

Remember to do what works for your family. Think about other activities or games that suit your kids' interests, such as making up stories, or watching as the "audience" while your older child sings, dances, or puts on a show. As long as the activities are safe and age appropriate, it really is up to you.

It might take a bit of time for you, your baby, and your older children to get acclimated to a new routine, but it will happen soon enough. In the beginning, you might feel a bit frenzied trying to split your time between an infant who needs to nurse and an older child or children who also crave your attention. Before you know it, though, if you continue to make your older children feel special and include them in your breastfeeding sessions and other times with the baby, you will begin to build new routines together that work for all of you!

Breastfeeding Affirmation

My baby and I will work out the quirks of our breastfeeding relationship.

CHAPTER
5

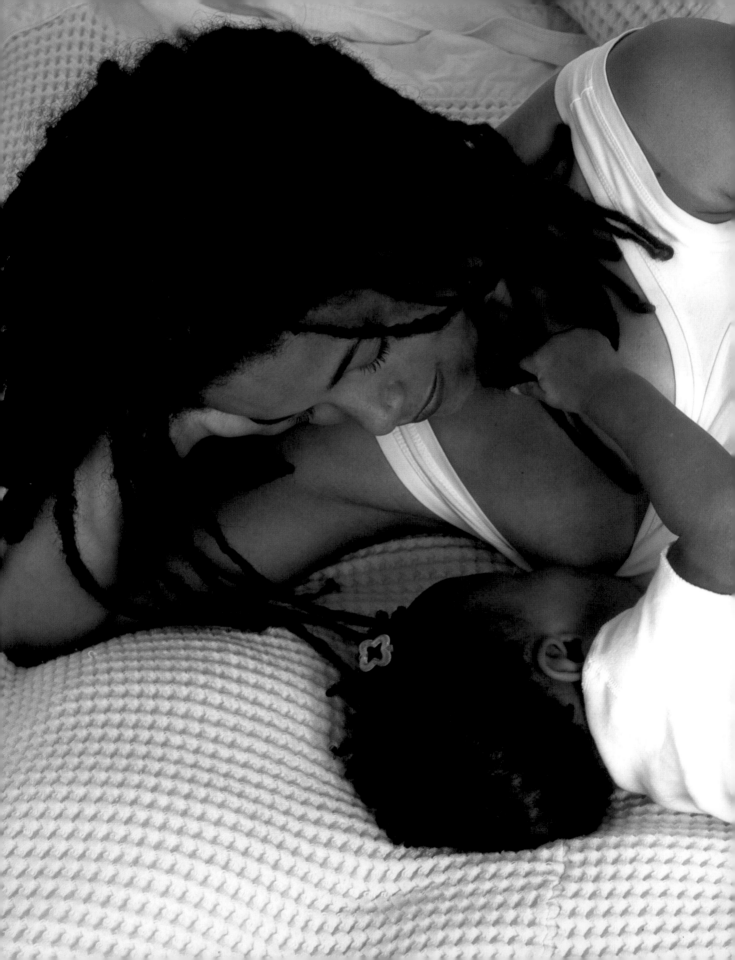

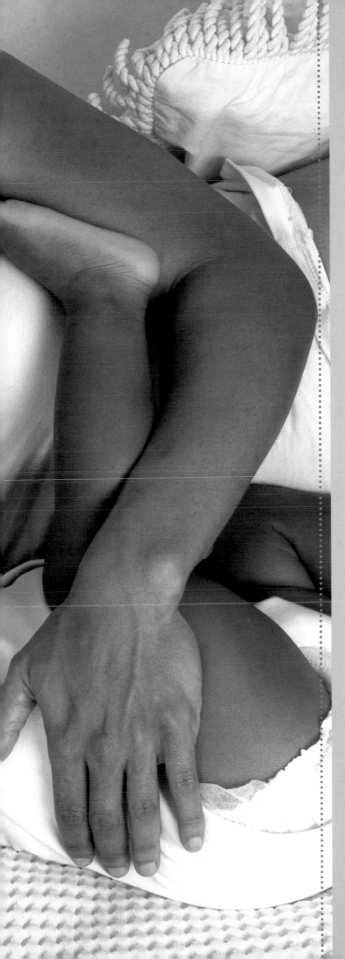

Living a Breastfeeding Lifestyle

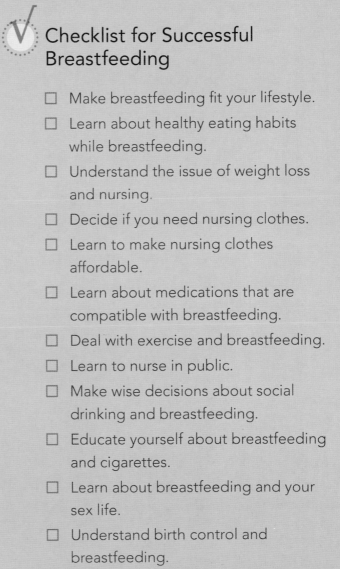

✓ Checklist for Successful Breastfeeding

- ☐ Make breastfeeding fit your lifestyle.
- ☐ Learn about healthy eating habits while breastfeeding.
- ☐ Understand the issue of weight loss and nursing.
- ☐ Decide if you need nursing clothes.
- ☐ Learn to make nursing clothes affordable.
- ☐ Learn about medications that are compatible with breastfeeding.
- ☐ Deal with exercise and breastfeeding.
- ☐ Learn to nurse in public.
- ☐ Make wise decisions about social drinking and breastfeeding.
- ☐ Educate yourself about breastfeeding and cigarettes.
- ☐ Learn about breastfeeding and your sex life.
- ☐ Understand birth control and breastfeeding.
- ☐ Be a breastfeeding advocate.

Weaving breastfeeding into your life is easy. By doing so, you can ensure that you are enjoying the most benefits from breastfeeding and the ease that it can add to your life. During pregnancy or as a new mother, you might have heard naysayers complain that breastfeeding is too hard or that it runs the show. Yes, feeding your baby should always be a priority, but breastfeeding is not something that should restrict your life. Rather, it's something that you can easily work into everything you already do.

Breastfeeding certainly takes a lot less time to prepare for than does bottle feeding. There is no mixing, measuring, heating, or washing involved. When your baby is hungry, you need only pause to latch your baby on, and the milk is instantly ready and just right every time. Yes, you must stop to breastfeed your baby several times a day. But the simple act of feeding your child is but one of many things that you must do for your baby every day, just as you would change diapers, give a bath, or perform any other task. Having a child alters your life and lifestyle in many ways. But the joys and benefits of breastfeeding—and having children in general—far outweigh those changes!

MAKE BREASTFEEDING FIT YOUR LIFESTYLE

One of the best things about breastfeeding is the portability of it. You can simply take you and your baby anywhere, and you have everything you need for feeding. You do not need to lug baby bottles, sterilizing equipment, liquids, washers, and so on. This ease of use makes breastfeeding wonderfully simple for most mothers.

That being said, you need to figure out what your lifestyle is and how breastfeeding fits into it. In what ways will breastfeeding affect your daily life? Do you need to calculate medications? Do you have any chronic conditions? Will you need to think about clothing that will help you to nurse discreetly? Will you be able to eat everything you want, or do you need to follow a special diet? What about exercise? Most of these questions can be addressed and then fully integrated into your life as you breastfeed.

One of the reasons many women cite for breastfeeding is they believe it will make their life with a new baby easier. This can be very true. But it is also important to remember that having a baby can be

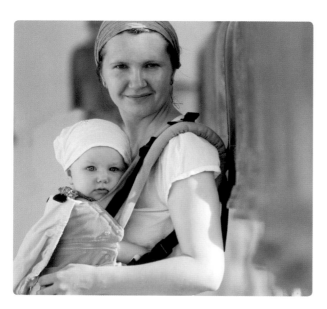

Breastfeeding fits into your lifestyle easily with very little modification. The benefits far outweigh the adjustments.

TIP

Multitask While Breastfeeding

During your breastfeeding sessions, plan ways to add your baby into the mix of things you are doing. Can you type while breastfeeding? Can you read a book to your toddler? Answer a phone? Breastfeeding does not have to be done to the exclusion of all else, all the time. Although sometimes taking a break to sit back and relax with your little one is the fun part!

difficult, breastfeeding or not. You might have good days and bad days. Sometimes breastfeeding gets a bad name and women start to pin all of their woes on it. They mistakenly believe that if they were not breastfeeding, life would be simpler. This detrimental thinking can be hard to take, particularly if you are really pro-breastfeeding. Of course, it's normal to think these things at times, especially if and when your baby has days when it seems like he wants to nurse constantly. But just remind yourself of the added problems and time constraints that you would have if you were not breastfeeding. As time goes on, and you and your baby become an expert nursing team, you will continue to reap benefits from breastfeeding, and you will enjoy it even more.

LEARN ABOUT HEALTHY EATING HABITS WHILE BREASTFEEDING

Unlike during pregnancy, there are typically no food restrictions while breastfeeding. The most important thing is to focus on consuming a well-balanced, healthy diet. This should consist of a variety of fruits and vegetables, whole grains, protein, and some fats.

What You Should Eat

The breastfeeding period is a unique time in your life. You have a very split focus. On the one hand, you are working to nourish a baby who is trying to grow at a rapid rate. On the other hand, you are focused on healing your body after pregnancy and birth, and this probably also encompasses some thoughts about losing at least a few pounds to get back toward your pre-pregnancy weight.

As your baby gets older and your strength comes back, you might wish to focus more on returning to your pre-pregnancy weight. While this is possible, you should take care not to severely limit or restrict your calories. Breastfeeding burns a fair number of calories. Some mothers find they are really hungry and eat through those calories fairly quickly. Limiting your calories too much will compromise your strength, but can also negatively affect your milk supply. You can, however, work on losing weight and toning your body. Incorporate a workout into your daily routine, even if that workout comprises walking the baby. There are no real restrictions on the type of exercise you can do, unless you have specific medical issues from the birth.

CHAPTER
6

Vital Nutrients for Infant Health

Breast milk is unique in that its value cannot be duplicated. In addition to breastfeeding, these nutritional guidelines for your baby stress the importance of a healthy, balanced diet and an overall picture of health. For further information, always discuss guidelines particular to your baby with your pediatrician.

NUTRIENT	SOURCE
Protein: Babies need protein to build healthy muscle which carries nutrients through the bloodstream and fights infections. Proteins are also a source of energy. A sufficient amount of protein is particularly important during growth spurts and in infancy.	Meat, fish, beans, egg, starting at 12 to 24 months
Amino Acids: Amino acids are the building blocks of proteins. The amino acids allow the body to build protein. The body can make all but ten amino acids. Babies need to get these specific amino acids from what they consume. They are significantly important for healthy growth.	Legumes, vegetables, fruits, and grains, starting at 6 to 12 months
Breast Milk: The amount of essential amino acids in breast milk is ideal for babies. It contains two types of protein—whey and casein. Whey is present in larger amounts and is easier for baby to digest.	Mom
Fat: Fat is a vital nutrient in an infant's diet. It is a source of energy for growing babies and an essential building block for myelin, the substance that surrounds nervous tissue allowing nerves to function effectively. As with amino acids used to build protein, there are fats that babies cannot formulate themselves and must be included in their diet to ensure healthy growth. The types of fat in breast milk are ideal for babies.	Egg yolks, cheese, and yogurt (coconut, rice, or soy) starting at 12 months
Iron: Iron is necessary for the creation of red blood cells which carry oxygen to muscles and the brain. The American Academy of Pediatrics recommends that infants receive between 0.15 and 3.0 mg/100 calories of iron for normal growth and development. Premature infants may have different iron requirements, so discuss your baby's iron needs with your pediatrician.	Iron-fortified cereal, dark green leafy vegetables, blackstrap molasses, starting at 6 to 12 months

NUTRIENT	SOURCE
Carbohydrates: Carbohydrates are an essential components of many body structures, but their most important function is as a source of energy. While infants can use protein and fat for energy, using carbohydrates for energy spares protein and fat to be used as building blocks for muscles, nerves, and other vital structures.	Organic brown rice cereal, pasta, legumes, potatoes, starting at 8 to 12 months
Vitamin A: Vitamin A is important for healthy skin and eyes. Vitamin A (also called retinol) is important in inhibiting infections. It was the first fat-soluble vitamin discovered, hence the name vitamin A. When consumed in recommended amounts, breast milk satisfies an infant's vitamin A requirements.	Dark-green and deep-yellow fruits and vegetables, and grain products, starting at 6 to 12 months
Vitamin D: Vitamin D encourages a healthy bone structure by promoting absorption of calcium and phosphorus, important components of bone, from other foods. This vitamin is unique in that it can be made in a baby's skin after mild exposure to sunlight. Some mothers' milk may have low levels of vitamin D. For this reason pediatric experts recommend that infants who are exclusively breastfed receive additional vitamin D as a precaution.	Fish and egg, and sunshine starting at 12 to 24 months
Vitamin E: Vitamin E is an antioxidant and provides protection against the damaging effects of substances in the body. Breast milk is an excellent source of vitamin E and satisfies a full-term infant's requirement. Premature infants may have the need to supplement vitamin E. If your baby was born early, discuss this particular need with your pediatrician.	Asparagus, avocado, sweet potato, leafy greens, soy beans, mango, and kiwi, starting at 6 to 12 months
Vitamin K: Vitamin K is essential for normal clotting of the blood. To prevent a bleeding condition that can occur after birth, newborns are routinely given a supplement of vitamin K.	Green, leafy vegetables, starting at 6 to 12 months

CHAPTER
6

This information was compiled from a variety of sources and based on generally accepted guidelines for infants and toddlers. See Appendix B, page 292. Always confer with your pediatrician for nutritional guidelines pertaining to your baby's specific needs.

The only food exceptions would be foods that you normally avoid. These could be foods that you are allergic or sensitive to in your own diet. You might also find that occasionally your baby is sensitive to foods and additives as well. For instance, caffeine might keep your baby awake or feeling jittery, in the same manner as it would do to you. These will be things you will want to use your best judgment on. Just observe your baby, and make minor adjustments based on your personal experiences.

While it is not common, some babies can be sensitive to some foods that you eat. First determine why you think your baby is reacting to your diet. Is it because of gas? Generalized fussiness? A runny nose? Diaper rash? Vomiting? While something you are eating might be causing these things, they might also have other causes as well.

If you think a particular food is bothering your baby, try keeping a food log. Mark down what you eat and mark down when your baby is upset. Then consider how that looks. Does your baby cry? Perhaps your baby gets really gassy? Does your baby have a rash?

Using this journal might help you to find a pattern and narrow down the offending food. All babies are different, but one of the most common issues is dairy sensitivity. This sensitivity can look different for many families, however. You might find that your baby fusses if you eat milk or cheese, but is fine with a tiny bit of cheese in something else, such as a casserole. These might be a sign of food allergies to come, or they could simply be something your baby outgrows.

To be sure that what you are eating is bothering your baby, most lactation professionals will recommend an elimination diet. This means you would cut out the food or foods that you suspect, one at a time, to see whether you notice changes in your baby. Generally, it will take several days before you can be sure that a certain food is what is bothering your baby.

Reduce Gassiness

Cruciferous vegetables such as cabbage, Brussels sprouts, broccoli, and cauliflower, as well as beans, can be tough on a young infant's digestive tract, as they tend to cause a lot of gassiness. Sometimes mothers notice their babies tend to get fussier after they eat these vegetables. Infant gas drops are available to alleviate such discomfort. But before you resort to giving your baby medication, consider taking gas pills yourself when eating these foods. The digestive enzymes in the pills will pass through your milk, and your baby will get the benefits. (You can confirm with your pediatrician or lactation consultant that it's safe to take these pills if you're at all concerned.)

This is not a sign that you need to quit breastfeeding. Chances are good that whatever is bothering your baby is most likely to be a cow's milk protein, and the same ingredients would be in other supplements. If your baby has milk sensitivity, as a breastfeeding mother you are actually at an advantage here because you can simply adapt your diet to include fewer dairy products as needed.

Caffeine and Breastfeeding Babies

Many women consume caffeine on a daily basis prior to pregnancy. Many women give up caffeine during pregnancy. Those who do not abstain from caffeine still tend to limit the amount of caffeine they consume each day. Caffeine consumption in pregnancy should be limited to about 150 to 300 mg per day.

If you have given up caffeine during pregnancy, you might simply stay on the anti-caffeine bandwagon for a while during lactation. This is typically just simpler for everyone involved. But if you are still consuming caffeine or if you start consuming caffeine, you will need to watch your baby for signs that it is bothering her. Although caffeine is approved by the American Academy of Pediatrics (AAP) as a "safe" drug for lactation, you should still attempt to limit your caffeine consumption. There are health benefits for you, such as being less jittery and able to sleep better when you do not have caffeine in your system, and these will probably hold true for your baby too!

That being said, not all babies are bothered by caffeine, even though it is a stimulant. But if your baby is bothered, you might notice wakefulness in

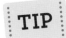

Spice Things Up

Mothers try to remove spices from their diets. While your baby will get tastes of food flavors and spices, babies do not seem to be bothered by these taste changes. In fact, mothers in other cultures rarely change their diets for breastfeeding, meaning that these babies are constantly able to try new tastes. Spicy foods, garlic, and lots of other tastes are common, and if you like them you should not avoid them while breastfeeding.

excess of normal. You might also see agitation or restlessness, even screaming. Cutting out caffeine to see whether the symptoms go away is the only real way to tell whether that is the source. The problem is that it can actually take days for you to notice a difference in caffeine reduction.

Caffeine is also something that your baby will grow to tolerate typically. So if your newborn is sensitive to caffeine, your six-month-old might not be so sensitive. This means you might wait to start your caffeine consumption.

Caffeine peaks in your breast milk in about an hour. How long it hangs out there really varies. For

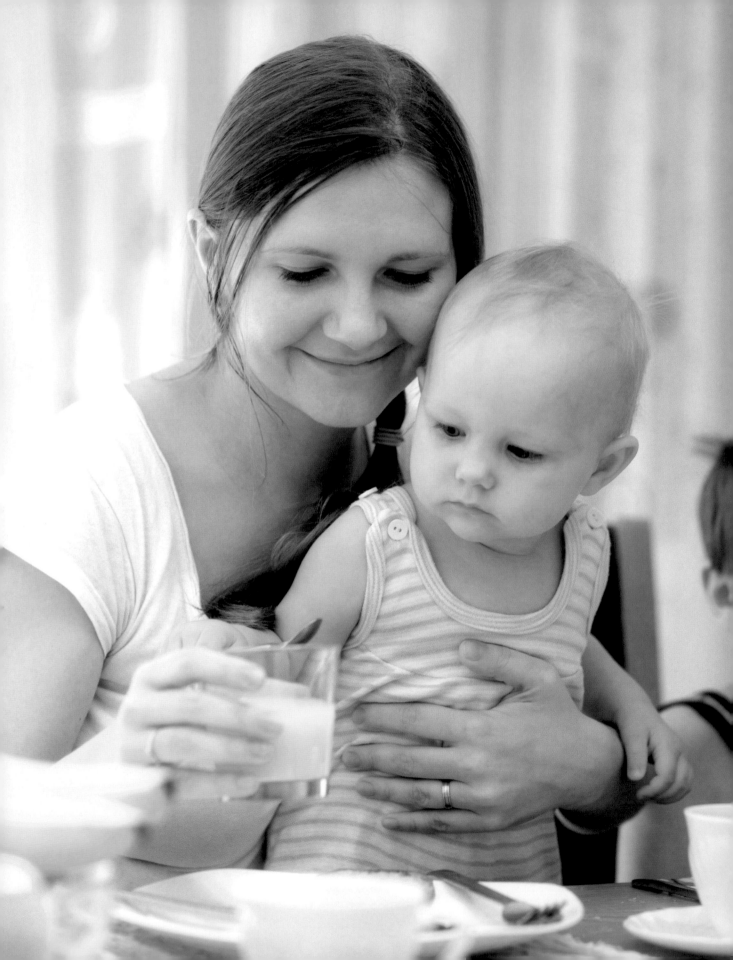

a newborn, the half-life of caffeine, or the amount of time it takes for half of the caffeine you have consumed to be gone from your milk, is up to four days. However, in a six-month-old, that time frame is closer to about two and a half hours.

Use caffeine wisely. Avoid it later in the day if you must consume it. Watch your baby for signs of sensitivity. And look for hidden sources of caffeine, such as chocolate, various foods, and teas.

Artificial Sweeteners

Nothing brings up a debate about safety and health concerns as do artificial sweeteners. Here's the deal: Not a lot of research has been done on all of the artificial sweeteners on the market today, particularly as it applies to breastfeeding. One thing you need to keep in mind is that all artificial sweeteners are not alike and should not be lumped together.

Aspartame (Nutrasweet): This is one of the most common artificial sweeteners. The biggest problem with aspartame would be if your baby had phenylketonuria (PKU), a genetic metabolic disorder. If your baby has not been diagnosed with PKU, aspartame is listed in the safest (L1) category by Dr. Thomas Hale in his book, *Medications and Mother's Milk.*

Saccharin: This chemical can build up over time in your breast milk. It is rated as moderately safe (L3) by Dr. Hale.

Sucralose (Splenda): Despite the lack of research on the subject, the makers of Splenda say that it is safe for nursing mothers.

Basically, artificial sweeteners are typically just a bunch of chemicals or are made from a bunch of chemicals. Limiting the amount that you consume is generally a good idea, whether you are nursing or not.

There are also more natural alternatives to artificial sweeteners. These can include natural products such as stevia, agave nectar, and honey, to name a few. Very little research has been done on the majority of these, but they are plant based. You will need to do your own research and talk to your practitioner about using these products.

UNDERSTAND THE ISSUE OF WEIGHT LOSS AND NURSING

In pregnancy, your body changed rapidly. One of the things your body did was to lay down some fat stores. These fat stores were for the express purpose of helping to support breastfeeding. If you are trying to lose weight and reduce these fat stores you will want to do this while maintaining your milk supply.

CHAPTER
6

If you are in good health, your diet does not need to be radically altered for breastfeeding.

Reducing Calories While Breastfeeding

If you are trying to lose weight, you will want to figure out how to reduce your calorie intake easily. It takes about 300–500 calories per day to breastfeed for most women. You should factor this in when you are figuring out how many calories you need to consume to lose weight.

If you try to reduce your caloric intake too suddenly, you could have a problem with your milk supply. You might notice a sizeable drop in the amount of milk you produce. This usually happens when a mother is not consuming enough calories, after previously having an adequate supply.

This does not mean you cannot reduce your caloric intake or diet. You just need to do so cautiously and safely. To ensure that you maintain your milk supply, watch what you are doing regarding your dietary changes, and be aware of how your milk supply is responding.

When Do You Lose the Weight?

If you are really interested in the weight-loss aspects of breastfeeding, you're in luck. Breastfeeding can help you to lose those stores of maternal fat that are specifically laid down in pregnancy just for the purpose of breastfeeding.

You might hear some mothers say that losing weight while breastfeeding is a myth. This could be because they expect to eat whatever they want, not exercise, generally not take care of their bodies, and yet watch the weight melt away. While some women do lose weight pretty easily while breastfeeding, this is not true for all women.

Some mothers feel like they did not lose their pregnancy weight until after their child was a bit older. This might be due to other hormonal effects of pregnancy wearing off. It could also be due to a change in the mother's or baby's eating habits.

The best plan for weight loss while breastfeeding is to eat to appetite the first two months. Do not focus on calories or exercise. Rather, focus on your new baby and recovering from pregnancy and childbirth.

After that period of time, you move into the two-to-six-months range for breastfeeding. During this time, breastfeeding mothers tend to lose more weight than mothers who are not breastfeeding, even when the breastfeeding mother is consuming more calories. The typical weight loss, without restricting calories or adding exercise, is about 1–1.5 lbs (.45–.68 kg) during this point.

If you add some exercise to this, you will burn even more calories. At this point, you can also consider reducing the number of calories you consume. This is not harmful to you or your baby. Only rapid weight loss is typically something that would affect your milk supply.

After the six-month mark, you will continue to lose weight from breastfeeding. The amount that you lose will slow a bit. This is normal for all mothers. At this point, the amount of time you spend breastfeeding begins to reduce as baby begins to add solid foods to his diet. Also, keep in mind that as you get closer to your pre-pregnancy weight, those last few extra pounds are always the hardest and slowest to come off. These might be some of the reasons behind the slowdown in weight loss.

I'm Hungry All the Time!

Breastfeeding is hard work on your body, and most nursing mothers find that yes, they are hungry all the time. (This is great news for those of us who love to eat!) For this reason, some mothers decide to focus on burning calories rather than reducing the amount of food they eat, because mentally and emotionally it can be difficult to remain in a constant state of hunger. The most important thing is not to ignore your body. If it says "Hungry!" then feed it.

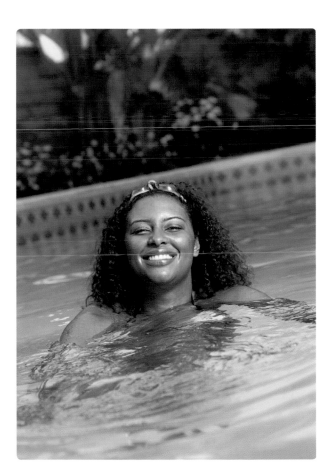

Exercise, in addition to breastfeeding, is a great way to help you achieve postpartum weight loss.

Instead of taking a deprivational approach to food, focus on ensuring that what you eat is worth the calories you're investing. Remember to eat foods that will boost your blood sugar and sustain it, rather than have you suffer from a sugar crash a few hours after eating.

Be sure that you are eating well, even if you are eating often. Remember that your body is working on trying to feed another human being. This takes energy. You need fuel, food, to produce that energy.

DECIDE IF YOU NEED NURSING CLOTHES

Clothes that are made especially for breastfeeding are not new. In recent years, though, the number of nursing clothing lines available has dramatically increased. This is good news, because you have lots of choices available to you. Nevertheless, don't be fooled into thinking that nursing clothes are mandatory for a successful breastfeeding stint.

Breastfeeding or nursing clothes have special openings that allow you to nurse or pump with ease. These are usually hidden openings that hide the rest of your body while you are doing what you need to do. Some work simply by moving fabric and others involve fasteners. The openings are discreet and are usually hidden with cleverly placed pieces of fabric or other designs.

While breastfeeding clothes have some great benefits, they are not necessary for everyone. Some women completely revamp their wardrobe and invest in lots of nursing clothes. Some women choose to have a few key pieces of nursing wear. And then there are mothers who have next to nothing when it comes to breastfeeding clothes. If anything, know that nursing clothes have more to do with your own perceived level of comfort than the reality of what people can see when you are nursing. There are ways to make almost any clothing—nursing or not—work to your advantage, if you are strategic.

You will find what works for you and your family. How many nursing-specific clothes you need will largely depend on how you nurse and what your lifestyle is like. For example, if you work out of the home and you have to breastfeed in your work clothes or use a breast pump, nursing clothes might be imperative. It can also depend on your baby. Some babies really hate anything touching their face while they nurse, even the edge of your shirt, making nursing with regular clothes a bit more difficult.

Nursing clothes come in nearly every form you can imagine. There are nursing tops, nursing dresses, pajamas for breastfeeding, and even bathing suits. This is where your lifestyle can also play a part. If you never go swimming, you obviously do not need a bathing suit. And if you do go swimming, there are also ways to make a normal bathing suit work. For example, consider a V-cut suit that crisscrosses in the front. Then, when your baby wants to nurse, you can simply throw a t-shirt on over your suit, pull down one side, and nurse easily. In this way, see what you already have in your wardrobe that is breastfeeding friendly and then fill in the pieces, if need be, from there.

If you think you will need multiple tops for the week, mainly for work, it would make sense to invest in some nicer breastfeeding shirts. Three to five blouses should be able to get you through the week. You can try to mix and match blouses with different accessories to create new looks. Or even cover up with a sweater when possible to give the appearance of a new outfit. Nursing tank tops are also a great option, because you can purchase just a few of these and then layer them under other clothing items to change up what you're wearing even more.

You can also purchase a nursing dress for special occasions or for work. A good nursing dress is really nice to have because it is nearly

Self-Care Tips

Nursing tops can make a lot of difference in how easy it is to breastfeed discreetly, but they also add comfort. You're probably sick of wearing the same two shirts that fit you at the end of your pregnancy, so splurge! Get a couple of really pretty nursing tops. They will help you with nursing in public and give you something that makes you smile when you wear it. Anything beats your maternity clothes! Look online for sales or even hit up consignment shops known for having maternity clothing.

impossible to nurse in a normal dress. While you could pair a shirt and skirt together to make it more breastfeeding friendly, that doesn't always look as dressy as you might like.

Sleeping in a nursing night gown or pajama top can make your night much easier if you are still nursing at night. This is true whether you are sleeping with your baby or not. Not having to struggle with your clothes in the middle of the night while feeding your baby or pumping is a blessing!

If you do not need a bunch of clothes but just want something for the occasional party or outing, try getting just a couple of shirts—perhaps a nice blouse and a t-shirt or two. These would help you to mix and match for nearly any event.

Types of Openings in Nursing Clothes

Once you have decided which type of nursing clothes you are looking for, consider which types of openings you are looking for in shirts. The openings to your nursing clothes will help you to access your breasts, so ease of use is important. Take these points into consideration:

- Breast size
- How many babies you are feeding at one time
- Breastfeeding or pump use
- Material used
- Manufacturer's reputation for cut

All of these things will play into which openings work best for you. For example, if your breasts are spaced farther apart or are not large, a middle cut

in your shirt will make it difficult to breastfeed or to use your pump without stretching your shirt or being uncomfortable.

Center Opening

A shirt with a center opening is designed with one single hole. It is usually large enough so that you can maneuver your breasts to come through the hole to feed your baby. This is done one at a time. The opening is usually covered with a flap of fabric.

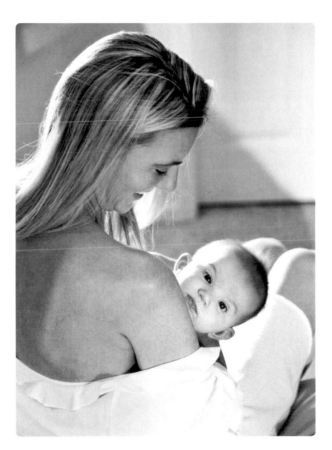

Nursing clothes are a great way to help you stay modest while nursing.

This type of opening works well for nursing but is not usually conducive to using a breast pump. This is also better for women with more breast tissue. Center openings are not as common as other openings. You are more likely to find this option in night clothes.

Slits on Either Side

Openings or slits on either side are much more common in breastfeeding clothes. The slit might be centered directly over the breast area or at the side, closer to your armpit. Many women prefer this style because it is easier to use for women with breasts that are large or small. Some women find they feel more covered when using this type of opening.

Pull Away

Pull-away fabric can be a bit trickier. This style usually works best for women with smaller breasts. Constant pulling can actually wear out the fabric. This will make your shirt not wear as well for as long as other opening types.

Other Considerations

Another thing to keep in mind is the make of the shirt or article of clothing. Some nursing clothes are made with double layers of fabric. This can make them warmer than you wish, or just right. The benefit here is that your middle is always covered.

In some of the less expensive brands, rather than having a double layer of fabric there is a large flap of fabric at the front, which is meant

A Breastfeeding Bra Is Key

Breastfeeding clothes are great, but they work best when you also wear a breastfeeding bra.

to lay flat and cover your abdomen as you nurse. This often can ride up, making your shirt or figure look bunched up. It also does not cover your sides very well.

Other Nursing Clothes

A few products are designed to help you make your regular clothes work as nursing clothes. They work with varying successes. They can help you save money when you find a product that works for you.

The simplest thing to do is to purchase several nursing tank tops in various colors. Then you can use the nursing tank as your base and layer over it with other clothes. Add a t-shirt over it for a casual look. A nice sweater or blouse also works over nursing tanks for a dressier look.

Some shirts and products are designed to help you do the same thing. Some are sold for use in pregnancy as a way to keep your pants up before your move to maternity clothes. Then they double during breastfeeding as a way to cover your midriff. You can also cut the breast section out of a t-shirt and then layer another shirt over it to keep your middle covered and give you easy access to your nursing bra.

One really simple way to create your own nursing shirt is simply to wear a button-down shirt over any other top, or skip the top altogether. You can unbutton the button-down shirt from the bottom and then pull the undershirt up slightly, revealing your bra. This can work really well in a pinch or as everyday nursing wear.

Other Nursing Accessories

One of the main reasons to wear nursing-friendly clothing is to keep covered. You might find there are other ways to do this. In general, the goal is to keep your breasts and your stomach from showing, and to do this without breaking the bank on breastfeeding specialty clothes.

Nursing Covers

One popular breastfeeding item is a specialty nursing cover. While many brands are available, all of them basically do the same thing: cover your breasts and your baby while you nurse. Most of these covers slip over your head and provide you access to your baby, However, not all of them allow you to easily see your baby without lifting the cover.

If this is something you might be interested in, definitely try it out. Consider waiting until your baby is here rather than registering for this item as a baby shower gift. Sometimes babies are really averse to using covers, or they prefer certain types. This can save you money.

Covers are great for totally hiding what's happening when nursing. The problem is that many women do not want to draw attention to themselves when they are breastfeeding in public. And a nursing cover screams "I'm breastfeeding under here!" So if that isn't the message you would like to send, think twice about using a cover for breastfeeding.

That being said, most people who use covers to nurse really like them. They find them easy to use with their babies. It's easy to pack a nursing cover in a diaper bag and have it handy anytime. But it is always wise to practice without the cover, in case you ever accidentally leave it at home.

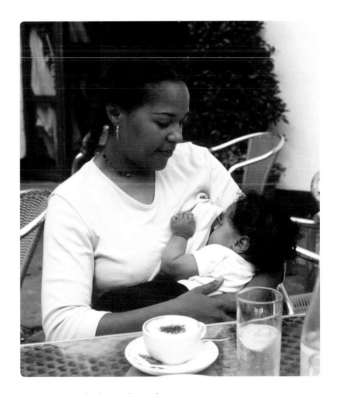

Practice breastfeeding in front of a mirror, you will find that you aren't showing skin. This may help you feel more confident about nursing in public.

Using a Blanket

Instead of a fancy cover, some women use a blanket to cover their babies while they nurse. This is a lot less expensive for most families. The problem comes in that it can be difficult to cover yourself up while holding your baby. A blanket can also slip off very easily or be blown away in a breeze.

These might not be deterrents for some mothers. You may decide to try a blanket first to see how it works for you and your baby. You might also find that when you forget the cover you would normally use, a blanket will work in a pinch.

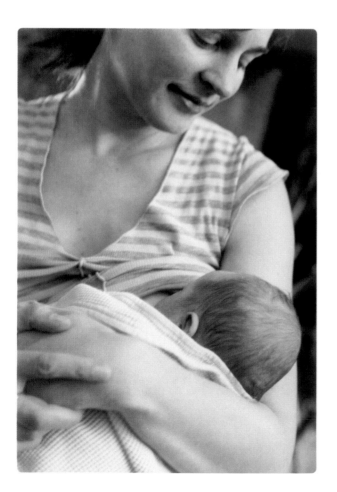

If you are caught in a pinch, you can try a blanket as a cover-up Talk to your baby so he will not be distracted by the covering and focus on nursing.

Other Ideas

Some companies are really thinking outside the box when it comes to nursing coverage. Mobleez is one of those companies. It has developed a wide-brimmed, soft hat your baby can wear. The brim is wide enough that it covers everything you could possibly need covered. The nice part is that it's great for babies who hate blankets and generally being covered. The downside is that you have to hope your baby is agreeable to wearing hats!

There are also a few products that can help you to convert a blanket into a nursing cover. They usually consist of clips attached to a ribbon. The ribbon then goes around your neck; you clip each end to a side of the blanket and use it as a cover.

What If Baby Doesn't Want to Be Covered?

Some babies will have nothing to do with any type of nursing cover, whether it is an actual cover designed for that purpose, a blanket, a hat, or anything else. No matter what, they will grab the edge and pull it away from their face. They might even refuse to nurse this way.

Practice at home with your baby. Consider holding your baby's hand to prevent this unwanted exposure. You might even make it a game and kiss your baby's hand as you hold it, telling her what you don't want her to do: "Let's not move the blanket!"

Talk to your baby and distract her while you are nursing, to keep her mind busy and not thinking about moving the cover.

For a baby who will not use a traditional cover, you might also consider an alternative breastfeeding cover. The baby hats made to hide your breast are one such idea. But you can also be creative and find what works for your baby. Perhaps your baby will be more amenable to using a cover if you nurse her while she is sleepy or asleep. Nursing in front of a mirror can also help you learn to breastfeed discreetly without a cover.

Nursing Pads

Nursing pads are handy items to have around. They are made from either reusable materials that are just washed and worn again, or of disposable materials. You can use breast pads to line the inside of your nursing bra. This lining helps to prevent breast milk from leaking onto your clothes.

Not every woman who breastfeeds leaks breast milk. And leaking breast milk is not an indicator of how much breast milk you have or do not have, although it is more common for women to leak larger amounts when they have an overactive letdown. Some mothers find they need breast pads for just the first few weeks. Other mothers find they feel more comfortable wearing breast pads the entire time they nurse. Once you have breastfeeding well established, you will know how your body works and whether you need breast pads.

When selecting a breast pad, consider the content of the materials. Washable breast pads are particularly green. They are made from various materials such as cotton, wool, or flannel. The initial expense for a box of three pairs of reusable breast pads might be similar to buying a larger box of disposable pads, but they last forever. Disposables are nice if you need to change your pads frequently, particularly when you are out. Just be sure to find a brand that works for you.

When you wear breast pads, you will need to change them when they are wet. Sitting in a wet breast pad for long periods of time can lead to fungal infections or sore nipples. This is particularly true of breast pads that are backed in a plastic coating to prevent leaks. Ensure that your pads are absorbable, but breathable. You can find breast pads wherever you buy nursing bras, and at most department stores and drug stores.

LEARN TO MAKE NURSING CLOTHES AFFORDABLE

Just as in any other fashion industry, nursing clothes can be expensive. That being said, there are some really well-made clothes that always look great and last through the births of many children. But if you are looking to minimize your breastfeeding clothing allowance, there are ways to ease into breastfeeding fashion.

CHAPTER
6

Make Your Own Nursing Clothes

If you are even slightly handy with a sewing machine or just a needle and thread, you can consider converting some of your old t-shirts into nursing clothes. You can actually buy patterns for nursing clothes or download some from the Internet. There are also simple, nonpatterned ways to make some shirts.

The easiest way is to take a t-shirt that has some give to the material and to measure about 6 inches (15.2 cm) vertically over where each breast is located. Center the slit over the nipple area. Remember, you can always cut more if you need to, but you will have a harder time repairing a cut that is too large.

Once you've cut your slits, stitch around the edges of the slit material. This will keep your shirt from fraying. Do not worry if you do not sew well. No one but you and your baby will see this area. If you absolutely do not wish to stitch this area, you

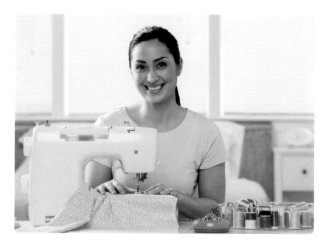

Altering your own clothes for nursing convenience is easy and affordable.

can get away with it, though some fraying might occur. Try to choose a shirt made of material such as a jersey knit, which will fray less than others.

Then, use this t-shirt as an under layer to any other shirt. It will provide easy access to your breasts for nursing or pumping. But it will also cover up your abdomen.

Apply this technique to old tank tops. Simply cut the area out around the breasts. Think of cutting a big U-shaped area out around your bra. Then the tank will not show at the top of your clothes, nor will you need to measure for slits. You should also stitch these edges to prevent fraying. You can do this with a needle and thread quite easily. Even if you're not handy with a needle and thread, you could probably have another mom or a seamstress do this for a lot less money than the cost of nursing clothes.

Borrow Breastfeeding Clothes

One of the great things about having friends who also have children is that you can borrow from each other. Ask your friends if they have any breastfeeding clothes you can borrow. While they might not be exactly the style you are looking for, they can supplement your wardrobe at least for now.

There are even women in play groups and mom's groups who pool their wardrobes together, either as a group or among a few friends. Sharing a bunch of nursing clothes does require a bit of juggling as well as proper timing when it comes to pregnancies and breastfeeding. But if you each invest a small amount of money, you might all gain a very nice wardrobe.

Consider Used Breastfeeding Clothes

You can look for used breastfeeding clothes in many places. First, try your local consignment stores. If you have one that specializes in maternity or children's clothing, you might start there.

Also look for places online, such as online auctions—perhaps eBay or something similar. You can also find some trading sites or places where you can make local purchases, such as Craigslist.com or Freecycle.com.

If you have the time or inclination, yard sales are also potential sources for good, used nursing clothes. Hit areas where young families live or where the sale ads include baby items or maternity items. These are more likely to have nursing clothes available. If you have a Mothers of Twins Club, be sure to see whether they host clothing sales. These sales can be a gold mine for nursing and baby clothes.

Once you have purchased some clothes, remember that they are an investment. The clothes you purchase now will last a long while. This often means you can buy nursing clothes with your first baby and then use them for all of your other children.

Use Clothes to Nurse Discreetly

Nursing clothes can help you to breastfeed more discreetly. There are ways to ensure that your clothing hides all parts of your breasts except for the part covered by your baby's mouth. The right clothes will

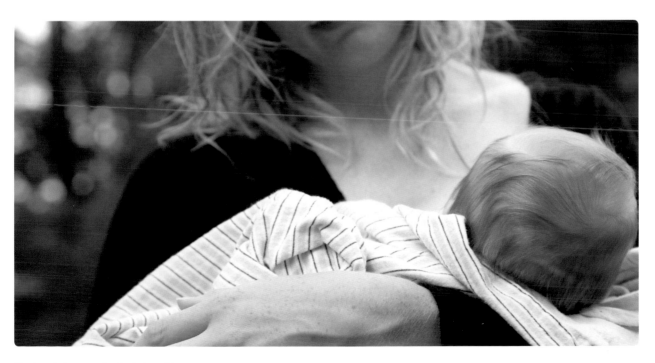

Having clothes specifically designed for breastfeeding will make nursing your baby easier, particularly in public.

also help to cover your middle, which often hangs out if you are not wearing a nursing top or making allowances for it.

There is a learning curve to using your clothing. This is why it is important to see which types of openings work best for you, your baby, and your body type. Once you get the hang of it, life gets much easier.

LEARN ABOUT MEDICATIONS THAT ARE COMPATIBLE WITH BREASTFEEDING

Medications and breastfeeding are a hot topic. The good news is that this area is currently being studied a lot. More information is available than ever before, and this makes it a lot safer for you and your baby to breastfeed without worry.

Nursing mothers routinely use many medications every day without issues. These include over-the-counter pain medications, medications for certain chronic conditions, and many other medications. Do not despair if you are worried about medications and breastfeeding. Chances are good that you will find out that a medication is safe or that there is an equivalent you can take.

Lack of available information is certainly not the problem in this department. The real issue concerns practitioners who are not all well versed in breastfeeding and medications. This often leads to nursing women being told they need to quit nursing or they need to pump their breast milk for a certain period, and dump it out before feeding their baby.

Many women who take medications on a daily basis to treat chronic conditions nevertheless breastfeed their babies. This is becoming increasingly common as this number rises for a variety of reasons. We have more mothers who have chronic conditions (older mothers, as well as those with knowledge about the safety of pregnancy and lactation with certain chronic diseases). We also have more knowledge about breastfeeding as it relates to medication.

Which Medications Are Safe?

Many medications are safe to take while you are breastfeeding.

Be sure that you and your practitioners can answer the following questions when trying to decide which medication is safe for you to take while nursing your baby:

- What is this medication?
- What is known about this medication and breast milk?
- How much of the medication will get to my baby?
- What effects should I look for in my baby if I take this medication?
- Will either my baby or I need special testing?
- Have studies been done on this medication and breast milk/breastfeeding babies?
- Where can I get this information?
- How old is my baby?
- How long will I have to take this medication?

- Is this medication the only one available, or is there a different but safer medication?
- Do I need to take this medication right now, or can it wait until my baby has weaned?

After answering these questions, you might have a better idea about the safety of a particular medication. Sometimes, however, there won't be any really hard and fast answers. You might be left with a clear view that a medication is safe, or you might get a mixed reaction and need to make a judgment call for yourself. It is rare that a need for medication would necessitate weaning, but it does occasionally happen. Be sure to talk to your lactation professional before doing anything drastic.

How Do I Research a Medication?

You can find information about medications from many sources. Some of those sources are not very breastfeeding friendly, however. The standard answer, if it is not known, is to label a medication as something you would not want to take when breastfeeding. This is often what drug manufacturers will do for medications that have not been studied.

For example, you can look at a medication, such as some antifungals, and they are labeled with warnings that they should not be used if you are breastfeeding. But then if you look deeper, you will see this exact medication is being given to premature infants. The good news is that in this case your baby would likely get a much lower dose after the medication is processed in your body.

Rating Breastfeeding Medications

Dr. Thomas Hale has written a breastfeeding medication book, *Medications and Mother's Milk,* and he updates it every two years. In this book, he has a scale for rating medications and their interactions while breastfeeding. When you have a specific question, you can refer to his book to find out where a particular medication falls in the categories regarding medication safety. Also, ask your doctor if he or she has a copy of Dr. Hale's book, should you need to take medication while nursing. Some doctors and pharmacists do not stay abreast of medications and their compatibility with breastfeeding. Often weaning is their suggestion, rather than looking into an acceptable medication. You will need to be proactive when researching this information.

CHAPTER
6

Consequently, using the inserts found with a medication might not give you the whole picture. As an alternative, you might also use the *Physicians Desk Reference (PDR)*. The catch is that this reference book often has nearly the exact same information as the drug insert, so it's not necessarily the best resource.

Dr. Thomas Hale's book, *Medication and Mother's Milk,* is probably the best reference to look up medications for the breastfeeding mother. You should be able to find this book at your pediatri-cian's office or with your lactation professional. Many local La Leche League chapters own copies of this book in their group library. If doctors who do not have the proper knowledge prescribe a medication for you, you should have them get the information on a particular medication from your pediatrician or your lactation professional. This can help to assure them that a medication is acceptable or possibly give them ideas for alternative medications.

Who Can Help Me to Determine Whether a Medication Is Safe?

You should talk to a whole team of people as you make your decision about the safety of a medication. Ideally, this team will involve medical practitioners and laypeople. Consider talking to:

- The doctor or practitioner prescribing the medication, herb, or supplement
- Your baby's practitioner
- Your lactation professional
- A pharmacist or herbalist
- Other families who have made this decision, when possible
- Your partner

All of these people will have valuable information to add to your decision. In the end, the decision is often left up to you. You will have the best answer for you and your baby. This is the truth about anything for your baby. You will have to have these hard conversations and decide what is right, be it ibuprofen or other medications. I advocate open and

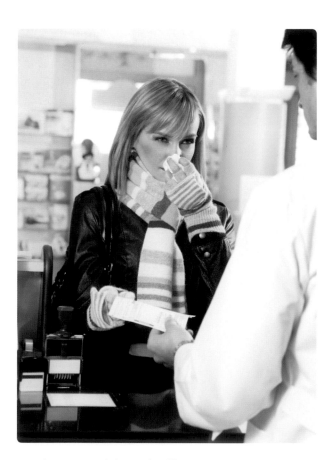

Your pharmacist can help you when filling prescriptions and give advice about medications and their impact when breastfeeding.

honest discussions with everyone involved before making a decision, Doctors don't make decisions for you. Ultimately, you are responsible for the decisions you make for yourself and your baby.

DEAL WITH EXERCISE AND BREASTFEEDING

Exercise is very compatible with breastfeeding. In fact, the combination of eating well, exercising, and breastfeeding is your best bet for postpartum weight loss. This trifecta of good health is what will really help you to get back into good physical condition and feel great while parenting your baby.

Exercise Safety

Breastfeeding and exercise generally are compatible with no risks. The first few weeks after you have a baby, you should limit your exercise to gentle stretching and walking. But as your body heals, you will get the go-ahead to add more exercise into your life gradually.

During the first few months, you might still notice some effects of pregnancy on your body. This might mean your center of gravity is still a bit off. Relaxin, a hormone designed to help your joints soften for an easier birth, might also still be present. This can make injury during exercise more likely, so be careful. But this, too, will gradually go away.

As the effects of pregnancy ease, your body will get back to normal—although this will be a new normal. The good news is that most breastfeeding mothers have no physical issues with breastfeeding and working out.

Breast Milk and Exercise

There has been a lot of talk about what exercise does and does not do to breast milk. Exercise is good for both the breastfeeding mother and her baby. Normal levels of exercise do not do anything harmful to a mother's milk. Nor does exercise turn your breast milk sour.

A study titled "Infant Acceptance of Breast Milk after Maternal Exercise," published in *Pediatrics*, showed that after extreme workouts, at nearly 100 percent intensity, there was an increase in the lactic acid in breast milk. Lactic acid is not harmful; it simply builds in the muscles as you work out. And it does not seem to make babies refuse breast milk, either from you, a baby bottle, or a substitute feeder. In fact, lactic acid disappears after 90 minutes in your breast milk.

What can cause babies to shy away from your breasts after working out is the taste of sweat on your breasts. If you are sweating, your breasts might taste salty to your baby. You can either shower or simply wipe off your breasts if your baby reacts this way.

Exercise Wear and Breastfeeding

Most breastfeeding mothers will not need to purchase special workout clothing. Just be sure that you have a great exercise bra to support your breasts, to avoid any painful bouncing. But other than that, specialty wear is best left for the professionals or if you will wear your workout clothes often in general. For instance, if you love to swim and you do so to exercise often, you might want to

CONFIDENCE CUE

One of the biggest lifestyle hurdles for new breastfeeding moms is nursing in public. Unless you intend to hide for months on end, at some point you will have to nurse near others. There is a huge secret to success here: Practice makes perfect. If nursing in public is worrying you, try to nurse discreetly at home, before attempting it elsewhere. You can even do it in the mirror until you're sure of who can see what. Once you've tried that, branch out. Start out nursing in the corner booth of a restaurant with friends to cover you if needed. Then keep trying more and more spots until you've conquered them all. Soon you'll be nursing in public like a pro.

invest in a nursing swimsuit. This can also double as your regular swimsuit as well.

What you might want to wear are breast pads. These will help to soak up any breast leakage you might have while you are working out. You might not leak at all or you might leak a bit. Until you know which category you fall into, a breast pad will help to protect you from breast milk spots on your clothing.

If you find that exercising with full breasts is uncomfortable, take care before you work out. Simply feeding your baby should make your breasts feel a bit lighter. You can also hand-express or use a breast pump if you are away from your baby.

If your breasts do not really bother you, it will not matter how you schedule your workouts. But remember, regardless of whether you will be feeding your baby while wearing exercise clothing, the most important thing is to have a good, supportive bra on to minimize the bounce factor.

LEARN TO NURSE IN PUBLIC

Breastfeeding in public happens all the time. Every day you pass someone who is nursing her baby, and probably just don't notice it. Most women are quite adept at breastfeeding discreetly in public.

If you are a first-time mother, you might have questions about how to nurse in public without showing off your breasts. You might want to figure out how to nurse with confidence. This is easy to learn, though it gets even easier the longer you breastfeed, simply because you and your baby's comfort levels and confidence increase.

You'll get your best advice for learning to nurse in public from talking to other mothers. Ask your friends who nurse in public for tips and advice to see what works for them. You might also ask if you can practice in front of them before heading to the mall food court. You might even practice by nursing in front of a mirror, so you can watch yourself. Really, try this—you'll be amazed at what a reality check it is. You'll quickly find that you can see a lot more of what is going on when you look down at your baby than others can when they look straight at the two of you. These practice runs will help you to feel more confident in your nursing style.

Nursing on Location

One of the easier ways to breastfeed discreetly is to use location to your advantage. If you are in a restaurant, sit in the back. This means fewer people will be sitting there to notice. You can also sit with your back toward the majority of people.

If you are in a mall or store, there are also places you can go to nurse. Many stores have really nice women's lounges; some are even equipped for breastfeeding mothers. Here, you will find nice chairs and couches to relax on while you nurse.

At the park or outdoors, you can sit on benches to get better support while you are nursing. A picnic

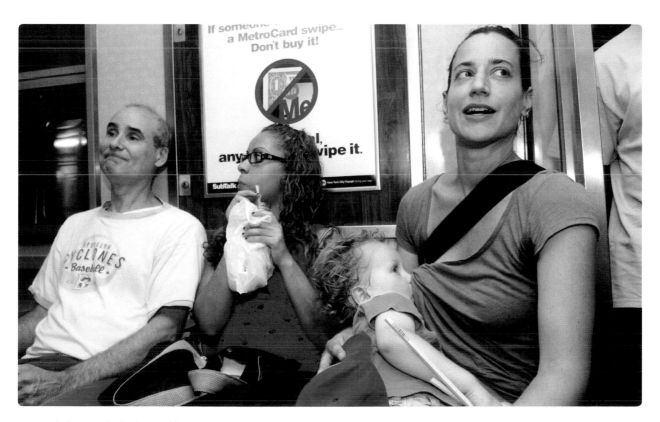

Having clothes specifically designed for breastfeeding will make nursing your baby easier, particularly in public.

CHAPTER
6

table can also work well, as you can support your baby with the actual picnic table if you lean forward. If weather turns nasty while you're outside, you can always return to your vehicle for a bit until the weather calms.

Movie theaters are also a great place to nurse while you are out. The even nicer part is that it's a great way to sneak in a date night with your baby. (Obviously not every baby will find this to be a wonderful experience, but if your baby likes to sleep while nursing in the evenings, this can be something to try!) Simply wait until the lights dim and the main feature starts! Then go ahead and nurse your baby. You might also try movies that are designed for new mothers and babies—many movie theaters have special showings every so often designed for this purpose.

MAKE WISE DECISIONS ABOUT SOCIAL DRINKING AND BREASTFEEDING

You are probably getting conflicting advice about drinking while breastfeeding. This might mean you have a lot of questions. Your best bet is to look at the hard facts and decide what works for you and your family.

Alcohol and Breast Milk

The amount of alcohol in your breast milk is directly related to how much you drink. It is also affected by how much you eat and how much you weigh. For example, the more you weigh, the faster you metabolize alcohol. And if you are eating, less alcohol is more readily absorbed.

When you drink alcohol your breast milk will also contain some of the alcohol. This amount will peak thirty to sixty minutes after drinking an alcoholic beverage. If you drank while eating, it can take longer—about sixty to ninety minutes—for that alcohol to peak in your breast milk. Pumping and dumping—expressing breast milk after you have had alcohol—is not recommended. It's a waste of breast milk, because usually, by the time you are ready to feed your baby again, there is so little alcohol in the milk that it is safe for your baby to ingest. If you are worried about your baby getting alcohol in your breast milk, feed your baby first and then enjoy your drink. Chances are good that by the time the next feeding comes around, you will not be feeling the effects anymore and your breast milk is considered clean.

Another factor to consider is how old your baby is when you are drinking. All the way to about three months of age, a new baby has a more immature liver. This means that even though babies are get-

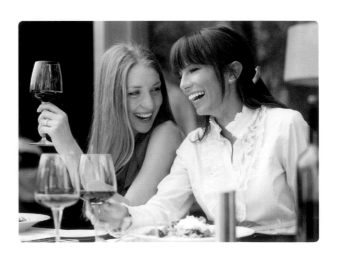

You can enjoy some alcoholic beverages in moderation when breastfeeding.

TIP   Pace Yourself!

Since you've abstained from alcohol for nine months while pregnant, you might find that one drink really affects you more than it might have before pregnancy. Be mindful of this when drinking.

ting reduced amounts of alcohol, it will take them about twice as long to process that alcohol. After that point, babies can metabolize alcohol much more quickly. So when it comes to consuming alcohol, the younger the baby is, the more effects you are likely to see.

How Much Is Too Much?

If you are drinking to the point of inebriation, you should not breastfeed while drunk. Once you are feeling sober, your breast milk will have almost no alcohol in it. As soon as you are not feeling the effects, your breast milk is considered clean. Breast milk does not store alcohol. If you are drinking to the point of inebriation, child care is a must.

The research that has been done on breastfeeding and drinking has been limited to small amounts of alcohol. Binge drinking or drinking on a daily basis does not have a lot of data behind it. Obviously, however, the more frequently you drink, the more alcohol your baby has to process.

Having a glass of wine or a drink occasionally is one thing. But a baby who is exposed to chronic drinking will show many problems. First, you might notice the baby begins to sleep more. He might have an ineffective latch, and therefore weight loss or lack of sufficient weight gain might be noticed. Slowly, you will see deterioration in the baby's growth patterns physically and developmentally. This is why daily drinking is not recommended for breastfeeding mothers.

Social drinking is considered to be fairly safe for your baby. This might mean having a glass of wine at a party or with your dinner. You might go out with some friends and have a cocktail or two. But know the facts about drinking and breastfeeding. There are a lot of factors to consider. You should keep in mind your physical ability to tolerate alco-

A Glass of Beer to Bring in Your Milk?

Alcohol has not really been shown to increase the amount of breast milk you make, despite the old wives' tales. You might notice that your baby breastfeeds more frequently, but research published by the journal *Alcoholism: Clinical and Experimental Research* shows us that they actually get less milk.

hol, your weight, what you've eaten, your baby's age and weight, the amount of alcohol in the drinks, and other factors that might influence the decision.

EDUCATE YOURSELF ABOUT BREASTFEEDING AND CIGARETTES

According to the American Academy of Pediatrics (AAP), it is safe to smoke while breastfeeding. However, breastfeeding infants whose mothers smoke are more likely to be fussy and are at an increased risk of respiratory infections, early weaning, and other issues. You might also find that smoking negatively affects your breast milk supply.

The effects of twenty or fewer cigarettes per day are minimal, but the more you smoke, the more your baby is exposed to nicotine and other byproducts. So if you are a smoker, you should try to limit the number of cigarettes you smoke per day. You should also avoid smoking just before or during a feeding to minimize the amount of nicotine passed to your baby.

Consider Quitting Smoking

Many products are available to help you quit smoking. Dr. Thomas Hale, breast milk and medications researcher, has found that many of the products available to help you quit create less of a problem than smoking does. This means products such as nicotine gum or replacement patches are generally considered safe during breastfeeding. You should talk to your doctor about a smoking-cessation program that fits your needs, which can include safe administration of certain medications.

Secondhand Smoke

Even if you do not smoke, you need to protect your baby from secondhand smoke. Being exposed to secondhand smoke is dangerous for your baby. These dangers range from increased risks of respiratory infections, asthma, and allergies, to a higher incidence of sudden infant death syndrome (SIDS).

Do not let people smoke in your home. Even once the smoke clears, the chemicals remain in your furniture and clothing. This can bother your baby too.

If you are planning to go somewhere where there will be smoke, reconsider. If you find you are already somewhere and people start smoking, stay outside when possible. Or see whether you can leave your baby at home with a babysitter if you know ahead of time that there will be smoking at an event.

If you are out and near smokers, you will have smoke in your clothes and on your body. Be sure to take a shower when you get home. Also change your clothes before holding your baby.

LEARN ABOUT BREASTFEEDING AND YOUR SEX LIFE

Breastfeeding and sex is often a taboo topic. That is really a shame. Breastfeeding should not have much of an impact on your sex life, though postpartum recovery certainly does!

Many things about the postpartum period can affect your sex life. During the first few months, it is about the physical recovery. Perhaps you are

TIP

Make Time to Touch

Touching is important to all your relationships. Be sure to find time to touch your partner, whether it is holding hands, playing footsie, or giving each other a real kiss at least once per day.

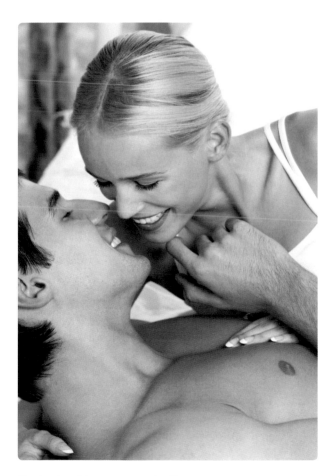

Nursing doesn't have to negatively affect your sex life. Remember to talk to your partner and move forward as you both feel comfortable.

recovering from having stitches on your perineum, or you are worried about a cesarean incision that must heal.

Once you have physically healed, you have other concerns. First, sleep deprivation is not sexy. Who has the time for sex when you're not getting regular sleep? Then you might also worry about the baby waking up. Most babies will sleep through anything for certain sleep cycles. Knowing your baby will help your timing. And many women worry about their bodies after pregnancy. Most partners are not concerned with the changes in a woman's body as much as you are. Be sure to have open and honest discussions on body image after birth with your partner; you might be pleasantly surprised.

Being "touched out" is another issue that new mothers might experience, and it can apply to how you sometimes feel about your husband or partner just as much as it applies to your other children. This comes from feeling like someone is always demanding part of you, particularly your body. This can be a difficult thing to explain to your partner. As your baby gets older and her physical demands on you diminish somewhat, this feeling should decrease.

Some mothers find that regular bits of time alone can help them to feel better about being touched. This is where your partner can be of great assistance. For example, if your partner agrees to watch the baby for thirty or forty-five minutes every evening so that you can have some alone time, you are likely to emerge feeling more recharged and ready to be together.

These are all huge issues that you will need to work through. Sometimes you can work with your partner to find a happy medium when it comes to baby-related issues as well as sleep issues. Remind each other about keeping the lines of communication open to discuss the changes that new parenthood brings to your sex life.

Orgasms and Lubrication

Orgasms are not harmful for a breastfeeding mother. The hormones released into your body during an orgasm are feel-good hormones, including oxytocin. Oxytocin is also known as the love hormone and is released during breastfeeding as well. (So, interestingly, the same hormone that helps to bond couples through sex also helps to bond mother and child when breastfeeding.) You do not need to have a waiting period after sex or orgasm before breastfeeding. Having sex or an orgasm does not affect the quality or quantity of your breast milk.

The best thing about orgasms is that they help your body to lubricate itself. Some women find they are a bit less lubricated in general while breastfeeding. This is a part of the normal changes in hormones. Be sure that you have an adequate amount of foreplay to help with this. An orgasm might also be all that you need to take care of this issue. But if you find you are still not as lubricated as you would like, you can use some of the lubricants that are made to help this issue, such as KY Jelly. Be careful using petroleum-based lubricants, as that might nullify or interfere with some forms of birth control.

Cope with Leaking Breasts

You might notice that your breasts leak during foreplay, sex, or orgasm. Your breasts might also leak if your baby begins to cry while you are in the midst of making love. This is normal. Most men are not bothered by leaking breasts; some men actually find it attractive or erotic. But, some mothers find the leaking bothersome. If leakage is a problem, you can either wear a bra to contain the leaking or keep a towel handy. If you place light pressure on your breasts, you can sometimes slow the flow of breast milk.

UNDERSTAND BIRTH CONTROL AND BREASTFEEDING

There are a lot of misconceptions about breastfeeding and birth control (no pun intended). Only you and your partner can decide which type of birth control you need or when you would like to add to your family again. Learning what you can about your birth-control options while breastfeeding will empower you to make wise choices.

Breastfeeding As Birth Control

There is a way to use breastfeeding as birth control. This is called the Lactational Amenorrhea Method (LAM). It involves very dedicated breastfeeding and parental knowledge. This method of birth control is not for everyone. It means that:

- You feed your baby on demand, day and night.
- Your baby takes no pacifiers and uses no bottles or other methods for feeding; all suckling is done at the breast.

- You do not use a breast pump.
- Your period has not returned.
- Your baby is not taking solids such as cereal.
- Your baby is less than six months old.

If all of these conditions are met, there is only a 1 to 2 percent chance of pregnancy. If any of these conditions change, it is time to find a backup birth-control method.

Barrier Methods of Birth Control

Barrier methods of birth control have been used for a long time. These do not include hormonal forms of birth control. This makes them very compatible with breastfeeding. Some barrier forms of birth control include:

- Condoms, male and female (88 to 90 percent effective alone)
- Diaphragm (90 percent effective alone, 95 percent effective when used with spermicidal jelly)
- Cervical cap (with spermicidal jelly, 84 to 91 percent effective for women who have never given birth; 68 to 70 percent effective for women who have given birth)

If you used a diaphragm or cervical cap for birth control before you became pregnant, you must be fitted for a new one after having your baby. These are prescriptive items that need to be replaced every year. More importantly, a diaphragm or cervical cap that fit you before you gave birth likely will be too small after you've given birth.

Some women favor these methods of birth control because they are used only when needed. If you are not having sex daily, this means you aren't thinking about your birth control on a daily basis. These choices also give you some control over when you use birth control.

These types of birth control do not affect breastfeeding at all. They will also not affect your milk supply. This makes them great methods for many breastfeeding families.

Hormonal Birth Control

Hormonal birth control must be prescribed by your doctor, midwife, or nurse practitioner. This type of birth control can encompass:

- Oral contraceptives (the Pill)
- Patches
- Injectables
- Rings
- Intrauterine devices or IUDs (with or without hormones)

(These methods are about 99 percent effective.)

Some hormonal methods of birth control contain estrogen and progesterone. This is meant to try to suppress ovulation. If ovulation does not occur, no egg is available to conceive. Some forms of birth control also render the uterine environment unfriendly should a fertilized egg make its way there.

Some women notice that hormonal methods of birth control negatively affect their milk supply, meaning they have less breast milk available for their baby. You should avoid all forms of hormonal birth control until you are at least six weeks post-partum so that you are able to build the best milk supply possible for your baby.

Many practitioners recommend that breastfeeding mothers avoid all forms of estrogen in birth control. Instead, they recommend the "mini Pill" or progesterone-only Pill, and some of the other methods of birth control that are progesterone only. The biggest benefit here is that you do not have to think about birth control often. Because of the potential impact on your milk supply, however, you might wait until further into your postpartum period rather than go ahead at the six-week mark. This might be a good, happy medium for your family. You can also back off on some of these methods should you see a negative impact on your milk supply.

Nonhormonal IUDs are another good alternative in this category, because you can be sure they will not affect your milk supply. They are about 99 percent effective—the same as oral contraceptives. Plus, once you are fitted and the IUD is inserted, you do not have to do anything with your birth-control method for several years. And if you want to get pregnant again, you simply need to have your practitioner remove the device, and you can begin trying immediately. However, IUDs work best for women who have had vaginal births. Full dilation is beneficial for a better fit and, thus, better birth-control protection. This is not an absolute, however, so talk to your practitioner about it if this is the type of birth control you desire.

Other Methods of Birth Control

Other forms of birth control are also available. Some are tough to follow, such as abstinence at particular times or not having sex at all. This is un-realistic for many families. But if not having another baby is that important, it is something that some families choose.

Natural Family Planning (NFP) is a natural extension of LAM. Though now you will need to monitor your basal body temperature, which is your body's baseline temperature. You should also follow your natural fertility signals, such as cervical mucous and potentially even cervical position. This method requires much attention to detail and is also not for every family.

NFP is something you would need to study and possibly even take a class in to help you get the most benefit. This method's effectiveness depends largely on you, based on how well you gather and interpret the data. So if you can't commit to taking your temperature every morning before getting out of bed, perhaps this is not the best method for you.

When choosing a method of birth control, you need to understand all the ramifications. Talk to your practitioner and your partner, and decide what is best for your family. No one else can tell you what is right for you. You might decide that what worked for you before having a baby is still the best method, or perhaps you will consider other methods now that you have had a baby. The choice is yours.

BE A BREASTFEEDING ADVOCATE

Being an advocate can mean different things to different people. When you decided to have a baby and became pregnant, you became an advocate for your baby as a parent. Likewise, when you decided to breastfeed you also become a promoter or supporter of breastfeeding.

While you might not think of yourself as a breastfeeding advocate, other women will see you and feel inspired. They will know they can come to you for answers to their questions about breastfeeding. They will be encouraged that breastfeeding is alive and well as they look at your healthy, robust baby. And they will see breastfeeding as the special gift that it is. And to think, you just thought you were having lunch at the mall with your girlfriends while you discreetly nursed your baby in the corner.

Breastfeeding Affirmation

With a little bit of flexibility, breastfeeding makes my life easier and saves me time.

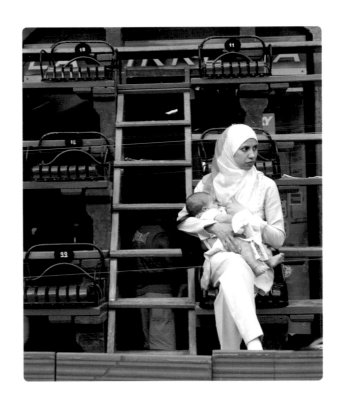

Be your own best breastfeeding advocate. It is not necessarily something you think about; sometimes it's just about feeding your baby.

CHAPTER
6

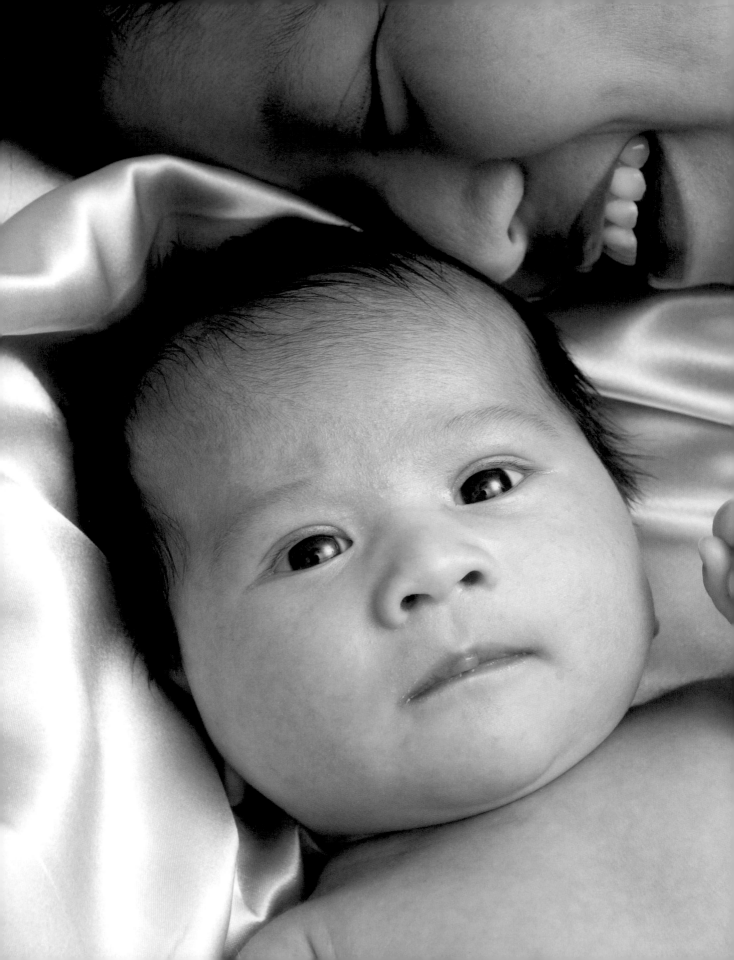

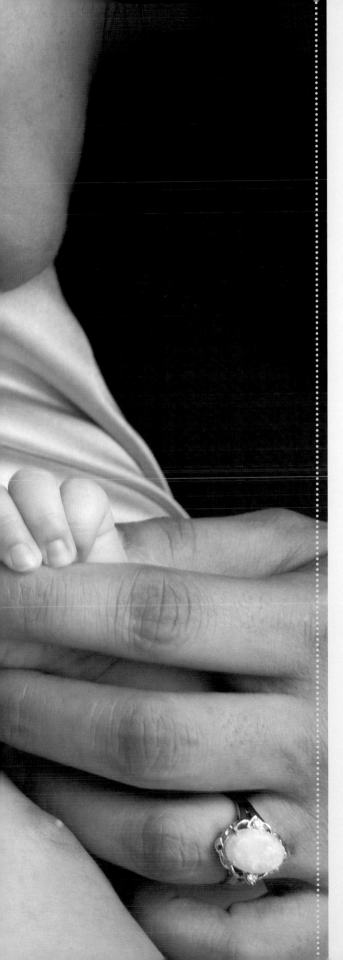

CHAPTER 7

Support for Breastfeeding Concerns

✓ Checklist for Successful Breastfeeding

- ☐ Define your breastfeeding problems.
- ☐ Prevent or treat sore nipples.
- ☐ Recognize the symptoms of mastitis.
- ☐ Know the challenges of breastfeeding after breast surgery.
- ☐ Increase your milk supply.
- ☐ Learn about breastfeeding aids.
- ☐ Figure out if and when you need a supplement.
- ☐ Remember that previous breastfeeding problems need not repeat.

Breastfeeding is natural, but we forget that we are not set up to know how to do it. This is partially because we did not grow up watching women breastfeed. Many of us did not have the advantage of seeing our mothers, aunts, or other relatives breastfeed. Plus, many issues can arise during childbirth or in the early postpartum period. Add to that other unpredictable events that are out of our control, including premature labor, and it's surprising that more people do not experience challenges with breastfeeding. Fortunately, if you are having trouble with breastfeeding, support is available to help you to overcome the challenges you are facing.

DEFINE YOUR BREASTFEEDING PROBLEMS

Breastfeeding can be a wonderful experience. But sometimes breastfeeding moms and babies can encounter bumps along the way. Perhaps you just have a general sense that something is not right. Or maybe you know specifically where the problem lies.

When you ask for help, you need to be sure you know what you are saying and what you are asking. This will help you and your lactation professional come up with the best care plan for you and your baby.

What Your Lactation Professional Needs to Know

When you call or visit your lactation professional, she will ask you a series of questions. You should be prepared to answer with as much detail as possible. Here are some of the questions you should be prepared to answer:

- Are you feeling pain?
  - ~ If yes, where?
  - ~ Does the pain occur at the beginning, middle, or end of a feeding?
  - ~ How long has this been happening?
  - ~ Does the pain move?
  - ~ Describe the pain.
- Is your baby having problems?
  - ~ How is your baby's weight gain?
  - ~ What was your baby's birth weight?
  - ~ What is your baby's most recent weight? (When and where was it taken?)
  - ~ Is there anything else in your baby's diet besides breast milk?
- What remedies have you tried?
- What was your birth experience like?
- How far along were you in your pregnancy when you gave birth?
- How old is your baby?

Being open and honest with your lactation professional is important. The more information she has, the better able she will be to help you find the right solution for you and your baby.

WOMEN'S WISDOM:

Pain is a signal that you need to stop and pay attention. This is true in breastfeeding as well. If the baby's latch hurts or feels weird, break the suction and try again immediately. It is normal to feel tugging while the baby nurses. Some mothers even report a tingling as they let down (although this is not true for everyone). But pain is not acceptable. Even one feeding with a bad latch can cause you days of pain. Nip pain in the bud, so to speak.

PREVENT OR TREAT SORE NIPPLES

Sore nipples are probably the number-one concern of breastfeeding mothers everywhere. No one wants to be in pain. And let's face it, nipple pain sounds really bad. And it can be. Fortunately, you do not need to experience nipple pain when breastfeeding. In fact, sore nipples mean something is not working quite right. If you do have nipple pain, you can do a number of things to relieve the pain and nurse successfully. It is a good idea to be familiar with these things, because although they work as cures, many are also preventive.

Causes of Sore Nipples

Sore nipples can be caused by multiple things. Thankfully, most are fairly easy to fix once you figure out what the problem is for you and your baby. This is where the help of a lactation professional is invaluable.

Bad Latch

How your baby latches on to your breast is the most important thing to pay attention to when it comes to sore nipples. Does your baby have enough breast tissue in his mouth? (It should be about 1 inch [2.5 cm]

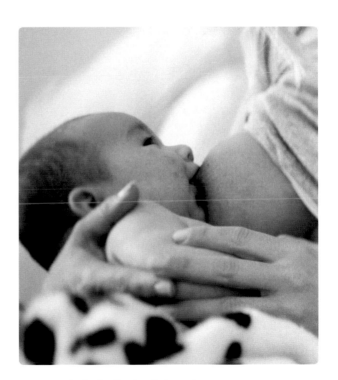

Preventing the first bad latch is the best advice.

CHAPTER
7

past the nipple portion of your breast.) Are your baby's lips flared out around your breast? Does your baby make any noises while nursing? Techniques to try:

Breast Sandwich: When getting your baby to latch, you should prompt him to get as much breast tissue into his mouth as possible. Try the breast sandwich technique. With your thumb at about nine o'clock on your areola and your fingers at three o'clock, bring your fingers toward your thumb, altering the shape of the nipple. The goal is to make it

longer, encouraging the baby to take more into his mouth. The key is to make the shape of the breast sandwich fit your baby's mouth in direction, meaning that if your baby's mouth is wide side to side, so should your breast be widest side to side. So if you alter the baby's position, you will need to alter your finger placement as well.

Wider Mouth Opening: The first trick is to show your baby how wide you would like him to open his mouth. About 8 to 12 inches (20.3 to 30.5 cm) from your face, hold your baby up. While supporting

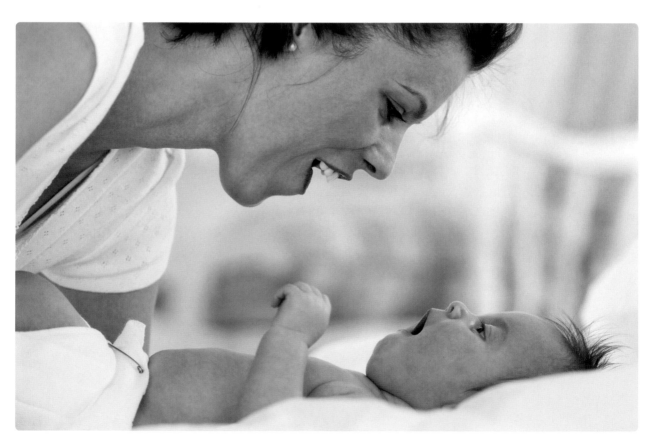

Your baby is amazingly responsive and will be very obliging to open to a wider mouth if you ask.

the baby's head, look at your baby and say, "Open!" Show your baby how to open his mouth. This can work wonders. If he is not practicing opening his mouth, you can gently encourage him to open up by pulling slightly on his chin.

Another trick to get your baby to open up wide is to actually use your index finger to help hold his chin down as he is latching on. It can take a bit of time to figure out how to do both at once. But it is a very effective technique.

Pulling Out the Lips: If your baby's lower lip is in the way or his lips are not flared out, your nipples will get sore. As your baby is nursing, look to see whether his top lip is flared out. You might need help watching that lower lip. If the lips are not flared out, gently pull them out while the baby is latched on. This will not hurt, and even this small difference can mean a big change in how your nipples feel.

Check Out Baby's Tongue: During breastfeeding, your baby's tongue should protrude over his lower gums. This not only helps with a good latch for a great milk supply, but it also acts as a protective measure for your nipple. A tongue in the wrong place can cause a lot of pain.

While you are nursing, pull your baby's lower lip back. You should be able to see his tongue at the bottom of your breast. If you do not see his tongue, you can try to relatch, having him open wider. This will usually cause him to pull his tongue into the correct position. A lactation professional might also advise you to encourage him to hold his tongue down by using something called suck training.

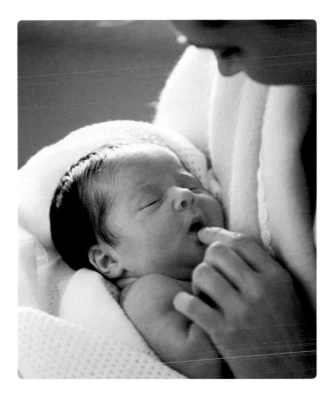

If you think your baby has a tight tongue check before jumping to conclusions. Your baby's tongue should protrude over his lower gum for successful nursing.

With suck training, first wash your hands. Just prior to a feeding, have your baby on your lap facing you, held up by one hand. With your other hand, insert your index or middle finger into your baby's mouth, nail side down. Have your baby suck on your finger. Then slowly roll the finger, nail side up. Using a bit of gentle force, pull your baby's tongue into the correct position while he is sucking. You can also give him verbal cues as you are doing this training. A lactation professional can also help you with suck training.

CHAPTER
7

If your baby is simply not able to bring his tongue out past his lower gum line, you might wish to have him evaluated by his physician or an oral surgeon. This might be an indication of tongue tie. Some babies with tongue tie never have a problem nursing, whereas other tongue-tied babies might need to have their *frenulum* clipped by a physician to free the tongue to be able to extend past that lower gum line.

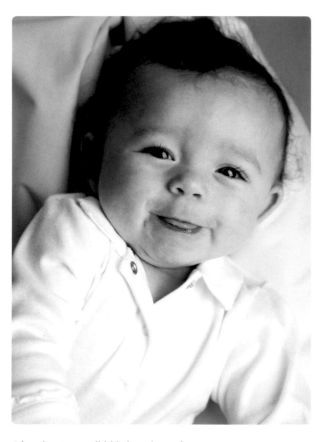

A frenulum is a small fold of membrane that extends from the bottom of the mouth to the midline of the underside of the tongue, also referred to as a tongue tie. Your physician can decide if it is necessary to correct this condition.

Poor Positioning

If you have gone over your baby's latch until you are blue in the face and cannot find anything wrong, it is time to look elsewhere. The next step is to look at your positioning while breastfeeding. This involves looking at both mom and baby.

Mother's Positioning: While breastfeeding, you should be sitting or lying down in a comfortable position. You should not have to lean toward your baby. Your feet should not dangle. Your shoulders should not be rounded.

Ensure that you have a comfortable seat. Get a nursing stool or ottoman so that your legs and feet are supported. Sit back into your seat properly. Remember, there's no need to lean—you can use pillows to bring your baby closer. It's always about bringing the baby to the breast and *not* the breast to the baby.

Baby's Positioning: Once you know you are positioned well, it is time to look at how your baby is positioned. For some babies, their position rarely matters. For other babies, 1 inch (2.5 cm) in the wrong direction makes all the difference in the world.

The first thing to check is that your baby's head is facing the nipple. Your baby should not have to turn or strain to latch on. Just as you would have a hard time drinking with your head turned to one side, so does your baby.

If you have larger breasts, you might find the extra breast tissue is pressing onto your baby's face. This can throw his latch off. Support your breast with the opposite hand if you think this might be an issue. Special support pillows are designed to help with this issue as well.

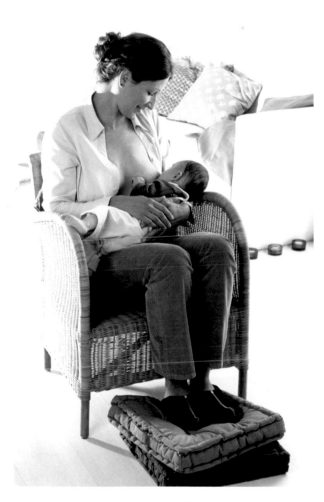

Don't hesitate to use cushions under your feet to help you get the best position for you and baby.

Yeast Infection

Occasionally, a yeast infection in your breasts or on your nipples can cause pain. This can feel like a burning sensation when you are nursing. You might notice that your nipple is red and shiny. And you might suspect it if your baby has thrush.

Talk to your lactation professional about treatments. Continuing to breastfeed is important. Ensure that both you and your baby are treated correctly depending on what type of yeast infection you have on your breasts. Sometimes oral medications are necessary and other times topical medication is used. (For more on thrush, see page 121)

Flat or Inverted Nipples

If you have flat or inverted nipples (see chapter 1 for information on this diagnosis), you might have some pain with breastfeeding initially, though not all mothers do. This pain can be caused by a poor latch or by the adhesions in your nipples stretching in the first weeks of breastfeeding.

Treatments to draw out your nipples, such as using a breast pump and the Evert-It, can help to reduce some pain on latch. Your baby is also really good at solving this problem, though sometimes it takes a bit of time to get the hang of it.

Try breast comfort measures that you would use for sore nipples of any origin. These are helpful in the case of inverted or flat nipples as well. Talk to your lactation professional often for advice and progress reports.

CHAPTER
7

Healing Your Nipples

Sore nipples can make you feel miserable. You might even have cracks on your nipples that bleed slightly. While prevention is best, sometimes soreness still occurs. If you already have sore nipples, you can do certain things to help heal them and make them feel better. This may take a bit of time, but be patient. Here are some of the best tips available.

Varying the position in which you nurse can be very helpful. So if you usually use a cradle hold, try a football hold at the next feeding. Any of the positions will work; just mix it up. This prevents the baby from putting pressure on the exact same spot on the nipple at every single feeding.

Nipple ointments can be very useful. Apply them after a feeding, and do not wash them off. Which brand you use is up to you, though sticking with brands that are known for breastfeeding promotion is probably your best bet. This would include lanolin products.

Another helpful trick is to heal your nipples with breast milk. After a feeding, gently express a tiny bit of milk. Rub this over the nipple, and allow it to air-dry.

You should generally let your nipples air-dry whenever possible. You do not need to wash your nipples, and even if you do clean them, do not use soap, which can dry them out. You can air-dry your nipples by leaving the flaps of your nursing bra down for a bit after feeding. If this makes your nipples rub against your clothes or is uncomfortable for you, a breast shell might be helpful. Also try drying your breasts after a feeding by using a hair dryer on the warm/low setting, though this does not feel good for everyone.

If your baby wants to comfort-suck, consider an alternative. This should be neither your breast nor a pacifier. A clean human finger works really well. It also gives your nipple a break.

Remember to feed your baby before he gets ravenous. If you start a feeding when he is only slightly hungry, he will be less aggressive on your nipples. If this is not possible, you can also consider starting on the least-sensitive side first. This can lessen the pressure on the sore nipple.

You can use all of these measures together to fix the original problem. They are very helpful at healing sore nipples fairly quickly. With the help of a lactation professional and some home-based work, you should be healed in no time.

Deal with Nipple Damage

Occasionally you might need to let a nipple heal after damage has been caused. You can choose to allow your baby to feed on the wounded side only once every few feedings. This will give your injured breast a chance to heal. If you choose to do this, be sure to use a breast pump to pump the breast that your baby does not feed from, to prevent a drop in your milk supply.

While feeding your baby on one side, do your best to ensure that he gets as much breast milk as possible. One way to do this is to use breast compression. As your baby is nursing, you will notice that he stops sucking at some point. This indicates that the flow of milk has stopped or has drastically decreased. Simply use one of the breast compression techniques listed on page 186 to get the milk flowing and the baby nursing again.

Some mothers find that numbing their nipples prior to a feeding can really help. A bit of ice or an ice pack can do the trick here. Do not expose your nipple directly to the ice or ice pack for fear of further damage.

Your lactation professional might also recommend a nipple shield at this point. This can help cover the nipple to prevent further damage or allow the nipple to be a bit less sensitive. Some studies show that this does not help as much as some believe, but if you have tried everything else, it might fall into the "What have you got to lose?" category. Whoever recommends a nipple shield should be qualified and observe the latch from beginning to end, or refer you to someone who can.

It might be that even after you have tried everything, you need to give both breasts some time to heal. This can take three to five days. During this time, pump your breasts to feed your baby and protect your breast milk supply. Avoid artificial nipples during this learning period and try to use an alternative to feeding your baby as described on page 65.

RECOGNIZE THE SYMPTOMS OF MASTITIS

Plugged ducts can cause mastitis, a breast infection. A plugged duct occurs when you have a blocked duct that is preventing breast milk from being expelled. You might notice a small area of engorgement or a small lump on one side of your breast. It might or might not be painful or red. Massaging the area and treating it with warm compresses can help alleviate pain and the blockage.

Some women get plugged ducts for seemingly no reason at all. In these cases, plugged ducts don't always lead to a breast infection. A breast infection can make you feel completely miserable. The good news is that breastfeeding can and should continue while you have mastitis, even if you are taking medications.

Signs of a Breast Infection

Mastitis is most common in the early weeks of breastfeeding, though it can happen at any point in your breastfeeding experience. It can also occur, but rarely does so, when you are not breastfeeding. Signs that you have mastitis include:

- Pain in your breast
- A breast that is warm to the touch
- Swelling in one or both breasts
- Feeling like you have the flu
- Fever of 101°F (38°C) or higher
- Redness on part or all of the breast

CHAPTER
7

Mastitis occurs when bacteria get inside your breast, either from a crack in the skin or through your nipple. The bacteria can come from anywhere, and can even include the bacteria that normally are on your skin.

While it is more common to see mastitis when there is broken skin (as in cracked nipples), it is possible to contract mastitis without broken skin. You might also find you are more likely to have a breast infection if you have a tight-fitting bra due to a restriction in milk flow. This restriction can also occur when your breasts are not properly emptied, which can be due to poor positioning of your baby or not changing positions when breastfeeding. Once you have had a bout of mastitis, you are more likely to experience it again.

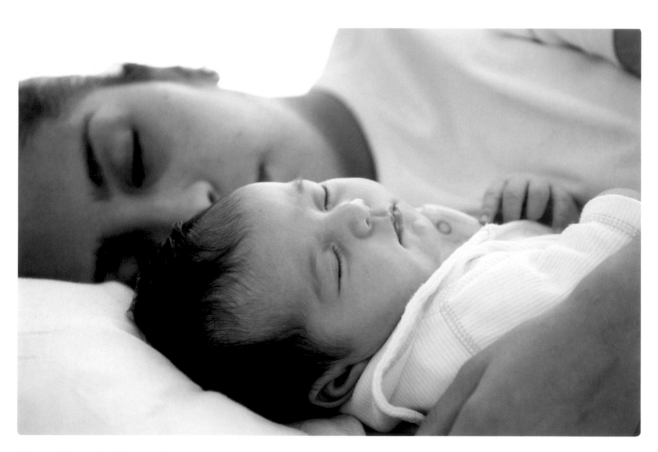

If you are diagnosed with mastitis, breast-feeding, sleep, and rest are an important part of your recovery.

Treatment for a Breast Infection

If you notice signs and symptoms of mastitis, seek medical care promptly. Receiving delayed or inadequate treatment for mastitis might be one of the reasons it is more likely to persist and/or reoccur. Get treatment as soon as possible to feel better.

Dealing with an issue such as mastitis is one of the areas where medical communication frequently breaks down for nursing mothers. Some obstetricians see all breastfeeding issues, even those that pertain to the mother, as things for which the baby's doctor should give care. If the mother is not a patient of the baby's doctor, it might be unlikely that the doctor will also care for her. Such instances are the perfect time for your lactation professional to step in and provide your breastfeeding-related care, but most lactation consultants do not have prescription privileges. If you are getting the runaround with your medical care, go to your primary care/family doctor for advice, even if you have to walk in. Anyone can provide you with this type of basic care for an infection.

A ten- to fourteen-day regimen of oral antibiotics is the main treatment for mastitis. You might also want to ask about care for yeast infections if you are prone to them when taking antibiotics. Also incorporate acidophilus into your diet, either in supplement form or in foods. Yogurts with live active cultures are also helpful to add to your diet during your course of antibiotics.

Call your prescribing physician within forty-eight hours if you are not feeling better. It might be a sign that the antibiotics are not helping you. Your doctor will have more advice if this becomes necessary, including, perhaps, a change in medication. The antibiotics frequently prescribed for mastitis are safe to take while breastfeeding.

In addition to the medical care you will receive, there are home-care treatments that will help you. Whenever you are sick, even if it is not mastitis, you will want to remember to head to bed with your baby. Try the forty-eight-hour cure. Do nothing but things that you can do from your bed. This means quiet nursing time; breakfast in bed; perhaps reading a bit. Simply spend time taking care of your body, your mind, and your spirit.

Breast Surgery and Milk Supply

Some women who have had breast surgery will have a full milk supply without much of a problem. Many will achieve full milk supplies with added work to encourage their supplies. Some women will never have a full supply. Defining your goal for breastfeeding might look differently than if you hadn't had surgery, but you can have a meaningful breastfeeding relationship.

Your antibiotics will usually kick in within a day or two. Until then, you can treat the fever with medication such as ibuprofen or acetaminophen. This will help reduce your fever, which will make your infection less painful. You can also use warm compresses on your breast if that feels good, and massage the affected area. You should also nurse, nurse, nurse. This can help you to feel much better. If for some reason you can't nurse or do not want to nurse, a breast pump can be very helpful. This helps to keep you comfortable and protects your milk supply.

Mastitis Prevention

The way to prevent mastitis is to be sure you are draining the breast milk from both breasts at every feeding. If you start to feel your breasts getting full, consider offering your baby a nursing session. Also avoid bras that are too tight or have underwire, as they can compress the milk flow as well.

When breast milk lingers, it can become thicker and harder to pass through the breast. This is when plugged ducts can creep up on you. Nursing frequently and with varied positions can drastically reduce the risks of mastitis and plugged ducts.

KNOW THE CHALLENGES OF BREASTFEEDING AFTER BREAST SURGERY

More and more women are having breast surgeries before pregnancy and lactation. This can include surgeries that increase or decrease breast size, biopsies, lifts, nipple surgeries, and more. While any surgery that involves the breast, particularly the ducts and the nerves, can affect how much breast milk you make, breast reduction surgery tends to have the most impact in terms of milk supply.

Get Your Medical Records and Talk to Your Practitioner

Before you have your baby and begin nursing, start by finding out exactly what you had done to your breasts. Even getting a copy of your medical records might help the practitioners you are working with now to figure out what your surgery was like. This can also help you to know what your chances are of building a full breast milk supply. However, nothing can be 100 percent for sure until you are actually lactating. A baby and a breast pump can go a long way toward making medical records prove nothing. Do not despair if you can't get your records; while it may be helpful, many mothers have nursed well even without this information.

Get a Lactation Consultant

Before you have your baby, try to find a lactation consultant who has worked with mothers who have experienced breast surgery. This will give you someone with whom you can discuss your options. A lactation consultant who is knowledgeable in these areas can advise you about what to look for before and after your baby is born.

You can talk to your lactation consultant about your fears and concerns, as well as your goals and dreams for breastfeeding. Your lactation support team can also help to put you in touch with someone else who has been in your shoes. Some places even have breastfeeding-after-surgery support groups.

Information Is Lacking

Most medical professionals do not have updated information on breastfeeding after a reduction or breast surgery. You will need to try to find this information as soon as you can, hopefully prior to pregnancy but definitely during pregnancy. This will help you figure out exactly what was done in surgery and how likely there is to be damage.

You will want to have access to a hospital-grade breast pump prior to the birth of your baby. It is also handy to have a supply of the medication domperidone or the equivalent on hand, should you have even a hint of low milk supply. This works by increasing the prolactin production in your pituitary gland. Your lactation professional, midwife, or physician may also recommend that you take an herbal galatagogue (milk production enhancer), such as Goat's Rue, with supervision, beginning at about the thirty-sixth week of pregnancy.

Know What to Look for Once Your Baby Is Here

During pregnancy your breast tissue will change. You will most likely experience an increase in your breast size; don't be too concerned. If you have had a reduction, you might be worried that you'll have larger breasts forever. A few months after birth, many mothers notice a decrease in the size of their breasts, bringing them closer to their normal size. After weaning, your breasts usually will go back to their original post-surgery size, if they haven't previously.

Since the time of your surgery, your breasts have been healing. Part of this healing might have involved reinnervation and recanalization. This means the nerves and ducts were trying to heal themselves to help you breastfeed. The extent to which this happens varies widely.

CHAPTER
7

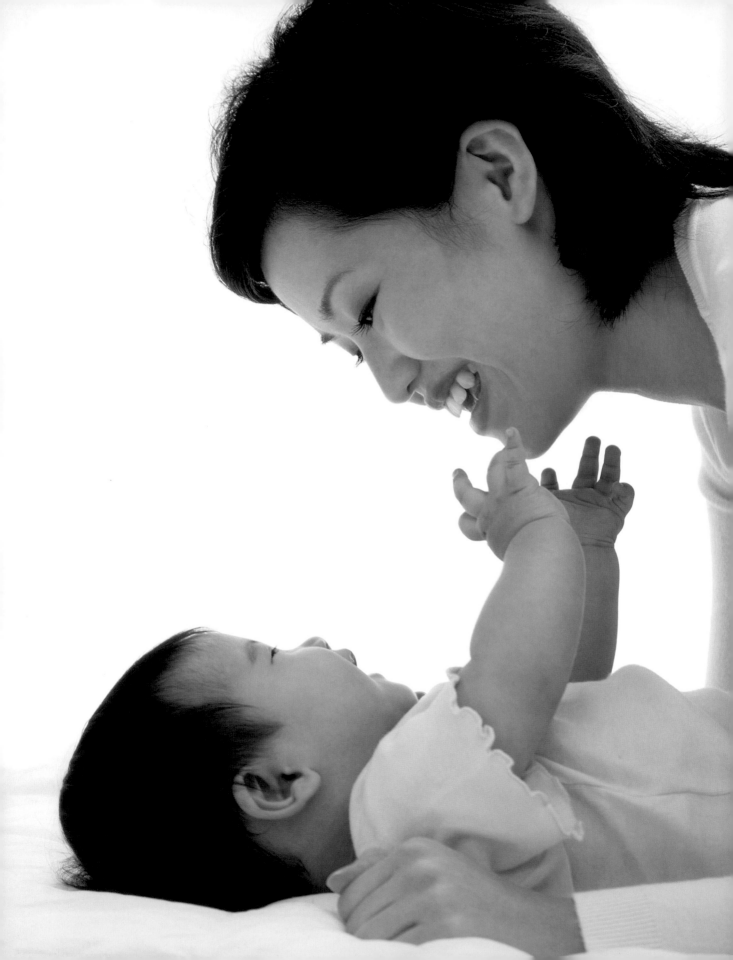

When your baby is born, spend the first two to three weeks emptying as much milk as possible from your breasts. This will help your body to get the signal that you need breast milk at a certain level. Even if your baby seems to be nursing well, using a breast pump to remove more milk is a good idea. You might not get much milk when you pump, which is fine. The goal is to tell your body that you need the milk.

Some sources will try to tell you that severed ducts are not allowing milk to flow out, thus causing inflammation, but this is not usually the case. You might experience engorgement when your baby is born. This is most likely caused by your milk ducts being full from the lack of breast milk removal. Normal engorgement can appear about the fourth day post-baby, slightly longer if you had a cesarean birth. If you have some milk ducts that are not able to excrete the milk, these ducts will stop making milk; this can take up to two weeks. After this period, the glands that do produce milk will continue to function normally. You do not need to have 100 percent of your ducts functioning in order to provide an adequate supply of breast milk.

While physicians have gotten better about talking to women who are undergoing surgery about the potential risks to their successful breastfeeding later in life, many women are simply not at a time or place to hear that information. Women sometimes make decisions without thinking them through, and then later wish they had considered more thoroughly. Try not to be harsh with yourself. There will always be times in our lives when we are not planning ahead and we make decisions we wish we could change. Just work on the positive side and move forward.

INCREASE YOUR MILK SUPPLY

Having a low supply of breast milk can feel devastating. Low milk supply can have so many causes. The cures take time. And meanwhile, you are frustrated and your baby is hungry because she is not getting enough milk. This is a very trying time. Fortunately, you can do lots of things to help increase your milk supply.

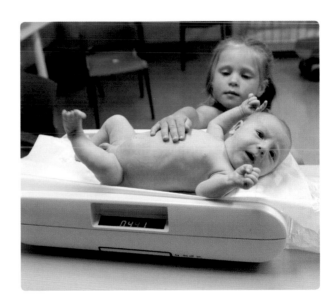

If you find that your baby is gaining weight slowly, you'll want to look for potential causes of low milk supply and assess your baby's breastfeeding technique.

CHAPTER
7

Don't Jump to Conclusions

Many mothers believe they have a low milk supply when in fact they do not. This is a fairly common concern, though thankfully it does not occur often. Some mothers experience slight breast engorgement from normal postpartum hormones or even swelling after giving birth that lasts for a few days or weeks.

Women make this mistaken assumption because their breasts will stop feeling as full after a few months of breastfeeding. At this point, milk isn't drying up; this change is simply due to the breasts' increased efficiency. Over time, your body learns how to make milk and how much milk to make, so your breasts tend not to feel full before feeding and feel soft afterward. This can confuse some mothers. As long as your baby is wetting her diapers, however, this normal adjustment should not cause any problems.

How Will I Know That I Have a Low Supply?

Typically, the first way you will know that you have a low supply is by watching your baby. If your baby always seems to want to be on the breast, yet is never satisfied, that can be a sign that she is not getting enough to eat. You might also think you have the best baby in the world because she doesn't take long to eat, and then sleeps a lot. This is also a sign that your baby is potentially not well fed.

You might also see the physical signs of low milk supply in the baby. One of the most important signs is not enough wet or dirty diapers. You might have been told that your baby is not gaining enough

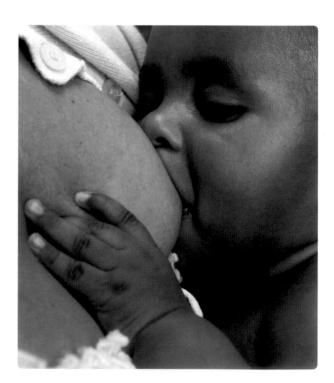

In most cases, frequent nursing, a latch check, support, and sometimes a good breast pump are all that is needed to boost your milk supply.

weight, or maybe she is even losing weight. While it is common for a baby to lose 7 to 10 percent of her body weight from the first to the third day after birth, from that point on weight loss is not expected.

Your baby will typically be expected to regain her birth weight by the time she is two to three weeks old. From that point on, your baby should gain about 1 ounce (0.03 kg) per day until she is near the three-month mark. At that point your baby should gain about half an ounce (0.014 kg) per day. If your baby is not gaining at this rate, you might have a milk-supply issue. But don't panic! Your baby might just have an alternate growth curve. Be sure to talk to your baby's doctor as well as your lactation professional.

If you have nursed a baby previously, you might also be worried about a low milk supply because of previous experiences. You must keep in mind that every breastfeeding experience is different. From one breastfeeding experience to the next you might notice that this time you are having no issues with supply.

Causes of Low Milk Supply

True low milk supply has many causes. Some are related to the process of breastfeeding, some to the physical attributes of the baby, and some to mom. Here is a list of potential causes for low milk supply:

- Scheduling feedings for baby
- Supplementing breastfeeding with formula
- Not letting baby end the feeding
- Using a nipple shield or pacifier

- Hormonal issues
- Nursing difficulties caused by oral differences in the baby (tongue tie, etc.)
- Baby not transferring breast milk
- Mom taking new medications (including hormonal contraceptives)
- Having a history of breast surgery

This is not a complete list of the potential causes

Self-Care Tips

Don't let breastfeeding drive you over the edge. The beauty of breastfeeding is that after a bit of time, you really don't have to pay a lot of attention to the logistics. Once you and your baby get a rhythm going, you can put it on autopilot. Don't worry about the details. If you are a list maker, find something to track other than the number of minutes you breastfeed. If you are a worrier, figure out how you're going to cope with some of that worry ahead of time as a preventive measure. Resist the urge to obsess over every little breastfeeding detail, and you'll save yourself a lot of unnecessary energy that you can then put to better use with your baby.

CHAPTER
7

of low milk supply. However, this list shows you how something as simple as using a nipple shield or pacifier can be detrimental to your milk supply. Sometimes low milk supply can be remedied fairly easily by removing the problem.

One of the most common causes of low breast milk supply is lack of breast stimulation. This can happen for many reasons, but scheduled feedings, particularly in the early days after birth, can lead to your supply being low. It can also happen because of a poor start to breastfeeding in addition to the lack of time at the breast. This can include a poor latch and ineffective milk removal, among other issues.

Some women also have physical issues that cause low milk supply. These vary widely by individual. It might be a hormonal issue or even a structural issue from a breast surgery.

Getting Baby to Work

One of the first lines of defense against a low milk supply is to correct any issues your baby might be having. This is where good lactation support really comes in handy. Having someone else to help you assess the situation is always a plus. Once a professional observes your baby nursing, then you can tell for certain whether you're really getting the good latch and milk transfer you believe you're getting.

Try various latching techniques to help you ensure that you find the best match for you and your baby. If your baby has a great latch but is not transferring milk as well, consider adding breast

TIP | **Power Pumping**

One pumping method is called power pumping. It involves leaving your pump out in the open where you can see it, which serves as a reminder to pump as often as you can. Do this drive-by pumping for about five minutes every hour. The goal is to stimulate the breast often, gathering what milk you can in the process.

compression to your breastfeeding routine. Breast compression is a simple technique to help your baby drain the milk in the breast fully. Although the compression itself does not directly make more breast milk, effective removal of breast milk in the first place does help to make more milk. Use this technique when your baby is latched on, but is not sucking because the milk has stopped flowing.

To perform breast compression, have your baby latch on normally. Form a C shape with your free hand. With your thumb on top of your breast tissue, fairly far back, compress the breast. Do not roll your fingers down toward the nipple as you do during hand expression; simply squeeze. Hold the compression until the baby stops sucking, or until your hand hurts. Repeat compressions as often as necessary, but only when the baby is not getting milk, as evidenced by a lack of swallowing/sucking at the breast. (Otherwise, if you use compressions while you are still having steady letdown, you are apt to flood your baby with too much milk, which might cause her to gag.) You might also switch breasts and repeat the technique on the other side. In some cases, it works really well to do compressions multiple times on each breast during a feeding. Breast compression is particularly helpful with infants who are quick to fall asleep. The technique is also beneficial when pumping.

Pumping and Breast Stimulation

Pumping is also a great way to help boost or alter your milk production in a beneficial way. Most mothers dealing with low milk supply use this method in some way, for good reason. Stimulating your breasts with a breast pump will help to increase your supply. Plus, you can completely control the breast pump, and you don't have to be concerned about whether the pump is hungry, sleepy, or sucking correctly for milk transfer. You should pump while also working to resolve any problems you or your baby might be having when nursing. The goal is to get your baby to latch well and enjoy the breastfeeding experience.

If you are dealing with the issue of low milk supply, you need to have the proper breast pump. A hand-held pump or even a high-end single-user electric pump is not designed to provide the right type of stimulation and suction for someone who is trying to build a milk supply. These pumps are designed to help you maintain a supply—which is not your goal here. Therefore, it might be time to rent a hospital-grade pump to maximize your efforts.

Once you have the right breast pump, you should allow your baby to nurse before pumping. When a feeding is over or if your baby is unable to latch or feed, pull out the breast pump. Try to use your breast pump in a way that mimics your baby as closely as possible. This means you will want to pump according to how you would be feeding your baby. So if your baby is a newborn, this might be a schedule of every two hours during the day and every three hours at night.

Freeze!

If you are pumping and your baby is not eating the supplemental breast milk, put it in your freezer and keep it for later. This is a great way to build up an extra supply for when you go back to work. Even if you're a stay-at-home mom, the extra milk you've stored in the freezer will come in handy when you are not available to breastfeed.

CHAPTER
7

Remember, the more stimulation your breasts get, the more milk you are likely to produce. Pump in conjunction with any other measures you are taking to resolve the reason behind your low milk supply, whether it is latch problems or milk removal, a physical difficulty you or your baby is having, or a hormonal support issue such as thyroid dysfunction, to give an example.

Pumping Strategies

The two most common strategies for pumping are to add extra pumping sessions between feedings or to pump right after you have fed your baby. Both ways are beneficial, although the theory and reasoning behind them are different.

Adding extra pumping sessions gives you the benefit of extra breast stimulation to increase your milk supply. You also can choose times when your baby is not nursing, such as an extra pumping session after your baby goes to sleep at night, in an attempt to collect extra breast milk. Later, you can feed this breast milk to your baby.

The problem associated with this method is that it can be hard to find the time to add a pumping session. With all of the care a new baby needs, you might feel overwhelmed already. Having someone support you by helping to care for your baby's other needs may give you that extra time you need.

Pumping right after you feed is the other option. This typically will produce less extra breast milk, simply because your baby should have gotten her fill. However, if you are having a problem with a baby who is not transferring breast milk well, this might be the perfect option. This method might also require that you have help, so you can pass the baby to someone else while you pump.

Some mothers actually manage to breastfeed on one side while pumping on the other. The plus here is that the baby helps to build your hormones and it can help you to pump more milk than you might have previously. The issue then becomes deciding whether you want to nurse on only one side per feeding, or whether you want to switch the baby and then pump during the feeding. Play with your strategy and see how your baby does or how much breast milk you get when you pump. You might also choose this method if you have one really sore nipple—use the pump on the sore breast and let your baby feed on the other.

How Long Should I Pump?

You might see a lot of arbitrary numbers when it comes to how long you should pump. Instead of paying attention to random numbers look at your needs and abilities. When are you pumping? If you are pumping after a feeding, you might not need to pump as long as you would if you were pumping to get as much milk as possible. The general rule of thumb is to pump until you have not seen any droplets of milk for two to five minutes.

Some mothers think that being able to pump for five minutes is not worth the effort. This may be what time you have to pump. It is okay to pump for just five minutes. Even if you do not get a lot of milk, you will still be stimulating your breasts.

Breast Milk Storage Guidelines

Storing your milk once you have pumped it is very simple. First, you need to decide how long you will be storing it. If you intend to feed the breast milk to your baby within about eight hours, you can pump it directly into the container from which you will feed her. The same might be true if you intend to use it within the week. Glass containers or hard plastics that do not contain Bisphenol-A (BPA) are your best bets. These are made to store breast milk. You will want to leave about 1 inch (2.5 cm) on the top to prevent spills because your milk will expand as it freezes.

If you intend to freeze your breast milk for more than a week, you might want to consider something less structured, such as special breast milk storage bags. Plastic or glass containers, while they work, will take up a lot of space and be rather costly if you decide to store anything more than a bottle or two. Special plastic bags are made for this purpose, although some mothers choose to use ice-cube–like trays with covers.

No matter how you store your breast milk, you want to think ahead. How much breast milk do you anticipate your baby will take at a feeding? To prevent waste, store your breast milk in small increments. It's much better to heat up two small bags of breast milk and have your baby drink all of it than it is to heat up one large one and waste part of it.

Breast milk stores differently depending on where you put it:

- Room temperature: four to eight hours (66–78°F, or 19–26°C)
- Refrigerator: up to eight days (less than 39°F, or 3.9°C)
- Freezer: six to twelve months (less than 4°F, or -16°C)

If the breast milk containers can be reused, you will want to wash them in hot, soapy water. Be sure to rinse them well, then air-dry them prior to use. Special drying racks are available, but you can also just leave them out on the counter to dry.

When Will I See an Increase in My Supply?

Typically, it will take a day or two before you will see an increase in your supply from pumping. This is because your body needs time to respond. Do not be upset if you are not immediately seeing a response to the pumping.

Natural Remedies

Several natural remedies are good at helping to increase your milk supply. One simple remedy is to try to add more oatmeal to your diet. Yes, some mothers report seeing an increase in their milk supply from eating a single bowl of oatmeal (not instant oatmeal) during the day. Some even say that anything with oats in it has increased their supply.

CHAPTER
7

Some herbs are also reported to be *galactagogues*, meaning they increase your breast milk production. These include:

- Anise
- Blessed Thistle
- Goat's Rue
- Fenugreek
- Milk Thistle
- Nettles
- Red Clover

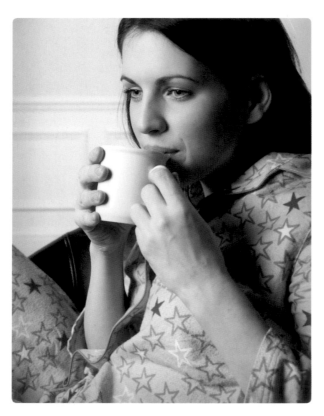

Talk to someone knowledgeable about herbs and their possible effects on lactation before using such remedies.

While you can certainly take these individually, the easier way to get these herbals is in a form that includes everything all together. A couple of supplments are available for nursing mothers that have combinations of these herbs in them. You might have also seen some teas and tinctures sold.

Herbalists, osteopaths, and many other practitioners can help you with your herb selection. Many lactation professionals also have training in herbs that are galactagogues. Be sure to seek help before attempting to use herbs as a remedy.

Medications

Medications can also be prescribed to help boost your milk supply. These are usually tried only after other remedies have not worked. These are typically domperidone (Motilium) and metoclopramide (Reglan). You would need to see your practitioner to get a prescription for these medications. The key here is that you should use herbs and prescription medications only in conjunction with all other techniques.

Metoclopramide has many side effects and domperidone is much more effective. However, domperidone is more difficult to find in the United States. Your lactation professional should be able to guide you to a source for domperidone. All prescriptions can have side effects. Know what the potential risks are in addition to the potential benefits before you begin taking any prescription medication. Since these are all prescriptions, you will be having a conversation with your practitioners about them. Be sure to ask questions at that point.

Avoid Artificial Nipples

While you and your baby are trying to overcome the challenge of low milk supply, it is best to avoid using artificial nipples of any sort. This includes pacifiers, baby bottles, and the like. The problem with artificial nipples is multifaceted. On the one hand, you have the fact that any sucking should be done at the breast for optimal time and stimulation to increase your milk supply. And yet, if you are using a breast pump and trying to give your baby the expressed breast milk, you might need to figure out a way to do so easily.

Using a pacifier might comfort your baby, but it presents two huge problems. It takes time away that your baby could spend nursing, even if it is for comfort. Using a pacifier also allows a baby to develop habits that are not conducive to breastfeeding, such as improper latching. If your baby learns to suck incorrectly on the pacifier, this can derail all of your efforts.

Baby bottles present similar issues. While bottles do give your baby the breast milk you've pumped, your baby could also develop habits that do not benefit breastfeeding. These habits can be hard to combat later. It is best to forgo baby bottles and artificial nipples at this juncture.

Don't worry if you need to feed your baby the milk you are pumping! Plenty of options and alternatives are available for feeding your baby. Talk to your lactation professional and your baby's practitioner about which is best for your baby. For a complete discussion of these alternatives see page 64.

The Emotional Strain of Low Milk Supply

Having a low milk supply might be very hard on you emotionally. You are trying your best, but for some reason, you are having trouble. This is a normal feeling to have when dealing with a low supply. No one wants to be told she is not making enough milk for her baby.

If you are having a hard time with these feelings, find someone to talk to, even if it's a friend. Someone in a breastfeeding group or your lactation professional is also a good choice. Be honest about your feelings. Cry if that makes you feel better about it, but then move on to find a solution.

This balance between feeling and action is important. It can be so easy to get caught up in your emotions because of the hormones flooding your body, particularly the hormonal changes that accompany childbirth. You need to be able to do both. Stuffing your emotions away is not helpful. In fact, it can be harmful. But failure to act will only make the problem worse.

If others around you are providing a constant strain because of the challenges you are facing, be honest with them. Explain that what you need most right now is help. You need emotional support to continue. You also need someone to support your physical needs with food, cleaning, and whatever other help would be appropriate. Generally, when people are given a job to do and they understand what is going on, they will quit being negative and start moving forward with you. If not, you will need to figure out how to find support from someone else or deal with the negativity.

CHAPTER
7

LEARN ABOUT
BREASTFEEDING AIDS

Plenty of products and gadgets are available for breastfeeding. Some are designed to help you overcome problems you knew you had; others seem to be solving "problems" no one even has issues with. Be leery if someone tells you to use something to fix a problem you didn't know you had. Just because we have a tool or gadget doesn't mean we should use it. Before you use any product, be sure to talk to your lactation professional about it and do your research. Some products can damage your breasts if you use them incorrectly, and some products shouldn't be used at all.

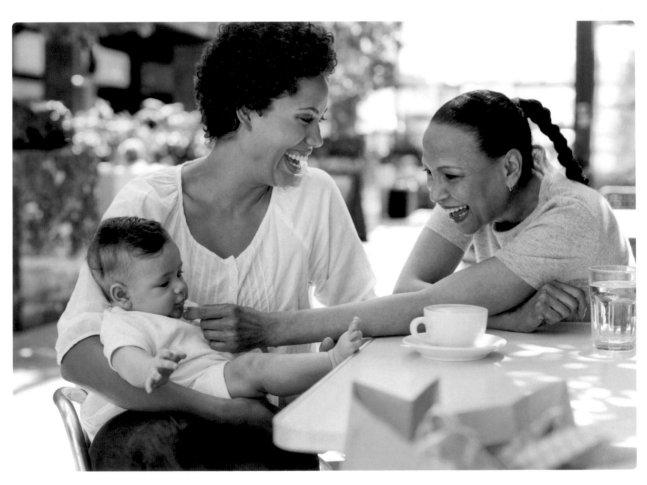

Be sure to find someone you trust to talk to about your feelings if you are having problems with or doubts about breastfeeding. This is just as important as a physical cure.

Nipple Shield

A nipple shield is a small, thin piece of plastic that fits over your nipple. It comes in two sizes, which are based on the size of your baby's mouth, not the size of your nipple. One size is for preterm infants and the other size fits full-term infants. If your nipple is larger, it might not fit in a nipple shield at all.

Nipple shields get "prescribed" for lots of reasons. Sometimes they are recommended to help a baby who has shown signs of nipple confusion. They are also used to help sore nipples heal, and to entice a baby to latch. Some hospitals or lactation support offices hand out nipple shields like a candy cure-all for breastfeeding problems.

While a nipple shield certainly has its time and place in breastfeeding, it is not for everyone. Some moms feel like they need six hands, but once they are past the learning curve they feel great seeing their baby satisfied at the breast. This means that on top of whatever problem you were using the nipple shield to fix, you might also have to deal with a resultant low milk supply.

Some babies really like nipple shields. A nipple shield can make it easier for some babies to latch, but then these babies can also become really attached to it. This means that if mom ever finds herself without the nipple shield, she had better watch out. This over-reliance can make weaning from the nipple shield a problem.

To wean your baby from a nipple shield, you will first need to ensure that your original problem, whether it is sore nipples, a positioning problem, or whatever, has been addressed. Help from a trained professional can be essential during this process.

Next, you need to ensure that you are using the thinnest nipple shield available. If you have been using something thick, such as a rubber nipple shield, switch to the silicone type. These are thinner, so it's harder for a baby to feel the difference.

The best time to try to remove the nipple shield is when your baby is sleepy or sleeping. Just try to slip your hand in, take off the shield, and pop the baby back on your breast. This trick can work well for some babies, but not for others. You might also try removing the shield once your milk has started flowing or when switching between the first and second breasts.

Evert-It

The Evert-It is a tool designed to help women who have flat or inverted nipples. This small, hand-held suction device creates enough suction to pull the nipple out a bit. When the nipple is pulled out, it should be easier to get your baby to latch on.

You can easily do this with a breast pump as well. Many mothers also manage to nurse well with flat or inverted nipples simply by allowing their baby to pull the nipple out. If that strategy is not working for you, this $10 (£ 6.7) gadget might be helpful. After using this technique for a while, you most likely will not need it anymore.

Breast Shells

Breast shells come in two parts. One part fits over the nipple area, exposing the nipple to the air, and the other half is a dome. This dome holds the bra off the nipple, allowing it to air-dry. This is often prescribed for women who are experiencing nipple pain and soreness.

If you find breast shells uncomfortable, air-drying can also be beneficial, particularly if a wet breast pad or bra is irritating an already-sore nipple. Just leave the flaps of your nursing bra down or take your bra off while you're at home, and cover yourself with a shirt. If this isn't an option for you because you are out of your home a lot, you might want to use the breast shells.

If you are using breast shells, be sure you are addressing the problem that is causing your nipple pain. A breast shell will not solve the problem or even heal the nipple all by itself. If you have nipple pain, seek the help of a breastfeeding professional.

Supplemental Nursing System (SNS)

A supplemental nursing system (SNS) is designed to deliver nutrition to your baby while also stimulating the breasts. These tools are typically used for babies who are learning to breastfeed when mom has a low supply, for babies who were adopted as mom builds a milk supply, and for other breastfeeding problems where you need breast stimulation to produce milk and you need to get food to the baby.

With an SNS, the mother wears a necklace that has a container attached. The container has two small catheter tubes that run out of the bottom. The mother attaches each catheter to her nipples using paper tape. The container is filled with expressed breast milk or other supplements.

When the baby latches on, she will get the nipple in her mouth with the tiny catheter extending just beyond the nipple. When the baby sucks, she is rewarded with milk. This allows the baby to nurse without the mother having to worry about whether the breast milk supply is adequate.

Despite the fact that this sounds like an ideal situation for moms and babies with issues, there are challenges. Namely, it is difficult to set up this system when you're alone, and this can add time to a nursing session. That being said, it is a great thing to have available for moms and babies who need it. When you are doing everything you can to breastfeed your baby, you will be thrilled to have this tool available to you.

If you need to use an SNS, ask for help in how to attach it. Get a lactation professional with a lot of experience to show you all the tips and tricks. Also get online and talk to other moms who use this tool. The knowledge base is huge, but often overlooked because people do not know it is available. These tips and tricks are what kept me using this product when one of my babies had breastfeeding difficulties.

Supplemental Nursing System (SNS)

The Supplemental Nursing System (SNS) is a tool to be used with babies who are having trouble nursing or when the mother is having trouble with her milk supply. The baby is able to be at the breast and nurse while there is stimulation of the breast to produce more milk. There is a bladder of supplemental milk providing instant gratification for the baby or serving as an additional source of nutrition, depending on why the SNS is being used. While you can purchase one of these devices without a prescription, it is best to use it with the guidance of a lactation professional.

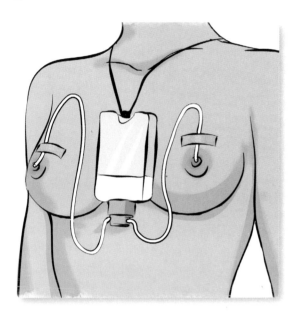

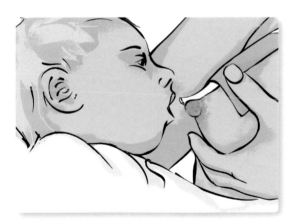

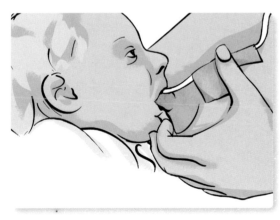

FIGURE OUT IF AND WHEN YOU NEED TO SUPPLEMENT

Breastfeeding is the best nutrition you can give to your baby. Breast milk is an amazing substance. However, sometimes your baby might need to be fed something other than breast milk. Thankfully, true issues are few and far between.

Supplementation might be necessary for several reasons, and it can occur in many forms. Perhaps your baby was premature and needs more calories. You might be asked to pump your milk and add a fortifier to it. This fortifier can help to boost your baby's caloric intake to allow the baby to grow faster (though some parents and medical professionals are now asking whether growing faster is really beneficial). Remember, all babies grow at different rates.

Supplementation can also be done using donor breast milk. This should be used in addition to the breast milk you are already providing. Donor breast milk can be used for entire feeding, or as a top-off to a feeding that you provide, either at the breast or with expressed breast milk.

On rare occasions, you should consider using artificial breast milk (formula). This should be done with the help of your lactation professional and your baby's doctor. They can help to steer you toward the best option for you and your baby. They can also help to ensure that supplementing is as temporary as you wish it to be. By and large, however, most breastfeeding mothers do not need to supplement their babies. Instances when supplementation might be necessary could include:

- Metabolic disorders, such as phenylketonuria (PKU)
- Unavailability of breast milk from other mothers

Schedule of Supplements

Once you have decided to supplement, no matter what type of supplement you are using you will need to figure out the best way to add this to your baby's diet. You will want to choose the timing that best helps you to overcome the challenges you are facing with breastfeeding.

Some lactation professionals recommend that you nurse the baby first and then add a supplement. This can be an ideal strategy. Don't wait until your baby is ravenous; you might not be able to have a good feeding because your baby is frustrated and hungry. This frustration can mean that you are unable to work with your baby as much because his need for food is too great. Try to start a feeding as soon as you see signs or cues of hunger. If it has progressed to the frantic stage, consider other options. If necessary, be open to providing small amounts of a supplemental feeding before you nurse. This can ease the stress on a hungry baby and make him more willing to try to nurse and to see it positively.

CONFIDENCE CUE

You know your breasts and you know when something is up. If you are worried about something and it's gnawing at your breastfeeding confidence, find help. You are a wise mama who can get help when needed. Listen to your instincts, and fix small problems before they get bigger. Pull out that address book and find a good, knowledgeable, breastfeeding person to bounce your concerns off of while they are fresh in your mind, and put your doubts to rest.

It is also important to point out that every baby is different. Even if you are met with the exact same set of circumstances, every baby is not *your* baby. You might be pleasantly surprised to find out that your new baby is not going to behave in the same manner as your previous child. This can be a relief when it comes to breastfeeding challenges.

Finally, do not overlook the emotional factors involved with a previous negative breastfeeding experience. Being able to calculate the differences intellectually or to detect a problem rapidly is not the same as dealing with a problem and finding a solution. Breastfeeding can be a very emotional experience, and emotional issues can really hold you back.

Whatever your feelings about past breastfeeding experiences, above all, acknowledge them and deal with them. Once you accept your emotions, then you can move forward and make things different the next time around. Remember, you don't have control of what happened in the past, but you can learn from your challenges and use that to your advantage now. Armed with more experience and the right information, you can make your current breastfeeding experience a positive one.

CHAPTER
7

The other alternative is to offer a supplement in one feeding. This is particularly helpful if you are supplementing with something other than your own breast milk. Someone else can do this feeding, while you use the time to get in a good pump session.

You must remember that supplements are a fast road to a low milk supply. It is imperative to ensure that you are still removing breast milk at a regular rate, if you intend to keep breastfeeding and to overcome difficulties. This is usually accomplished with a combination of breastfeeding your baby and using a breast pump.

Using a Lactation Aid

A lactation aid, such as an SNS or a Lact-Aid Nursing Trainer, can help you supplement at the breast. It can be a blessing for mothers who are working

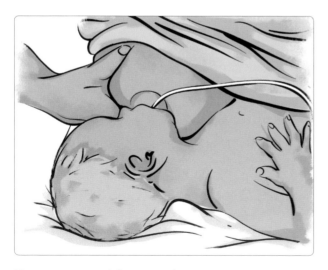

Having to use items to help you nurse, from a simple nipple shield to an SNS, can be depressing. Remember that these tools are temporary and help you move toward your breastfeeding goals.

hard to nurse but still have a very low milk supply. Lactation aids are not the easiest devices to use, but they can be helpful for feeding your baby while you are building your milk supply. If you think this tool might be a good option for you, talk to your lactation professional about using a lactation aid.

Cross Nursing and Breast Milk from Other Mothers

The idea of wet nursing is an age-old concept. In the past, women with children were actually paid to come in to households and breastfeed other babies. Since the 1930s, there has been little talk of wet nurses in the United States, though it is quite popular in other parts of the world. The bigger risk now is that you need to worry about illnesses and infections such as HIV being transmitted in breast milk that has not gone through a milk bank.

That being said, many mothers take matters into their own hands. They offer pumped milk to other women who are having issues with low supply. They might offer breast milk in extreme cases where the mother has taken very ill and cannot pump or is no longer alive to nurse her baby. People can and do make this choice often; it is just not commonly discussed in today's world.

Some women also are able to "borrow" a nursing baby to help them overcome an issue they are having. Perhaps their baby is in the neonatal intensive care unit (NICU), and they are having milk supply issues. In a case such as this, a baby is much better than a breast pump! Maybe you have heard stories of mothers on cross-country trips. One drives while the other nurses in the back seat, hanging over the car seats until it is time to switch. Keep your eyes and ears open. You will find your own instances of cross nursing when you look around. If you decide that cross nursing is an option for you, be sure that you are aware of the mother's health status before you begin.

Weaning from Supplements

As you begin to wean your baby from supplements, you should monitor your progress by watching your milk supply to overcome any difficulties. As your milk supply builds, you can start backing off of supplemental feedings. Do this gently so that you do not disrupt the balance of your breast milk supply and your baby's health. Do this by watching your baby's diapers. The wet and dirty diaper count will be your best guide as to how your baby is doing.

When eliminating outside sources, the first thing to remove is artificial supplements, followed by banked breast milk. Finally, remove your expressed milk until you are completely feeding your baby at the breast. You should do this in increments of 1 ounce (30 ml) at a time. For instance, take away 1 ounce (30 ml) of supplementation for the first day. Then stay at this level for three days. So if you were giving a supplement of 10 ounces (296 ml) total per day, start with 9 ounces (266 ml) for that day. If your baby's diapers indicate that things are going well, move forward.

The second reduction will also be 1 ounce (30 ml). Wait for two or three days. Watch the diapers and then make your decision. If for some reason you feel like there is a question about whether to move forward with the next reduction, stay at the level you are at for a few more days.

As you are removing supplemental feedings, remember to nurse your baby more frequently. If he still seems hungry, offer the breast again. This will help your baby to be in control of his feedings.

REMEMBER THAT PREVIOUS BREASTFEEDING PROBLEMS NEED NOT REPEAT

Sometimes it can feel as though you have a baby and everything that can go wrong does. For whatever reason, you might have had a breastfeeding situation that was less than ideal or in some way could have been better. Perhaps you are worried that this experience, however negative, will affect your ability to breastfeed the next time around.

Fortunately, most breastfeeding problems are not doomed to repeat themselves. And some of the issues that came up the first time around, you are now more knowledgeable about. You might even have more control over them the next time. As such, you'll start from a much better place than you started with your last breastfeeding relationship.

If you have had previous problems, be sure to talk to a lactation professional ahead of time to have a game plan for your next baby. Try to look back and see whether you can pinpoint some of the

CHAPTER

7

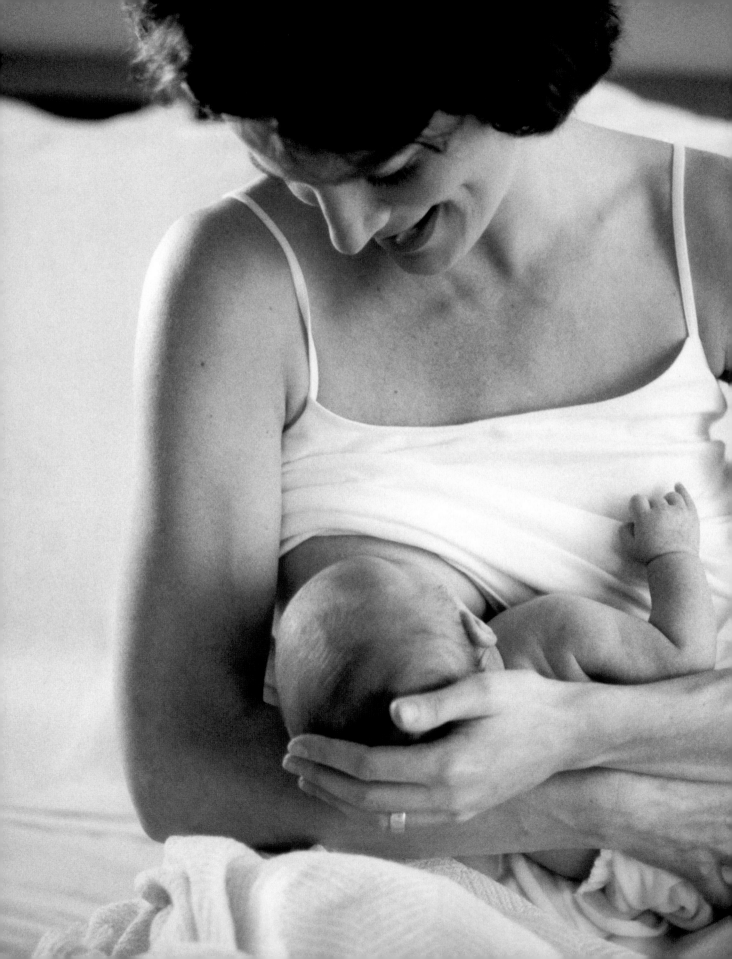

issues that plagued you last time. Consider some of the things you might do differently. Once you have this game plan, you can begin to enact the parts that might occur before your baby's birth and, thus, prepare for when your baby is here.

Even if circumstances were to set themselves up similarly to your previous breastfeeding experience, there would likely still be a huge difference. The next time around, you will be more aware and knowledgeable. And sometimes being able to recognize a problem faster or with more precision is important. Other times, the rapid response is critical to solving or resolving the issue.

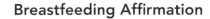

Breastfeeding Affirmation

Breastfeeding might have challenges, but my baby and I will work to overcome them.

CHAPTER
7

Confidence in breastfeeding is important. Problems you have heard about or have previously experienced should not be of concern. Move forward with an optimistic mindset and a positive plan.

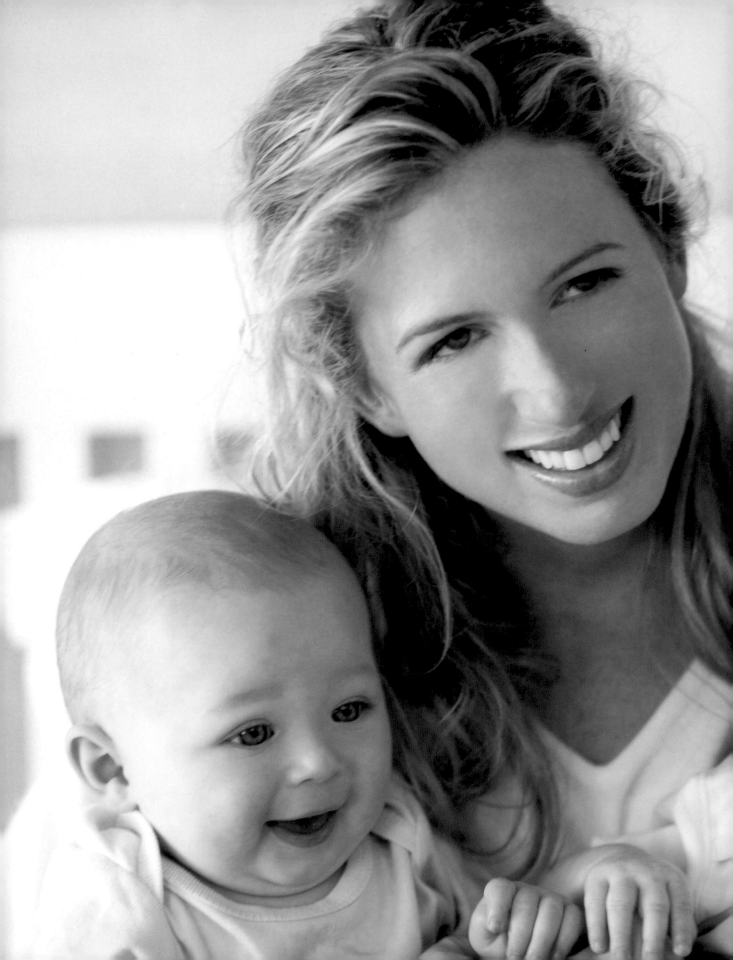

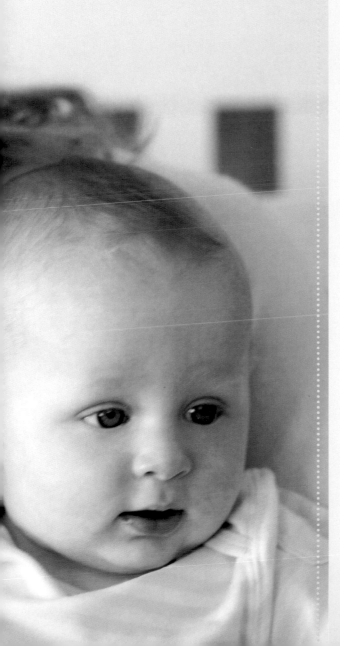

CHAPTER 8

Advice for Preemies, Multiples, and Other Special Nursing Needs

 Checklist for Successful Breastfeeding

- ☐ Learn the challenges of breast-feeding the near-term baby.
- ☐ Nurse your premature infant.
- ☐ Learn how to feed twins and other multiples.
- ☐ Find help for breastfeeding a baby with special needs.
- ☐ Understand the benefits of adoptive nursing.

Certain circumstances can lead to extra challenges in breastfeeding. Breastfeeding books often overlook these circumstances, despite the fact that many mothers experience them. You will need knowledge and support to be able to tackle breastfeeding and caring for an infant or infants who need extra attention, even if it is only in the short term. Fortunately, if you create the right circumstances you can be successful, just as with nursing any other baby.

Late Preterm Infants and Elective Delivery Rates

Hospitals and medical practices that have high elective induction or cesarean rates frequently have higher numbers of late-preterm infants. This is because the baby's actual due date might have been incorrect, making her birthday a bit earlier than expected. The American Congress of Obstetricians and Gynecologists (ACOG) and the March of Dimes are working to crack down on these early births and the obstetricians who are inducing them.

LEARN THE CHALLENGES OF BREASTFEEDING THE NEAR-TERM BABY

A near-term infant is defined as a baby who is born typically between thirty-four to thirty-six weeks' gestation (with full-term being defined as thirty-seven or more weeks' gestation). This is the fastest-rising segment of the preterm birth population. While these babies generally fair much better than their smaller and earlier counterparts in all measures, they still have significant problems in a few key areas, namely breathing and feeding.

While you might have a baby who is not ill and comes immediately to your room, other problems might arise. For instance, a baby born slightly early has less neurological development than a full-term infant. This usually means the baby's ability to suck can be delayed or it might not be quite right. This can make breastfeeding more challenging as your baby learns.

Frequently, help from the lactation consultant or counselor on the hospital staff is necessary. It is truly helpful if you have someone who is used to helping mothers who have preterm and near-term infants, because of their special needs. They can help you come up with the best plan to help you feed your baby, in spite of the challenges ahead.

Infants who are born even slightly early are more likely to require a stay in the neonatal intensive care unit (NICU). This is most often on account of breathing difficulties, although sometimes other issues are at hand as well.

Neonatal care units cause a variety of other unforeseen issues that often don't have to be dealt with for full-term infants. For instance, schedules and policies can make it difficult for mothers to be close to their babies around the clock and, thus, can inhibit early breastfeeding. Parents also must deal with IVs and other precautions and therapies being used.

NURSE YOUR PREMATURE INFANT

Breast milk is particularly important for premature infants. Their bodies are susceptible to many issues, including disease and complications due to prematurity, but breast milk can help prevent many of these problems for your baby. In fact, your body knows the point at which your pregnancy ended, and your breasts will respond with specialized

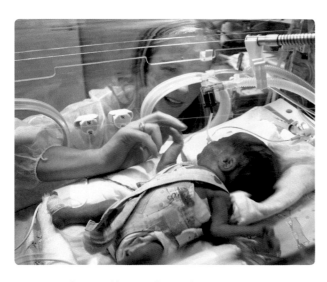

Premature infants need breast milk urgently for its healing, preventative, and nurturing power.

breast milk made for your premature baby (the milk in this case is higher in protein and contains the antibody sIgA to help fight infection). You might have many challenges when nursing a premature baby, though lots of mothers successfully navigate these waters with support from lactation professionals and other parents who have been there.

Building a Milk Supply and Feeding Your Preemie

Building a milk supply is the first challenge when feeding a premature baby. You will need to do this with a hospital-grade breast pump. Your neonatal intensive care nursery should have access to a specialized lactation professional. She can help you choose a pump and plan when and where to pump.

Most nurseries have a special area where you can pump. Many will allow you to bring the pump into the room with your baby. (For more on breast pumps, see chapter 9.) You may need to follow specific protocols regarding milk storage. Be sure to ask questions as often as necessary to get the proper information.

Typically, your premature infant will receive breast milk via a nasal gastric tube or gavage feeding (nasogastric tube feeding). This gives your baby the full advantage of the breast milk without the work of nursing at the breast. This saved energy will hopefully mean your baby is able to grow faster.

Getting to the breast is an issue for premature infants. While your baby might not be ready to feed, spending time on your chest is important for his

CHAPTER
8

growth and development. It also helps you. When your baby is ready to breastfeed, you might have many thoughts going through your head. You might be excited and nervous. This is fairly common.

Remember, your baby will have to learn to nurse at this point. How well he comes to the breast will depend on a lot of factors, including whether he has been using artificial nipples for feedings, his age (corrected and otherwise), his weight, your breasts, and other factors.

For those first feedings, remember: Your goal is to have him experience the breast as a pleasant place. Don't let him sit there and scream at the breast. If he appears upset or frustrated, calm him before continuing your nursing session. This won't be your only chance for him to nurse.

Even if your baby does nurse a tiny bit, most likely at first he will not be getting all he needs from the breast. This means you will still need to pump to help keep your milk supply up. This dance of pumping and nursing might take a while to figure out. But as your baby increases his time at the breast and transfers milk well, you can decrease your breast-pump use.

Avoiding infection is critical for premature infants. Since their immune systems are immature, they are more susceptible to infection. And when they get infections, you are more likely to see severe reactions and complications. Breast milk will help to combat infection. The American Academy of Pediatrics (AAP) recommends breast milk for all babies, including premature infants.

What Is Kangaroo Care?

Kangaroo care (the term for skin-to-skin contact as used in the NICU) means using skin-to-skin contact to help your baby stabilize. While it is often used with premature babies, kangaroo care is recommended and beneficial for all new infants. Being skin to skin with your baby can help him regulate

WOMEN'S WISDOM:

Special babies have special needs. While breastfeeding is the perfect food, sometimes it can be hard to get your milk supply established or create a good feeding pattern due to your baby's needs. This doesn't mean you shouldn't breastfeed or provide breast milk. And don't be placated and told that your baby will be fine without breastfeeding. If you think you're having an issue, get help. Some professionals are stumped when it comes to helping with breastfeeding special-needs babies—even doctors and nurses. If you need help breastfeeding or pumping for your special baby, ask someone who helps mothers in your situation with breastfeeding on a daily basis, not someone who just happens to be free at the time. All nurses' stations should have a list of people that you can call for specific breastfeeding help.

his body temperature, breathing, and other body mechanisms. Babies who are allowed skin-to-skin contact via kangaroo care tend to grow faster and have fewer complications. It can also increase your parenting confidence, as babies who stay in close contact with their parents tend to fuss and cry less. Babies typically also soothe more quickly because this proximity to their parents means their needs are met more promptly. Kangaroo care can be done with mom, dad, or anyone old enough to hold the baby skin to skin.

Kangaroo care is standard in many NICUs. Talk to your nurses and practitioners about the hospital's protocol for kangaroo care. If a protocol does not exist there, ask what you need to do to implement kangaroo care for your baby.

At What Age Can Nursing Start?

If a baby is born quite prematurely in terms of development, nursing might not be able to start right away. This is because these babies might expend too much energy sucking and trying to get milk. But as reported in "Persistent Beneficial Effects of Breast Milk Ingested in the Neonatal Intensive Care Unit on Outcomes of Extremely Low Birthweight Infants at 30 Months of Age," published in *Clinical Perinatology*, being able to supply your baby with breast milk will help him to grow more quickly so that he hopefully will be ready to breastfeed sooner. Building your milk supply will help you to be ready for when it is time to bring your baby to the breast.

Some babies are ready to breastfeed sooner than others. Generally speaking, your nursery staff will tell you that your baby can be expected to begin breastfeeding near his due date. This may be before or after his due date, depending on your baby's health and growth.

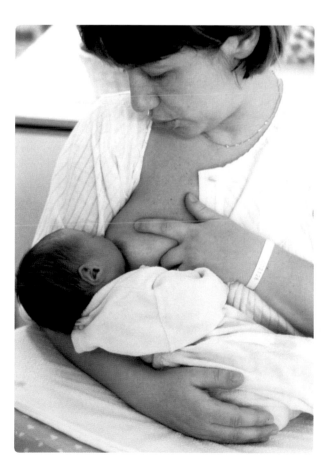

Your first nursing sessions after birth are likely to be exciting yet challenging for both of you. Hang in there as you learn together.

CHAPTER
8

TIP

Preemies Need to Suck

Sucking in a premature infant is a necessity. A pacifier can help a preemie cope with pain and discomfort from medical procedures. It can also be given with other feedings to help associate sucking with food. For this reason, using pacifiers for this specific group is recommended by lactation professionals for comfort and health.

What about Weight Gain?

Weight gain is typically the key to when your baby will be able to come home. Your baby's doctors will give you a weight goal. They'll also explain what feedings should look like before you will be able to go home. Typically, you will be able to go home at or near your original due date. Having good support for breastfeeding will help your baby gain as much weight as possible.

Some babies who are in a NICU will need additives or supplementation. This can be done with human breast milk fortifiers and breast milk from the human milk bank if you would prefer this to standard infant formula supplements. The benefits are that you retain the protection against disease and necrotizing enterocolitis (NEC) when using human milk supplements.

Finding Support

The breastfeeding challenges you will experience with a premature infant are greater than those the average mother will typically have. This means you will likely need greater support, in terms of both the amount you receive and the quality of knowledge those support people can share with you.

Many NICUs have registered dietitians, lactation professionals, and social workers on staff. Together, these teams can help you to get the care you need, particularly as it relates to having a premature infant.

You can get specific breastfeeding advice for your baby's medical needs. Your nurses and lactation professionals will help you through nursing, particularly when it comes to moving machines and tubes to help you get close to your baby.

LEARN HOW TO FEED TWINS AND OTHER MULTIPLES

Having twins and other multiples is becoming increasingly common. Even better is that there are more mothers of multiples who successfully nurse their babies. Some great role models are available to talk to about breastfeeding more than one baby at a time.

Myths about Breastfeeding Multiples

Plenty of myths circulate about breastfeeding in general. But armed with facts, you should be able to pick apart most myths before they can work on your confidence level. Here are some of the more common myths about breastfeeding multiples:

- You can't make enough milk.
- All you will do is feed the babies.
- Bottle feeding is easier when you have more than one baby.

These statements are false! Mothers of multiples make plenty of breast milk for their babies. The key to good milk production is the same as with any singleton: Nurse early and often, and follow cue feeding for all babies when possible.

Feeling like all you do is care for your babies is a normal way to feel with multiples. This statement might appear true, but you also have to change diapers, eat, sleep, and bathe. So while you will spend the bulk of your time caring for your babies, you will spend only a portion of that time feeding the babies. In other words, caring for multiples is a lot of work no matter how you slice it. Breastfeeding will not make or break you.

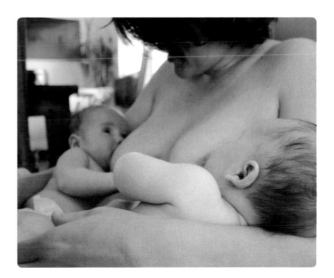

Nursing twins and other multiples is possible. Many moms are very successful, with some patience and adaptability.

CONFIDENCE CUE

Breast milk is such an amazing substance. It is the perfect temperature, contains the right amount of fat and calories, and even has knowledge of your baby in that your body knows how to make special milk for preemies or babies with other problems. Don't let the fact that your baby has special circumstances alter your plans. You can provide your baby with breast milk and love. At first, this might look different from what you had planned, but it can be done. Be sure to find other moms who have been where you are and have goals like yours. This can make your breastfeeding journey much easier. If you don't know where to look, ask a social worker, a lactation professional, or even a staff nurse.

CHAPTER
8

You might be told that bottle feeding is easier with multiple babies. But the truth is that breastfeeding is the perfect lay-down-on-the-job activity. You simply latch on and feed your baby. You can multitask if you choose. But in general, there is nothing to prepare, nothing to wash, and nothing to purchase—times two or more.

Know that there are always people you can talk to about breastfeeding multiples. Finding support from other mothers of multiples is a great idea. Also look for a lactation consultant who has worked with mothers of multiples before you.

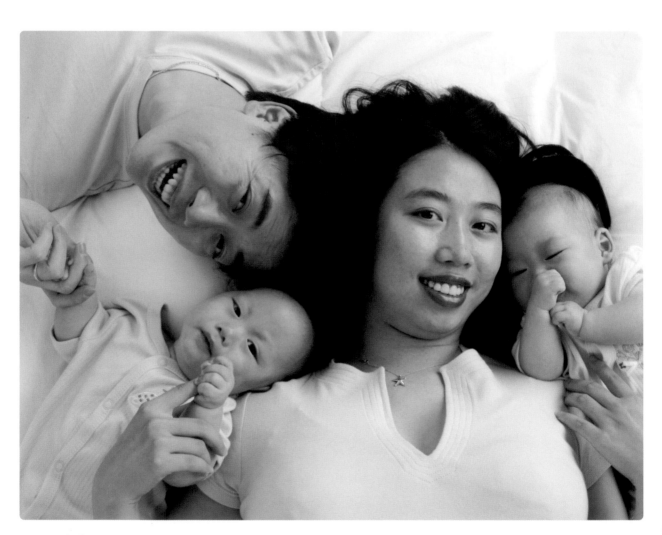

Having multiples can be a huge transition. Family time helps calm frayed nerves and bring joy to your lives.

What Challenges Do Multiple Babies Present?

Although the statements in the list in the preceding section are myths, that's not to say that breastfeeding multiple babies isn't challenging. Some challenges you might have no control over, such as the gestational age at which they are born. Twins are more likely to be born early and are more likely to require interventions at birth. These are two known factors that can increase the risk of having breastfeeding difficulties.

In some ways, you will need to think of your nursing experience as simply nursing two babies at the same time. It is really not the collective nursing situation that most people think of when they think of breastfeeding twins and other multiples. Even if you have identical twins, they will still have different issues when it comes to nursing. Learning these differences will help you in your quest to breastfeed. An example might be that one baby has an issue with tongue tie, while her twin nurses just fine. You might also see one baby has a different nursing style or pattern than her siblings. This can be challenging when it comes to figuring out when and how to feed your babies. But patience and help will go a long way toward deciphering this pattern.

If prematurity is on the list of things you're concerned about, you might need more help with breastfeeding from your lactation professional. And remember, even slight prematurity can make a big impact on your baby's nursing abilities. You can overcome these challenges with time and support.

TIP | Managing Twins' Feeding Patterns

If you are feeding on demand and both babies prefer opposite schedules, you will have to figure out how to handle this situation. Some mothers choose to allow both babies to maintain whatever schedule they naturally prefer. Others try to gently mold their babies' schedules closer together.

Having more than one infant at a time brings other issues as well. You have two hands and how many babies? This means you might have to do some baby rotating in terms of how you feed them and when. For a while, you might need help during feedings to ensure that you can get each baby latched well and nursing (and to help with those issues that come up during a feeding, such as someone needing a diaper change!). As you get past the first weeks, this will become much easier.

Should You Feed Together or Apart?

This is one of the most frequently asked questions when it comes to breastfeeding multiples, and you will probably go back and forth with your answer.

CHAPTER
8

Some mothers find it easier to nurse one baby at a time. This takes longer to accomplish and might leave you feeling like you do nothing but feed babies all day. It also requires more help, because you simply cannot nurse one baby and care for two or more alone if you really intend to feed.

Feeding both babies together, while it offers you the chance to save time, might be harder for a while. Particularly at first, as you are learning your babies' styles, cues, and patterns, you might not be able to hold and latch both babies adequately. Having someone there to help you can be beneficial, but it might also make things a bit more hectic. And a hectic mom means nervous babies, which in turn means the nursing session is getting off on the wrong foot.

The ideal solution is to nurse sometimes together and sometimes apart. As you and your babies get to know each other, nursing can become simpler. You might find your babies actually help each other to nurse. Twins are often known to pat one another to give comfort. Or if you have one baby who might be having a harder time latching, let the first baby get the flow going, and then suddenly your other baby will be nursing like a pro!

How Do You Manage Your Breasts?

You might have heard that mothers of multiples spend a lot of time trying to decide which breast to use for which baby at which feeding. While it is possible to keep track of this information, it might not be wildly necessary. Some mothers try to relax by simply assigning a breast to a baby.

For example: Baby A gets the right side for the first half of the day, switching to the left after six o'clock in the evening. Baby B starts on the left and switches to the right. This ensures that your milk supply is built in the same manner for both sides. Remember, babies nurse differently. Other parents rotate per day, some per feeding. The system you choose really is up to you.

The rotation gets a bit trickier when more than two babies are being fed. Fortunately, most mothers of triplets or more say that once you learn a rotation, it is simple and actually can help to keep you sane while trying to feed multiple babies. For example, start Baby A on the right and Baby B on the left; rotate Baby C to the right and Baby A to the left; then rotate Baby B to the right and Baby C to the left, ensuring that each baby had each breast at each feeding. Obviously, you can start in any rotation. Some mothers do one baby at a time, while others prefer multiple babies at a time.

Breastfeeding Positions for Multiple Babies

How you hold your breastfeeding twins or multiples is not vastly different from nursing a singleton. However, there are some things to consider, particularly as the babies get older. Here are some examples of nursing positions for multiples.

Cradle Hold for Multiples

This is a very basic way to hold your baby when nursing. It is what most mothers think about when it comes to breastfeeding. For multiples, you will need to do it slightly differently.

Breastfeeding Positions for Multiple Babies

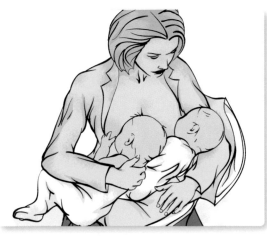

Cradle Hold for Multiples

The cradle hold is a great way to hold newborn twins who are nursing well. It can also be a great position to start with one baby and then add the next as you're learning to nurse.

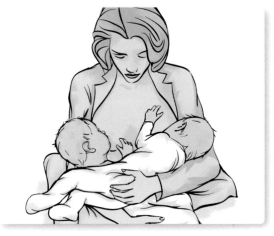

Cross-Cradle Hold for Multiples

The cross cradle is helpful when you're needed to give your baby's head better support. It is also a good position to start with one baby and then add another baby when nursing two.

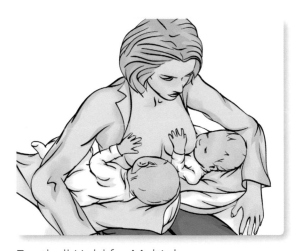

Football Hold for Multiples

The football hold is perfect when learning to nurse twins, particularly after a cesarean birth. You can look down and see both babies, particularly their latch, and there is little pressure on your incision.

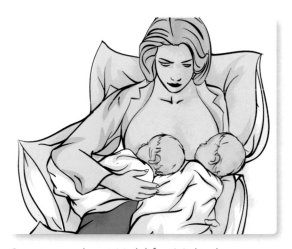

Semirecumbant Hold for Multiples

Semirecumbent is a great position to try to get ome rest while you nurse. It can also be a good way to reinforce skin-to-skin contact for your babies.

TIP | **Healing a Nipple Wound with Twins**

If you experience sore nipples while breastfeeding multiples, it might be more difficult for your nipples to heal because of the added time that your breasts are in action. Talk to your lactation professional. She can help you devise a way to find time to allow your breasts to heal. The solution might involve pumping for a while to get your wound under control. Obviously, prevention is the first step.

Each baby will lay from left to right or right to left, according to your preference. The baby at your right breast will be supported by your right forearm, with her head nearing the crook of your right arm. The baby at the left breast will lay on her sibling, supported slightly by your left hand. A pillow can help to prop the babies up. Use your right hand to help latch the left baby and your left hand to help latch the right baby.

Once the babies are latched, feel free to move until you're comfortable. As you become more familiar with nursing your ability and comfort level will increase dramatically. Some mothers choose to latch the first baby on alone and then add the second baby.

Cross-Cradle Hold for Multiples

The cross cradle is similar to the cradle hold. The difference is that you want to support the baby's head with your hand on the opposite side you are feeding, rather than your arm. So if you are feeding from the left breast, you would use your right hand. This provides you with more control.

Trying the cross cradle with twins might also mean using a different angle than you might with a singleton. Part of this will depend on your dexterity. Figure out what is most comfortable for you and your babies.

Football Hold for Multiples

The football hold is great for multiples, but some mothers find it more difficult to use. However, it's great for viewing your babies' faces and keeping babies off your abdomen if you had a cesarean birth.

Another nice perk is that both babies can lay there while you spend an extra minute or two getting one baby latched on at a time. A pillow can be helpful for propping the babies up. You will probably want a pillow under each baby. Remember to bring the baby to the breast and not the breast to the baby. You do not need to add a sore upper back to the mix right now.

With this hold you can also use the cross-cradle type of support on your baby's head. Place your palm just below your baby's neck, on your baby's upper back. Use your hand to help your baby maneuver to the breast and attain the best latch.

Side-Lying Hold for Multiples

This is a breastfeeding position that most mothers of multiples want to hurry up and learn. This is because you can try to get some rest while nursing if you can make this work. Truthfully, breast size can be an issue here. The larger your breasts, the easier it is to use this position.

Unlike with a singleton, you will want to lay on your right side, and then tilt backward slightly. Use a pillow to prop your body in place. With your right breast, nurse one baby lying sideways and facing you on the bed. Your other baby will be nursing lying with her face toward your left breast and her body lying on your body, feet to feet.

Tips for Breastfeeding Multiples

There is no doubt about it: Breastfeeding multiples is worth it! The minor challenges that can occur for every mother are likely to be increased simply because more babies are involved. Here are some tips for breastfeeding multiples successfully:

- Get help for your home. Let someone else worry about the dishes and dinner.
- Get connected with your local mothers of multiples group.
- Find a lactation professional who has experience with multiples.
- Consider a postpartum doula who has experience with multiples.
- Remember to sneak away, even if it's just for a shower.

- Be sure you are well hydrated and well fed.
- Consider renting a breast pump to help with milk supply, particularly if your babies were born early.
- Remember to ask for help whenever you need it.

Breastfeeding multiples is one of the hardest things you will ever do, but the rewards are great. Later, as you get familiar with what you are doing, you will be able to do it in your sleep (hopefully, literally!).

If you are feeding on demand and your babies prefer opposite schedules you will have to figure out how you want to handle this situation. Some mothers choose to allow their babies to maintain whatever schedule they naturally prefer. Others prefer to gently mold the schedules closer together.

Breastfeeding Can Relieve Your Stress

Breastfeeding a baby with special needs can help both you and your baby to stay calm in a medically complex or hectic environment. All of the time spent in the hospital, beeps from machines, and medical people around can make life feel hectic and crazy. When nursing, you and your baby can get some much-needed peaceful time together.

CHAPTER
8

FIND HELP FOR BREASTFEEDING A BABY WITH SPECIAL NEEDS

Sometimes your baby might have special needs that will affect your breastfeeding relationship. This might involve a physical issue, such as low muscle tone. It might be a congenital difference, such as a cleft lip or palate. Perhaps your baby needs surgery, or even has a genetic condition such as Down syndrome. Some babies will face many of these issues at once.

While your baby might have a harder time nursing depending on the circumstances of the special need, he might also nurse very well when given the chance. Know that breast milk is still the best thing for your baby. In fact, breast milk might be even more important for a baby who has special needs or is facing surgery. With breast milk's antibiotic-like properties, you'll find your baby is less likely to have problems with infection because he is breastfed. This will also help to protect your baby in a hospital environment.

That being said, you might have to deal with things you didn't expect. Perhaps your baby has physical issues that make nursing difficult. Finding support from people who are knowledgeable about breastfeeding and the specific issue you are facing is key.

You might be dealing with a baby who has latch issues. You might need help with positioning for a baby with surgical wounds. Be sure that you are open to doing something other than what you originally thought you would do. For example, although this book previously discussed nursing positions, most of those won't prepare you for nursing on all fours as you hang over your baby who is in traction from surgery. But being open to trying new things will help you.

Talking with other mothers who have been where you are is even more helpful when you are dealing with a situation that is out of the normal scope of most of your social support. You can also find various places for referrals and support. For example, La Leche League International has several information pamphlets for coping with special needs, such as nursing with Down syndrome, cleft palate, and more.

Galactosemia

The only condition that would bar a baby from breastfeeding is the metabolic disorder galactosemia. Galactosemia prevents babies from breaking down the simple sugar, galactose. You will know quickly whether your baby has this condition. A test is done as a part of states' newborn screening processes.

UNDERSTAND THE BENEFITS OF ADOPTIVE NURSING

If you have adopted a baby or will be adopting a baby, you might be interested in adoptive nursing. Breast milk, in any quantity, is so beneficial that the American Academy of Pediatrics (AAP) recommends breastfeeding to adoptive mothers. Mothers who choose to breastfeed their adopted children have varied successes with breastfeeding.

Some mothers can create a full supply for their babies, while others are able to build only a partial supply. Remember, any breast milk is good breast milk! But planning ahead and having a good, supportive team on your side will make all the difference.

If you know ahead of time that you will be able to get your baby at a specific time, you can begin the process of making milk. Typically, this will involve pumping with a hospital-grade breast pump. You should work with a lactation professional to help you figure out the best schedule to meet your needs.

Sometimes medications or herbs are used in the process, such as fenugreek or fennel. These can be helpful for some women, while others do not find them helpful at all. Your practitioners will help you to figure out what your best chances are at building a good milk supply and which type of medicinal or herbal support (if any) is best for you.

Once the baby is with you, you can begin nursing, even if you don't have a lot of milk or any milk. A supplemental nursing system (SNS) is beneficial because it allows the baby to breastfeed and stimulates the breasts while providing the calories necessary for your baby's health. Even if your baby is not able to get breast milk, having the baby at your breast can be a good option for some mothers. For more on SNSs, and on the Lact-Aid Nursing Trainer in particular, see pages 195 and 198.

Get Support from Others for Your Choice

Hopefully, your decision to breastfeed your adopted baby has been met with joy; if not joy, then at least acceptance and support. There is no greater place to find that support and joy than from other families who have been there.

Self-Care Tips

Breastfeeding a baby with special needs, even needs that are not life threatening, can be a strain. Remember to ask for help and figure out how you can make it easier on yourself. If you are pumping, perhaps you need help with older kids, your home, or even just occasional meals. Be sure to have a high-quality hospital-grade pump on hand to build your supply. If your baby is in the hospital, remember to leave occasionally, even if it's for a walk around the parking lot.

CHAPTER
8

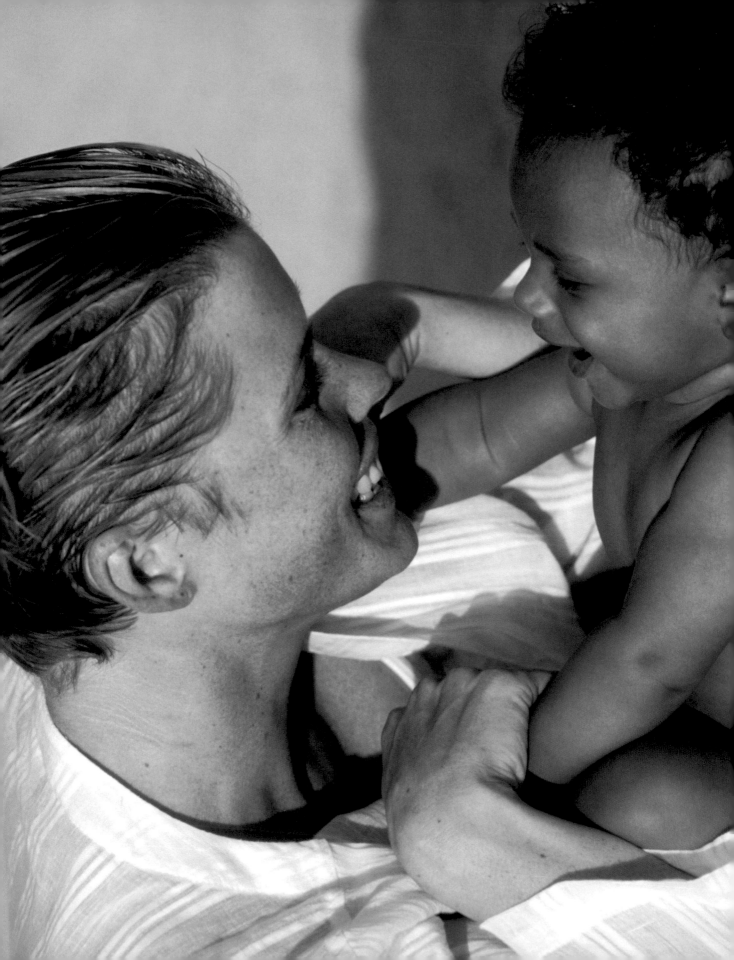

Breastfeeding Affirmation

*I am up to the unique challenge
of breastfeeding my baby.*

You might have a problem finding an adoptive breastfeeding mother across the street, but you can find someone locally. Start making connections through local adoption support groups. Even if you do not already know someone who has nursed a baby, you are likely to find someone who knows someone who has nursed.

You should also ask your La Leche League leader for names. She might be a good resource when it comes to finding another mother to talk to about the issues of adoptive nursing. She might even have a graduate in mind to pair you up with as you go along your journey. Other places to ask include your pediatrician's office; online support groups; and adoption groups, either those you are a part of locally or others elsewhere.

In addition to finding support for yourself, you might also find support for other family members. This might mean someone for your partner to talk to about the hows and whys of adoptive nursing. You might even find someone your extended family can talk to that would help to provide them with the confidence to support you in your decision.

Whatever the outcome of your efforts to nurse an adoptive child, you should know that you've made an amazing and worthwhile choice. Whether you produce a little or a lot of milk, you are giving your baby an incredible gift that will affect her in many beneficial ways throughout life. And even if you are unable to produce any milk, never underestimate the power of breastfeeding in terms of sheer emotional bonding. Whatever time you spend nursing your adopted baby at the breast, be assured that you will be fostering a close, nurturing love that will set the tone for your relationship together.

CHAPTER
8

Breastfeeding your adopted child in any amount can be a real option. The health benefits and bonding experience provides a great start for you and your new baby.

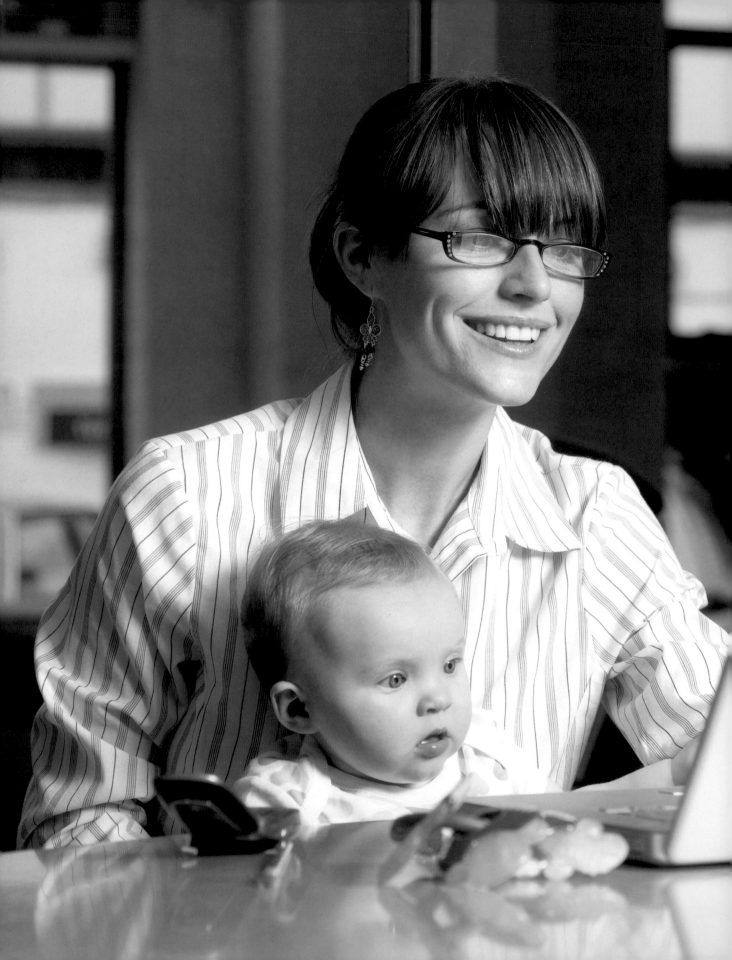

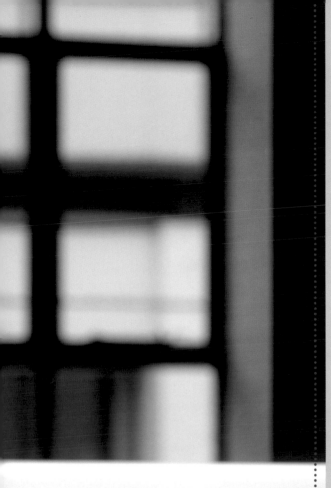

CHAPTER 9

Breast Pumps: Casual and Constant

 Checklist for Successful Breastfeeding

- ☐ Choose the right breast pump.
- ☐ Learn to hand-express your breasts.
- ☐ Make arrangements to pump at work.
- ☐ Figure out how you pump best.
- ☐ Find a location for pumping.
- ☐ Investigate your breast milk storage options.
- ☐ Make a decision to pump exclusively.
- ☐ Wean from pumping.

Using a breast pump is not always necessary. The breast pump can add an element of convenience to your life if you are working outside the home or are away from your baby, even if it is for only a short period of time. A breast pump can also be a blessing when breastfeeding challenges arise. Whether and how often you use a breast pump will depend on many factors, including:

- Your baby's gestational age at birth
- Your childcare situation after your maternity leave
- Your body's milk supply
- Your baby's ability to nurse
- Your baby's health

Realize that just as you have choices about breastfeeding for varying lengths of time, you also have choices in how much breast milk you provide and how. Some mothers choose to provide only breast milk and only by using a breast pump, while other mothers decide to use a breast pump as well as to breastfeed to feed their baby.

CHOOSE THE RIGHT BREAST PUMP

So many breast pumps are on the market. One of the biggest problems is choosing the wrong breast pump. It's not hard to make a bad decision when it comes to breast pumps. The advertising is confusing. The designs are amazing, and you probably feel pretty overwhelmed after spending just a few minutes among the boxes of breast pumps.

As you are shopping around, be prepared to ask some tough questions about the breast pumps you consider. Also know which answers you are looking for when you ask these questions. Before you can even begin to find the right pump, you need to figure out what type of pumper you will be by asking yourself these questions:

- How often will I need to pump?
- How long will I have to pump?
- Do I need to be able to double pump?
- Does my baby or I have any issues that might require a medical-grade pump?
- Will I be using this pump for more than one child?
- What is my budget?
- Can I use flexible spending account (FSA) money on the rental or purchase of a breast pump?

The answers to these questions will help you to determine which breast pump is best for your needs. The general rule is that the less you intend to use your breast pump, the smaller the breast pump you will need. If you don't plan to be pumping a lot, you can generally purchase a pump with fewer options. If you intend to pump once a week, for instance, you might be more tempted to buy a single pump that is powered by hand or by batteries. On the other hand, if you need to pump multiple times per day, nearly every day of the week, a more powerful electric pump might be in order. A word of advice: Buy the

CHAPTER
9

TIP

Be Sure to Have a Backup

A backup breast pump can be a good idea. In fact, it's nearly mandatory for mothers who pump on a daily basis. This way, you'll be covered just in case you are out without your pump or if you have a pump failure.

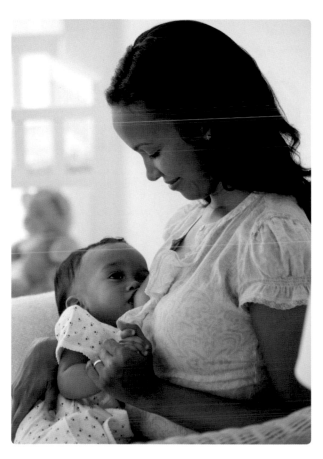

A breast pump is never as good as your baby but don't worry if you need to pump— you and your baby still have an amazing relationship.

best breast pump you can afford. This means that even if you intend to be a once-a-week pumper, buy the high-end, single-user double pump. The reasoning is that you do not know what changes might come your way—whether you might get a job down the road, or how many children you plan to breast-feed via pumping your milk.

Do some research before you head to the store to buy a breast pump. Know what is available. Read user reviews online and talk to other mothers you know who have pumped. This will give you a better idea about what's available and help you to narrow down the choices. You might even want to talk to your lactation professional to get her opinions on breast pumps. Remember, just because it's called a breast pump doesn't mean it is effective or that it can't damage your breasts if you use it incorrectly.

Here is what you need to know about choosing a breast pump:

- What is the pump most commonly used to do? (Recreational pumping or heavy-duty pumping?)
- Is it a single-user or multiuser pump?
- Can you double-pump? (Pump both breasts at the same time?)
- Does it require any special kits to go with it?
- How is it powered?
- How long can you expect it to last?
- How do you clean it? (Which parts, etc.?)
- Does this pump come with any accessories?

Talk to the women you meet at your La Leche League meetings or at your other breastfeeding support groups, as well as at breastfeeding and baby-care classes. Get their advice on which breast pumps are out there and how they work. Other mothers will be a great source of reviews, positive and negative.

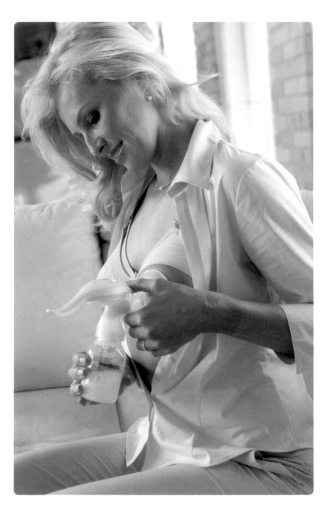

Having a back-up breast pump is important if you depend on your breast pump for success.

If you are registering for a breast pump for your baby shower, you should know that they are fairly expensive. Do not be tempted to ask for a breast pump model that is lower in price simply because you do not want to frighten people. Your choice of breast pump is very important and should not be based on cost alone. If the pump you choose is more expensive, perhaps several people will get together to buy it for you. Or you might use gift money you receive to buy it later on.

Beware of Free Breast Pumps

You might find that various places will offer free breast pumps, including your hospital, baby stores, and even formula/pharmaceutical companies. Remember, the key here is that you get what you pay for: nothing.

Typically, a free breast pump is a hand- or battery-powered breast pump. Most are low-end pumps that are not very effective at what they are supposedly designed to do. These pumps have been purchased at very low prices to entice you to do something, whether it is to give birth at a particular hospital, buy products from a certain store or manufacturer, or something else.

Some women who have used these pumps have been disappointed that they did not plan to get a good breast pump. Nothing is as frustrating as thinking you have a great pump and finding out that you do not. Some moms have actually been harmed by poorly made, low-quality breast pumps. Be very leery of these free breast pumps.

When to Rent a Breast Pump

Rental breast pumps are typically expensive, hospital-grade, multiuser pumps. These breast pumps have the motors sealed off to prevent milk contamination. This makes them safe for multiple people to use, in succession, though not at the same time.

A rental breast pump can be handy if you have a baby who is having problems nursing or if you are having problems with your milk supply. For example, if your baby is born early, even by just a few weeks, he might not be a great breastfeeder at first. This means that using a breast pump might be key for you to build and maintain a breast milk supply for your baby. It will also provide him with breast milk for however he is taking his feedings. It also protects him, particularly if he is having issues with his intestines.

CONFIDENCE CUE

Using a breast pump can be challenging. The challenge is not to get sucked into the hysteria of calculating milk quantities or worrying about how much of a freezer stash you have on hand. Remember, breastfeeding moms don't keep stashes around. But the challenges of pumping are worth it. Pumping is an added layer of love on top of your dedication to breastfeed. The work is hard, but your baby appreciates it. Be sure you find a good cheerleader, whether you're pumping for one feeding or twelve. Someone to cheer you on no matter what is always a good thing!

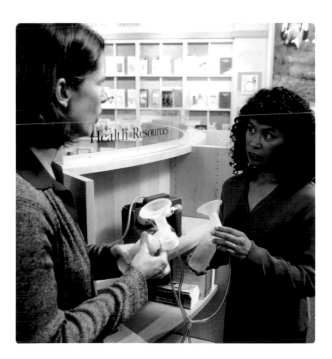

Finding the right lactation professional to help you choose the right pump will save you money and pain later.

To do this type of pumping, you need a hospital-grade pump. This is the big grandmother of all breast pumps. That is because this type of breast pump is designed to build and maintain a breast milk supply. Even the really cool and expensive breast pump you got for your baby shower will pale in comparison for this purpose.

If you are considering pumping to provide your baby with breast milk while you work on a regular basis, you will want to know what is involved. Consider a better pump, though it does not have to be a hospital-grade breast pump. You can make do with an electric breast pump in the $200 to $400 (£175–£350) range. Although this is expensive, remember, this pump will be an investment in your baby.

If you wish to pump only occasionally, you can use a manual or hand breast pump. This is not to say that a more expensive breast pump is not helpful; just that it's not as necessary. In fact, women in this category can often simply hand-express their milk without using a breast pump.

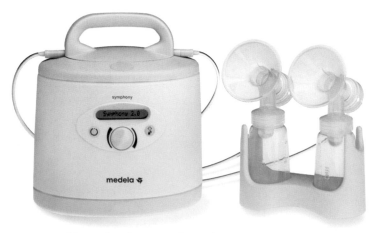

A hospital-grade pump can be your best choice depending on your needs.

When you're choosing a breast pump for your situation, think wisely and plan accordingly. Here are some questions to ask yourself about your needs:

- Are you likely to have a premature baby?
- How often will you need to pump?
- How much breast milk do you need to get from each pumping session?
- Do you want the ability to double pump?
- Do you need an electric or battery-operated pump?
- Do you have a disease or condition that might make your breast milk supply low?
- Have you had a previous baby with breastfeeding issues?
- How long do you intend to use the pump?
- How many children do you intend to have?
- Are there breast-pump rental facilities near you?
- Does your insurance cover the rental of a hospital-grade breast pump? Do you need a physician's note for a medical issue with mother or baby?
- Are you having twins or higher-order multiples?
- Do you need a breast pump with any special functions?
- Do you know what size flanges (the part of the breast pump that goes on the breast) you need for your breast pump?

If you are not sure which type of breast pump you will need, you can either wait to purchase one or go for the bigger, more powerful pump. Having a pump that does more than you need is far better than trying to make a lesser-powered pump pull off something that it is just not designed to do.

Borrowed Pumps

Borrowed breast pumps have received a lot of controversy over the past couple of years. Because higher-end pumps cost more than lower-end pumps, it is natural to try to get the most for your money. This can mean sharing a pump with a family member or a friend. The problem is that most breast pumps are not meant to be shared with others.

The average breast pump has two major flaws that prevent it from being shared easily. First, the motor is not as powerful as hospital-grade models. This means it will quickly wear out and not function as well. You might not even notice, despite the detriment to your milk supply.

Second, breast pumps sold in stores are not closed systems. This means it is possible to contaminate such pumps, particularly the motors, with droplets of milk. So while you might think you are safe because you bought new tubing, you are actually contaminating the new tubing and your pumped milk.

This is why the Food and Drug Administration (FDA) has come down against sharing breast pumps other than multiuser-specific pumps. Multiuser pumps are designed differently. You can purchase them, but the price is astronomical, even compared to the prices of the expensive breast pumps sold at stores.

LEARN TO HAND-EXPRESS YOUR BREASTS

Sometimes hand expressing breast milk is all you need to do. Depending on their body and how well they hand-express, some mothers never use a breast pump at all. Hand expressing can certainly save you money on breast pumps, parts, and rental fees if you are able to do it easily.

Putting the Pump On

Placing your pump properly is fairly easy. The most important thing is to ensure that you have the right size breast flange. Center your nipple in the flange. Select the speed and suction, if you have the ability to control these two items, and turn on the machine or begin hand pumping. You should not feel pain when pumping. If it is uncomfortable, try adjusting the placement of the flanges.

If you have a machine that has a two-phase pumping system (an initial letdown phase, followed by the full-pumping phase), it will automatically switch to the second speed after some length of time, depending on the breast pump. If you experience letdown before this preprogrammed time, you will be able to switch sooner.

CHAPTER
9

How Much Milk Should I Expect?

The amount of breast milk expressed will vary from mother to mother, day to day, and hour to hour. An average is ½ to 2 ounces (15–59 ml) per pumping session. This number is a combined number from both breasts.

To increase the amount of milk you get when you are pumping, be sure to try breast compression. Some mothers also find that changing the flange size of their breast pump can help. Remember, all breasts are not alike and the flange that comes with your breast pump might not be the correct size for you. Your lactation professional can help you to measure for the correct size. A variety of flanges are available for sale wherever breast pumps are sold.

One of the most effective techniques for hand expressing is called the Marmet Technique, named for lactation consultant Chele Marmet. To begin hand expressing, you should start by washing your hands. Then find a comfortable space. Bring whatever you will need: a small towel, a milk collection receptacle, and so forth.

Using the hand on the same side as the breast from which you are expressing, place your thumb above your nipple with your index and middle fingers under the nipple. They should be about a ½ to 1 inch (12.7 to 25.4 mm) away from the nipple, but not necessarily completely off the areola. Your hands should make the letter *C* with your fingers at noon and six o'clock, as though your breast were a clock. You should not cup the breast.

Once you have your fingers in place, pull straight in toward your body, keeping your fingers together. If you have larger breasts, you will want to lift your breast and then pull inward. Once you've pulled inward, you will then compress the milk reservoirs and empty them by rolling your fingers and thumb forward on the nipple. Repeat this motion, but move your fingers so that the noon or six o'clock fingers would now be at one and seven o'clock. Repeat the pull, roll technique. Continue rotating until you have come full circle. Keep doing the same thing until you have expressed as much breast milk as you can.

You will probably want to express your breast milk directly into the storage container. Some women use glass containers, whereas others use plastic bags expressly made for breast milk storage. You can also use any other container that can be sealed or covered to protect your milk from leakage and temperature damage.

When you are using the Marmet Technique, be careful to avoid injuring your breast tissue. Do not squeeze your breasts at any point. This is not effective at removing milk and can injure your breast. You should also avoiding pulling or tugging at the nipple for the same reasons.

One of the benefits of hand expression is that you completely control the experience. You can feel your breasts and know exactly how much pressure is required. You can move at the speed that works best for your body.

Use Hand-Expression Techniques with a Pump

One of the best-kept secrets about producing more milk when pumping is the use of hand expression in conjunction with a breast pump. To do this, hook your breast pump up, then use your hands to massage your breasts. Start at the back of your breast tissue and massage toward the breast pump flange and your nipple. Many mothers say this expression technique works wonders when they are pumping. When doing something this simple helps, why not do it? This technique can also give you something to focus on besides the clock.

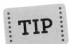 **Check the Small Parts**

If you notice a decrease in your output while pumping, check to see whether any of the smaller parts of your pump, such as the seals, need to be replaced. Depending on how often you use the pump and how you wash it, you might need to replace such parts as often as every three months.

MAKE ARRANGEMENTS TO PUMP AT WORK

Many women who return to their jobs intend to use a breast pump at work. However, the setup at companies around the United States varies widely. Some companies have amazing accommodations for nursing mothers who wish to pump at work. Other companies have no idea what to do when someone asks about their breast-pumping facilities.

Investigate Your Options

Before you make a formal inquiry at your place of employment, it is often best to scope out the situation first. Try to talk to other recently nursing or pumping moms. Ask them what they found out or were told about pumping on the clock. Did they meet with any resistance? Where were they told to pump? What were the breast milk storage options?

CHAPTER
9

The Marmet Technique

This technique is designed to help you get the most amount of breast milk with the least amount of effort. It is a very effective technique and used by women all over the world. It is a simple pull-and-roll technique. For more on this technique, see page 228.

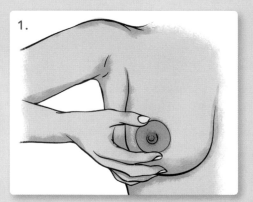

Grip with thumb and index finger.

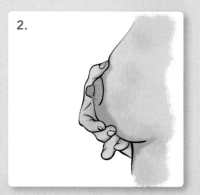

Push into chest wall.

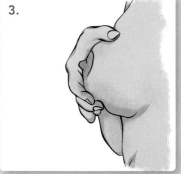

Roll.

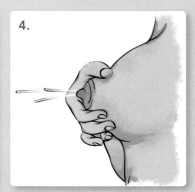

Finish roll.

If what you hear seems acceptable to you, you can talk to the friendly folks in your human resources department. Or if you have a smaller setup at work, you can discuss things with your supervisor. If what you are told is not acceptable, think about it. Do you have an idea for a more acceptable plan? Can you write it up into a formal proposal so that the people in charge will have something to look at when you make your case?

If you can't talk to other mothers or your research doesn't provide you with much in the way of information, you can always look to your supervisor for answers to tough questions. Questions that you will want to ask include:

- Where are the pumping facilities?
- Does the company have a relationship with a company that supplies certain pumps?

- What types of breaks will I be allowed to take for pumping?
- Is the room private? Is there a lock on the door?
- What are the breast milk storage facilities?

Your human resources department might also be a wealth of information for you, particularly in terms of finding out what options are available to you at your workplace. They might not have the answers immediately, however, and may need to get back to you. If your company does not have a lot of experience dealing with such issues, your human resources department might not know what the answer is or even what it should look like. This could be your chance to help them craft the ideal or close-to-ideal situation.

Aim for Your Ideal Breast-Pump Station

Having the ideal place to pump is not the standard, but it never hurts to shoot for the stars, particularly if you are advocating for something new where you work. The ideal space would have comfortable seating, plenty of electrical outlets, privacy, a sink, a microwave, and perhaps even someplace for storing milk.

In the real world, you will likely have to work with an acceptable solution as opposed to the ideal. This does not mean you should give up the ideal, but simply that you might not have time to wait for the ideal, at least with this baby. Being an advocate for an ideal space, even when it will not benefit you, is a wonderful act of breastfeeding advocacy. Your efforts will pave the way for other moms to

Keep Things Clean

Having a sink near where you pump is a must. It's a place to wash your hands, rinse off your pump parts, and keep your pumping area clean.

have a good work/breastfeeding experience. There are places to turn to for help in designing your nursing space if your company should want the information. Many of the pump companies have professionals who can help you, as well as various suggestions online.

Negotiate a Pumping Schedule

How often you need to pump will depend on how much milk you will need to pump and how many pumping sessions it will take to achieve that goal. For example, if you need to pump 12 ounces (355 ml) while you are at work, you will need to figure out how long that would take and in how many sessions. Are you a super pumper who can knock that amount out in one thirty-minute session? Or do you need three sessions of fifteen minutes each?

Depending on the work you do, it might or might not be easier to fit pumping in during regular breaks. For example, a mother who works in an office will have a vastly different experience than a mother who works on an assembly line.

CHAPTER
9

You will have to figure out your schedule with your co-workers and boss. Perhaps you need to work with your office to figure out the best way for you to pump. You might need to have your own plan, because you are likely to know more about pumping than your office manager or even your co-workers.

The first thing to do is to present the benefits for your company. You can give them data showing that workers who are breastfeeding having fewer

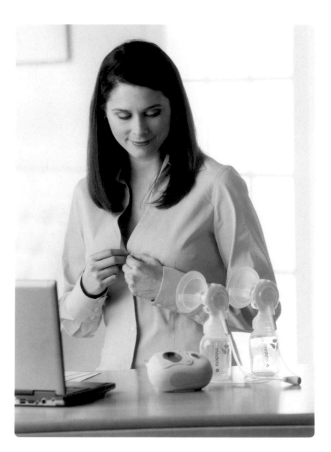

Setting up where you will pump can be the key to a comfortable and successful session of pumping. What do you want or need at your pumping station?

missed workdays for sick children. The Department of Health and Human Services even has a free tool kit online (www.womenshealth.gov/breastfeeding/programs/business-case). This can also lead to use of less health care coverage, as well as lower copayments for that health care. It also can help you to stay mentally healthy. When you feel like you are better able to provide for your baby, you are more focused at work and apt to waste less time (even unintentionally) worrying about your baby's care.

Hopefully, your company is willing to work with you and your schedule. Since your employers are not likely to know what you need, it is helpful to go to them with an available solution to the challenge. They might not accept your solution as is, but your plan will provide a starting point from which to work as you negotiate.

Where to Store Your Breast Milk at Work

Figure out ahead of time what your storage options are for keeping your breast milk cold during the day. Obviously, a refrigerator is the best bet, but not every workplace has that option. You might also need permission to store breast milk in the company refrigerator.

Some moms choose to purchase a very small refrigerator for their desk—one that holds about a six-pack of soda. Or you can also look into a dorm-size refrigerator. Other mothers make do with ice packs and insulated bags.

Enlighten Wary Co-Workers

One of the things you might not have thought about with pumping is the possibility of negative responses from or beliefs of your co-workers. Some women have said their co-workers were upset because they take pumping breaks.

Know that you will not make everyone happy. That is not your job. Your goal and your job here is to provide your baby with breast milk and to foster your bond with her. Breastfeeding is the ideal for her and for you. Pumping at work will help you to accomplish your goal. Having a supportive boss can go a long way toward assuaging any negative comments your co-workers might be making. If your boss presents a united front, you will have fewer problems with your co-workers.

There are two ways to deal with the issue of complaining co-workers. The first is education. Wherever possible, try to explain what you are doing, why you are doing it, and why you need the break time to pump. Be sure to also include how you intend to get your work done.

Your second option is to simply talk directly and frankly to the person who has issues with your breastfeeding breaks. Ask him or her to explain the problem. Once you hear your colleague's answer, you might be able to respond and help to alleviate the tension. It could be a misunderstanding. The sooner you address the issue, the more likely you are to find a peaceful resolution.

Where to Go When You Have Problems or Issues

If you are having problems with your co-workers, first try to address the issue yourself. Talking to other breastfeeding and working mothers can be helpful, as they might have advice based on something that has worked for them. Sometimes dealing with the issue yourself works beautifully, and other times it does not.

If you are having persistent problems with your co-workers, your supervisor is the next obvious step. Occasionally, however, the person complaining may be you supervisor. In that case, your human resources department is the most likely source of assistance.

If these options do not solve your problem and you are being harassed at work, you might have further options. Some women turn to their baby's physician for a note of medical necessity, with the doctor stating that pumping is necessary to get breast milk for the baby. This can alleviate the fight, but not necessarily the ill will. The other option is legal recourse, although this is probably a last resort. Most women choose choose to avoid this step.

What to Do If You Can't Pump at Work

Some women decide for a variety of reasons that they simply cannot pump at work. If your situation falls into this category, you will be unable to supply your baby with breast milk while you are gone. It simply means you will have to come up with a more creative pumping solution.

CHAPTER
9

Some mothers have a milk supply that is flexible enough that they can pump enough milk while they are at home—in the morning, at night, and on the weekends. In this way, they store up enough breast milk to allow their baby to have enough during the workweek. Other mothers will pump on one side while they nurse their baby from the other during certain pumping sessions to express milk. You may also be able to pump while you're commuting to work. You might be able to use a hands-free pump while driving or while you're a passenger in a car.

If you do not pump during the day, your milk supply will regulate itself so that you are not producing as much milk during the day as you were before. Your body can adjust to this situation. If you plan and work it out, you can manage to breastfeed and pump while you are at home or on the weekends to supply enough milk for when you are away from your baby.

Think in new ways, and a creative solution might be available. You simply need to experiment and decide what works best for you and your baby. Talk to other mothers—it can be a big help.

FIGURE OUT HOW YOU PUMP BEST

Using a breast pump can be very different from nursing your baby. Since your baby will always be more effective than a breast pump, you will want to figure out a way to maximize your pumping time so that you're able to express the most breast milk possible.

Timing

Timing refers to the timing of your pumping, meaning the times of day when you pump. It can also refer to how long to pump. Both are important keys in the scheme of using a breast pump.

Everyone has a hormonal clock. That clock will dictate which hormones are peaking when. While we can make general statements, such as more milk tends to be available in the mornings due to standard hormone levels, this might not be true for you. Your first step is to try to pump at various times of the day to see what works best for you. Do you get more milk pumping mid-morning versus early morning? If so, you should pump mid-morning.

If you are pumping at work, you might need to factor in when you are available to pump. It is best to have a slightly flexible schedule. If you are able to better match the times of day when your baby would naturally be nursing, you will simply have a better milk supply from which to draw. However, this is not always possible in a work setting.

You might need to take scheduled breaks at work. Many mothers will pump during the workday at least once, typically during their longest break. If you can find a way to multitask while pumping, it will help you to feel more productive, rather than sitting there and simply watching your milk collect, which can drive some mothers batty.

If you can check emails or do some other type of work while pumping, that's even better. But even if you're on a break and are not working, pumping is a good time to read a book, to eat your lunch, or even to engage in a mindless computer game, if possible. You can do this with a hands-free pumping bra or bustier. This hands-free blessing is an amazing thing and could radically change your outlook on pumping. (See the section on hands-free pumping on page 237.)

The key to pumping at work is timing. If you can pump at the same time every day, you and your milk supply will be better off and you will likely make more milk. Of course, consistent timing is not always possible, but it is ideal.

How Long Should You Pump?

There's no magic number for how long you should or should not pump. This might be a moot point if you have time limits set at your workplace regarding how long you can pump. It might also not be an issue because you have physical limits even when there are no time restrictions. Remember, the clock, in general, is not your friend when it comes to breastfeeding or pumping your breasts.

Some women will pump for a few minutes and get lots of breast milk, while other women get less milk in more time. You will figure out how your body responds as you begin pumping. Most women fall somewhere in between. Even if you do not have time to pump a lot or you don't get a lot of breast milk during a pumping session, the breast stimulation is always good and beneficial.

You will need to experiment to figure out how long you need to pump. Double pumping, when possible, is typically going to be your fastest method of

What Is Reverse Cycling?

When you initially set out to feed your baby you were probably thinking of nursing him more during the day, and then encouraging him to sleep more at night. But when you are using a breast pump, whether it is occasionally or many days per week, it usually means you are away from your baby for hours during the day. This is where reverse cycling comes in. Reverse cycling means that when you are with your baby, typically in the evening and at night, you should nurse more frequently to make up for nursing sessions you missed while you were away.

Reverse cycling is usually an easy way to nurse your baby. Both you and your baby have missed the physical contact and bonding that come with nursing, and your baby will likely be eager to nurse when he is with you. Reverse cycling can be particularly handy with some babies who are reluctant to take bottles of expressed milk while their mothers are away. With this technique, the baby can actually make up for missed feedings when mom gets home. You can also use reverse cycling to help build up your milk supply.

CHAPTER
9

expressing breast milk. The hormones are already present, meaning you do not have to worry about initiating the letdown process twice, and you are able to do both breasts at one time. This means that if you need to, you can actually get more breast stimulation than if you were single pumping.

Consider If You Have Time Restrictions

It's no big surprise that the amount of time women have to pump varies greatly. Some women can sit down in a relaxed way, think about their baby, and pump what they need in no time. Other women know they need to pump with whatever time they have available, but could still use extra time to pump some more.

Some women produce milk quickly when they pump, while others need a bit longer for their milk to flow. For example, if you have twenty or thirty minutes to pump, you might spend the entire time pumping. Or if you are able to produce milk rapidly, you might need only ten of those minutes to produce a certain amount of breast milk or to pump until the milk stops flowing readily.

Experiment with your time. What helps you to pump more? Spend a couple of days trying a few different methods, but try for two or three days before switching your technique. You also want to keep notes.

For example, say you have thirty minutes to pump. The first thing you might try is double pumping for twenty minutes and then having your lunch. Next, you might try double pumping the entire

time, while eating your lunch. Your third shot might be double pumping for ten minutes, eating your lunch for ten minutes, and then double pumping for another ten minutes. Everyone is different—you don't know how your body will best respond to pumping and to your various "schedules" until you test things out.

If you are not pumping against a time restriction, think of things in terms of your milk supply. How long does it take for you, on average, to get most of your milk out? This can vary; some mothers are able to pump more quickly than others for a variety of reasons, and it might not take as long as you expected.

What If You Do Not Have Much Time to Pump?

There might be days when your life or work does not go as planned. Maybe your lunchtime vanished because of a meeting, or you're not at your normal work station. Whatever the reasons, some women will skip pumping if they feel like they do not have the full allotment of time. Do not be tempted to skip a pumping session.

Even if you have just five or ten minutes to pump, it is beneficial. Some breast stimulation is good, even if you do not have the time to complete a milk removal as you might normally. While missing one pumping session will typically not alter your supply, you cannot control tomorrow's events, and missing two days in a row might alter your supply.

Hands-Free Pumping

Hands-free pumping is the ability to pump without needing to use your hands often. This can be accomplished by using a special bra or a special halter top. The bra simply has an added flap that comes down much like your standard nursing bra. It can be used both as a normal bra and your hands-free pumping bra. This extra flap actually holds your pump parts up while you pump. The halter is something that you wear. It fits tight against the body. This is what holds the pump parts on.

Hands-free pumping is a way to make pumping much less of a chore. You can do more, giving you the opportunity to send an email, read a book, flip channels on the television, or play with your baby. If you need to pump during the night for any reason, it also prevents you from falling asleep and spilling milk when your hands drop.

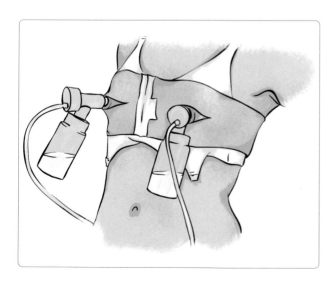

A hands-free setup for pumping can give you some sanity for pumping times and may actually increase the amount of time you pump.

How Often Should You Pump?

How often you should pump depends on a lot of factors. The biggest factor will be why you are pumping. If you are pumping while you are gone or away from your baby for a normal work shift, you would pump differently than if you were pumping to build your supply or pumping to supply your baby with breast milk because the baby has not yet been able to nurse at the breast.

If you are pumping because you and your baby are separated during the day, you will want to closely mimic your baby's nursing schedule if possible. This means that if you nurse your baby just before you leave him, after you get to work, you would pump the next time he would be ready to eat. This might be anywhere from two to four hours later, depending on your baby's age. You would pump again according to when he would nurse later in the day, and so on, until you are together again.

If you are pumping to supply your baby with breast milk completely (no supplements), you likely have gotten a recommendation from your lactation professional. Typically, this also will mimic your baby's normal routine but might include a more structured approach, particularly if you are trying to increase your milk supply. Since babies are much better than pumps at producing milk, it is not uncommon to see the two go together.

This type of pumping protocol is usually fairly intense. You will likely pump every two hours during the day. At night, you might go back to three or four hours, depending on your specific needs.

CHAPTER
9

WOMEN'S WISDOM:

Every single pumping session is important. It can be tempting to sleep in or skip a pumping session, "just this once." Don't blow off a chance to pump during the day if you can help it. Skipping it once can make doing it twice very easy. Then it can be a slippery slope toward losing a part of your milk supply. While missing an occasional pumping session will not harm supply for most women, miss the same session two days in a row and it will. If you're feeling down or tired about pumping, tell yourself to get started and pump for just a few minutes, then reassess.

FIND A LOCATION FOR PUMPING

Where you pump can make a huge difference in how well you pump, how you feel about pumping, and nearly any other thing you can imagine about pumping. When you are pumping at your home, you will have more control over your environment. Using a breast pump while you are at work might be a different story. Regardless of where you pump, it is ideal to think about your space and do a bit of preparation to make your area as comfortable and useful as possible.

Pumping Preparation

Preparing to pump does not need to be a major undertaking. First, get your pump and everything you will need ready. Things you might need while pumping include:

- Breast pump
- Power supply
- Collection items
- Other items you might need, such as food, drinks, a book, and so on

The other items you might need may relate to your break. Perhaps this is when you eat lunch; if so, bring it with you. It might relate to your work. If you are pumping using a hands-free system, you will want to ensure that you have your computer or other work that can be done during your pumping time. Or perhaps you have a bit of free time. Then you might bring a book, a puzzle, or a pen and paper to write a letter. You also might just use the time to relax.

Pumping at Home

When you pump at home, you should try to set up a spot where you can be extremely comfortable, particularly if you do a lot of pumping. Moving around at every pump session can be stressful; in addition, it increases the likelihood that you will sit down to pump, only to realize something is missing.

The goal for your environment should be to maximize comfort and relaxation to increase and maximize your breast milk output. This can usually be achieved nicely in your home. You have your stuff, you know where it is, and you do not need to move everything back when you are done pumping. So, for example, if you have a picture of your baby to look at while pumping, it can stay right there.

Set aside an area at home, even if it's simply a place to sit with a small basket for your things. You should be near an outlet if you need one for your pump. Make sure you are able to relax. Are you sitting in a rocking chair and pumping quietly? Are you pumping while reading and sending email? Or you pumping while you watch television and catch up on your shows? You will want to arrange your location so it's convenient for whatever you choose to do while pumping.

Pumping at Work

Most women find it harder to create a positive situation when pumping at work. While more and more businesses are creating pumping stations or lounges, your workplace might not have that luxury yet. As mentioned previously in this chapter, if you are feeling up to it, start advocating for a pumping station while you are pregnant. Try to get others who are pregnant or nursing to advocate with you for a shared space that can be used as a nursing lounge.

If that is not possible in time for you and your baby, you will have to make do with what you have. If you have your own office, you can work within that space. Do you have a door? Does it lock? What about windows to the office? Can these be covered

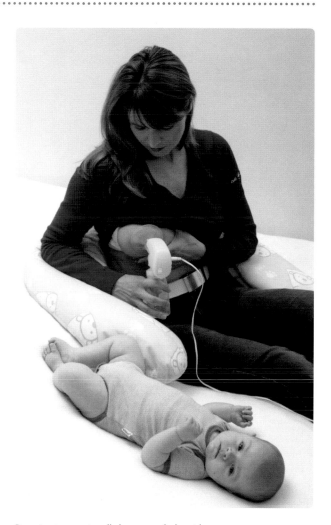

Pumping to occasionally leave your baby with someone else may seem daunting, but pumping a few minutes at the same time of day can be helpful to build a few ounces (milliliters) of breast milk to store in your freezer.

CHAPTER
9

if needed? Sometimes this scenario is as simple as you going in and locking the door while you pump.

If you need a lock, ask maintenance to put one on your door. If for some reason you cannot have a lock placed on your door, use a sign to indicate that people should not come in. What should the sign on your door say? Some mothers go the straightforward route: "I'm pumping!" Other mothers write: "Please knock first." What you write will depend on you, your work space, and your co-workers. Some mothers also move a chair or something in front of the door to prevent it from being opened accidentally.

If you do not have an office, you need to figure out which spaces might be available to you. Does one of your co-workers have an ideal office that she might consider lending to you a few times per day? Is there any shared space, such as a conference room, that might be workable? If you are having trouble determining where to pump, seek other mothers who have older children. They might have some tips that you might not have thought about yet.

Pumping in the Car

When all else fails, the best fallback option for some mothers is their car. It's not difficult to purchase car adapters for electric pumps. You can go out into the car and pump while you are alone. You can listen to the radio and eat lunch there as well. While it is not perfect, it might be your best option, depending on where you work.

The car is also perfect if you have long commutes or when you're on a road trip. You do need to be smart about how you pump when driving. Be sure you always put your hands-free pump and parts together and on when you are parked in a safe place, not while you are driving. You can turn on the pump and drive again. When you are done pumping, either you can pull over and remove the pump and parts, or you can wear it until you stop or get where you are going.

A lot of women pump in the car. It's private. It's handy. You can have some sense of ownership over it. But you will need to pay attention and avoid doing anything that isn't safe—putting on the pump while driving, or trying to manage the pump while driving, Once the parts are in place, you really shouldn't have to think about or do anything else

Think about Baby

Another trick to use when pumping to increase your milk supply is to think about your baby. Some mothers use a photo of their baby to help them visualize the nursing process. Other mothers bring an article of their baby's clothing to aid them in pumping. Often, you can actually feel the letdown when you have this added stimulus of thinking of your baby. It can be quite effective.

with the pump. The benefit to pumping this way is that for some women, it takes their minds off the process, and as a result they are able to produce more milk.

Pumping in Other Places

When you are at a hotel for business or pleasure, you can usually get everything you need to have for pumping. Some mothers prefer to pump on the bed, while other women really prefer to sit at a desk. This choice might be determined by how you handle your "free time" while pumping. There is not a wrong or right answer.

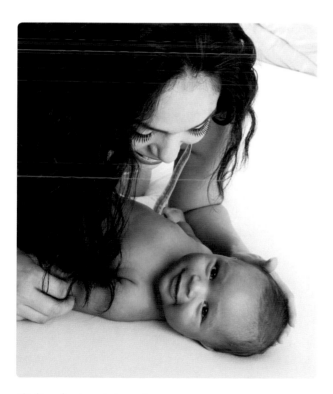

Thinking about your baby can be a great way to promote the let-down reflex when you need to pump.

If you are spending time at someone else's house, you will need to talk to your host about having some personal time and private space. This might be easier with some people than others. It might also depend on how long you will be staying. For example, being with your in-laws might be very different from staying with your best friend from college.

INVESTIGATE YOUR BREAST MILK STORAGE OPTIONS

Storing breast milk does not need to be complicated. Decide how much you need and how long you plan to store it. This will depend on your milk supply and part of it will depend on your baby's appetite.

Even with a vast supply of breast milk, if you are pumping daily, simply rotate the fresh breast milk out with the frozen. This way, your frozen milk supply will never be more than a few months old. This can take some coordination. You must remember to label your breast milk container every time and remember where to put the "newer" breast milk in terms of storage. Some tracking programs can actually track each individual bag of breast milk.

Freezing your breast milk does cause it to lose some of its beneficial properties, but it is still superior to other options. Many mothers give a combination of fresh and frozen breast milk to their baby each day. This allows your baby to have the best of both worlds.

CHAPTER
9

Storage Containers

How much and how long you store your breast milk will guide you in what containers you should use. If you are storing breast milk in the refrigerator overnight or for less than a week, you might simply want to store it in plastic or glass breast milk storage containers. Anything more than a week and you will have to freeze the milk. Some products are meant to save some storage space, even when using these cylindrical containers.

Using plastic breast milk bags can help you to save space and allow you to store breast milk flat in the refrigerator or freezer. These bags come in a variety of styles. Some are easy to attach directly to your pump. Other bags actually stand up when you are using them.

When choosing a breast milk storage bag, choose the one that works the best for you. You might want to know whether the bags contain BPA or other chemicals. You might want a bag that has a double seal. You might simply be better off trying a couple of types of bags until you figure out which style works best for you.

Where to Store Your Breast Milk

If you intend to store breast milk for longer than three or four months, you will need to have a deep freezer. This can be a small one kept in your basement or garage. Deep freezers are designed to handle long-term storage and they are not opened as frequently as regular freezers, thus keeping the breast milk safe. However, in reality, most women do not need to think in terms of this long-term storage.

TIP Hands-Free Pumping Option

Foot-controlled breast pumps are available for women who cannot use their hands or prefer to use their feet. Like the hand-held pumps that are activated by the use of hands, these pedals help to produce the power for pumping.

Typically, you will be using your refrigerator for short-term storage. As mentioned in previous section, you can keep breast milk in the refrigerator for up to a week. Your freezer is handy to use as storage for up to four months. Which form of storage you choose will depend on whether you have built up a stash of breast milk. A stash is not a requirement, but it makes some mothers feel more confident.

Heating Breast Milk

When it comes time to use your breast milk, you will need to be careful when heating it. Remember, breast milk is a living substance. You want to be careful to keep it in optimal shape. This means you should not use a microwave to heat the breast milk. Not only will a microwave kill some of the beneficial organisms, but it can also lead to hot pockets which can scald your baby.

The proper way to warm breast milk is more slowly. Let frozen or cooled breast milk come to room temperature. You can also warm it in a luke-

Pumping Sounds

"Pumping Secrets" is a collection of sounds on a compact disc meant to be used when pumping. The sounds of a baby nursing and suckling are supposed to help stimulate you to make more milk. It has been helpful for many mothers and might be something to consider trying.

No matter why you might choose to exclusively pump breast milk, you will need to be prepared for the experience. This will take some planning ahead on your part to make everything go as smoothly as possible. It would be a wise idea to talk to other mothers who have exclusively pumped for their babies.

You will need to decide which type of breast pump you require. In the beginning, it is recommended that you rent a hospital-grade pump to build up your milk supply. Once you have achieved a good breast milk supply, usually within a month or two, then you can switch to a slightly lower grade of breast pump to help you maintain your breast milk supply.

warm bath of running water. Products are available to help you do this, but an extra-large cup and your sink typically work just as well.

MAKE A DECISION TO PUMP EXCLUSIVELY

Some mothers have to exclusively pump breast milk for their babies. This is frequently because of an issue with the mother or the baby that makes breastfeeding difficult. However, a small but growing number of mothers are choosing to exclusively pump for their babies.

Choosing to exclusively pump breast milk is a big decision. Many things go into making the decision and it should not be made lightly. Some mothers choose this option because they believe it will be easier than breastfeeding. Some mothers choose it because they do not wish to nurse for a variety of reasons.

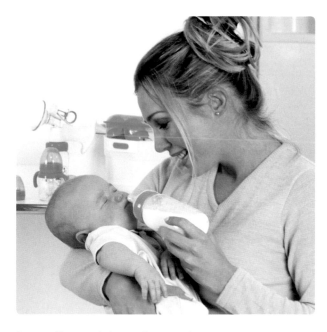

Breast milk can easily be stored in your refrigerator or freezer, depending on the intended length of time, for later use.

CHAPTER
9

You will also need to decide how you want to feed your baby. One risk that is often discussed regarding the issue of not breastfeeding is an increase in ear infections. This can occur, even when giving breast milk, if you are using a baby bottle. That being said, you can help to prevent this complication by using a vented baby bottle system as well as holding your baby upright while you feed her.

You should never prop a bottle for a baby. This is dangerous not only because of a risk of choking, but also for others reasons. One is an increased risk of ear infections.

That being said, bottle feeding is the preferred method of feeding a baby who is not breastfed. However, your baby might have issues that preclude bottle feeding, such as certain facial or oral malformations, or the inability to suck. If this is the case, alternative feeders are available. (See chapter 2.)

Once your baby is born, you should begin pumping as soon as possible. Wait no longer than four hours if possible. You will need to pump every three to four hours around the clock as you're building your supply. You might need to use the breast pump even more frequently if you have a low milk supply or any pumping difficulties.

In the beginning, you will most likely get only a few drops of colostrum. This is fine. Your baby does not have a large need for calories in the first few days. This first milk will help your baby to pass her meconium and prepare for more milk. You can use this milk easily with alternative feeding measures such as a dropper or finger feeder. Do not be tempted to throw this first breast milk away. Some health care professionals will try to convince you that it is so little in quantity that it is not worth saving, but it is exactly what your baby needs in the first few days of life.

Consider using some system to track both the breast milk that you pump and the breast milk that your baby eats. This can help you know how much breast milk your baby takes in per day versus how much you are pumping. It will also help you learn to manipulate your pumping schedule to get the best milk supply with the least pumping.

Tracking can be as simple as a notebook and pen, or it can be as complex as a spreadsheet. Some prepared spreadsheets are available at online groups such as Pump Moms at Yahoo! Groups. You can also use a variety of tracking programs, including Trixie Tracker, available online and for your mobile phone. These programs help mothers to stay on track with how long it's been since they have pumped and how much they have pumped. They can even track their breast milk through the storage process.

If you are going to be exclusively pumping, tracking will be of benefit to you. Some mothers find they actually enjoy tracking, feeling a sense of pride or accomplishment, while other mothers are completely overwhelmed and even annoyed with tracking.

If you find that tracking is not helping your mental or emotional state, track only occasionally. For instance, pump and track for a few weeks until your supply is established. Next, randomly check in and record a day every week for a few weeks, and then go to it every so often. You might consider tracking if you notice a change in what your baby seems to be taking in or in what you seem to be putting out.

How Much Will You Get When You Pump?

It is important to remember that everyone pumps differently. You will find moms who report they can pump about 30 ounces (887 ml) of breast milk in three or four pump sessions. And then you will also find moms who pump ten times per day and get only 20 ounces (591 ml). Pumping early and often will help you to build your best milk supply. That is because during those first few days, your body is primed to respond the best to building a supply. If that does not happen for whatever reason, do not panic, all is not lost.

Statistically speaking, pumping in the early morning is most likely to yield the most breast milk. Many mothers find this is true for them. However, if you find that you are more likely to get milk at a different time of day, that is what you should do.

Keeping Your Breast Pump Clean

Keeping up with your milk supply and the baby can be hard work. Exclusive pumping can be like working double duty. That is because you will be pumping, cleaning your breast-pump parts, feeding your baby, and cleaning your baby bottles. That is not to say that these are not reasons to do this double duty, and many moms would do it over and over again.

Think about how to make your life a little easier. Purchasing a microwave sterilizer can be a real benefit and help you to lighten some of your workload. These are simply large containers to which you add water and pump parts or baby bottles, and microwave for a few minutes. The larger ones can hold all of your breast-pump parts and several bottles as well.

Travel microwave sterilizing bags are also available. These are perfect for work or life on the go. While they do not hold as many parts, which makes you have to use them more frequently, they do a nice job. Cleaning wipes can do the trick in a pinch. The problem with the wipes is they can get very expensive. Keep some in your diaper bag or breast-pump case for times when you simply do not have access to a microwave.

Having a baby bottle drying rack can also be a good thing. This is simply a handy place to store all of your feeding supplies, from baby bottles to breast-pump parts. It also helps them dry so that you aren't hand-drying each individual piece. Having a few nipple brushes around is a good idea too. They are great for cleaning the nooks and crannies of breast-pump parts!

It can be handy to have a spare set of breast-pump parts for times when you want to run one set through the dishwasher. It also helps if you forget to clean one set right away and then discover it is time to pump again.

Some mothers also store their pump parts in the refrigerator between pumping sessions. The thought behind this is that they can then reuse the same breast-pump parts without the hassle of cleaning them every single time. This is a personal decision.

If You Have to Pump Exclusively

Sometimes breastfeeding your baby directly will not work out. Thankfully, this is a very rare occurrence. But when it happens to you, it can feel very overwhelming, particularly if this is not what you had planned.

CHAPTER
9

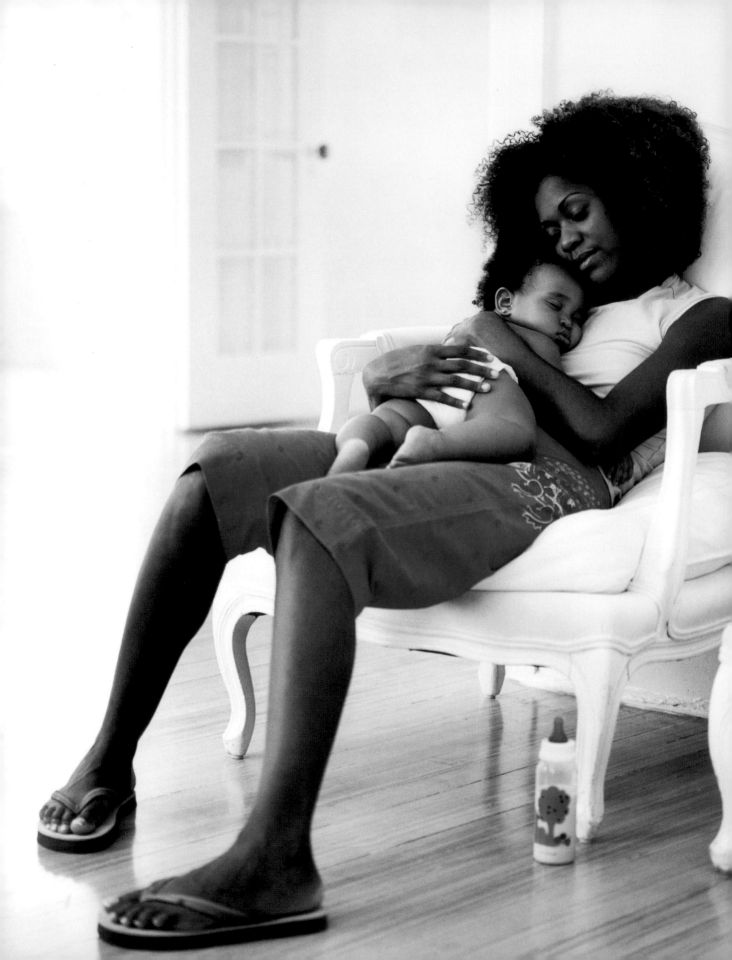

You might need to look at your breastfeeding goal and ask yourself whether it still holds true. As you walk the path of exclusive pumping, you might decide to stick with your goal, revise it, or simply take it day by day. The day-by-day approach is probably the most realistic, at least in the beginning. This is not to say that you will not reach your original goal. But because of the added work of exclusively pumping, thinking about it over the long term might be overwhelming.

Perhaps you feel forced into pumping exclusively because of your situation. That can make for a stressful life. Living ounce to ounce or feeding to feeding can be an awful thing to do. Having a small stash of breast milk in the freezer for emergencies is a nice feeling, but is not possible for everyone.

While it is not the case for everyone, you are more likely to have issues with your milk supply if you are exclusively pumping, simply because the pump is never as good as your baby. A good pumping schedule and support will go a long way toward helping your confidence and your breast milk supply.

Others might tell you that pumping exclusively for your baby is not worth it. They might encourage you to give up breast milk partially or even altogether. Only you can decide when you are ready to change what you are doing. Be sure to tell your companions how they can best help you in your goals for providing breast milk, including having faith, having confidence, and being supportive.

Providing your baby with breast milk is a great gift, no matter how it gets to your baby.

There is also something to be said for not giving up the hope of getting your baby to the breast. Even older babies, nearing one year of age, have decided to come to the breast for the first time. Encouraging your baby in any way that you can—providing her with love, support, and breast milk—will go a long way. Pumping is certainly not the easy path, but giving your baby breast milk despite all of the obstacles is an amazing gift.

WEAN FROM PUMPING

Weaning is a hot topic. But weaning from a pump is something that most people do not even think about. There are reasons why pumping sessions get dropped and there are ways to ensure mom's health and safety when that occurs.

Why Wean from a Pump?

Most pumping centers on pumping breast milk while you are away from your baby. The most common reason would be work, followed by illness of you or your baby. That being said, a pump is a very poor replication of a baby.

If you have been pumping at work for your baby and now you find that you no longer need the pumping session, you may consider dropping that session. Sometimes you might find you have built your milk supply so much that you can pump a large quantity of breast milk at fewer sessions than when you first started pumping.

Another reason to drop a pumping session might have to do with solid foods. If your baby has begun to eat solid foods, you may have less of a

CHAPTER
9

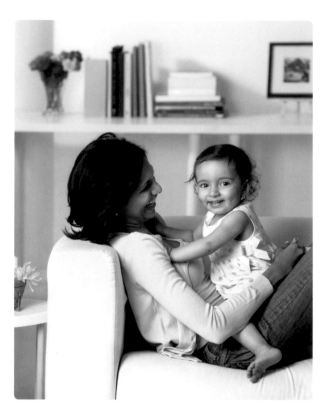

Weaning gently from a pump is not too terribly difficult because you decide when to pump and when not to pump. Your baby can help you ease any discomfort from engorgement.

Breastfeeding Affirmation

Every drop of breast milk I provide my baby is important.

need for expressed breast milk. This means that after a while, you might actually drop one of your pumping sessions because of the decreased need. This is typically not one of the first things that happen when you begin solids, but it does come rather quickly after that point.

Dropping a Session

The best session to drop is the pumping session that is either the hardest or, if you are concerned about your milk supply, provides the least amount of breast milk for the effort. If you are pumping at work, this might be a session that you drop, depending on how well you are doing and what arrangement you have at work for pumping. You might, instead, choose to drop the late-night pumping session.

Basically, you will want to phase out one pumping session at a time. Monitor your breast milk output to ensure that your overall milk supply is not dropping. Does your baby still seem satisfied after nursing? Are other pump sessions similar to what they had been prior to dropping the session?

Weaning When Exclusively Pumping

Weaning from the pump can be very different from weaning from your baby if you are exclusively pumping. You will want to ask yourself when you want to stop providing breast milk for your baby. Depending whether you are pumping exactly what your baby needs every day, or whether you have a built-up supply, the weaning experience might be very different.

Quitting the pump cold turkey is not advisable. If you simply quit pumping, you run the risk of painful complications, such as plugged ducts and mastitis. It is wiser to slowly wean from pumping.

Typically, you can drop a pumping session every three to four days. If you do this enough times, you will eventually get down to no pumping sessions per day. While you still might produce breast milk, you can try wearing a tight bra and avoiding breast stimulation for a bit. This includes even hot water and showers.

Your breast milk stash might last awhile longer. How long will depend on how much you were able to pump and store for your baby before weaning. The feeling of pulling out the last packet of frozen breast milk might seem a bit odder than you had planned. It is okay to feel melancholy about the last breast milk serving, but try to focus on the positive.

Find a way to celebrate that moment, even if it's something quiet and personal. Taking a few minutes to snuggle with your child and reflect on the gifts and journey of his life is one possibility. Some women choose to write poetry or take a photo. Remember, every drop of breast milk you have pumped has been of great service to your baby's health. The love and care it took to pump the milk was an amazing gift for your baby.

Self-Care Tips

Whether you are pumping for a few feedings during the workday or for every meal for your baby, you will want to monitor your breast milk supply. In addition to keeping a general eye on what you need, it will also help you try to predict the best pumping schedule for you. What seems to increase your pumping output? What seems to decrease it? A simple chart might help you to follow up on these leads. This can make for more efficient pumping and, perhaps, a bit of stored breast milk too.

CHAPTER
9

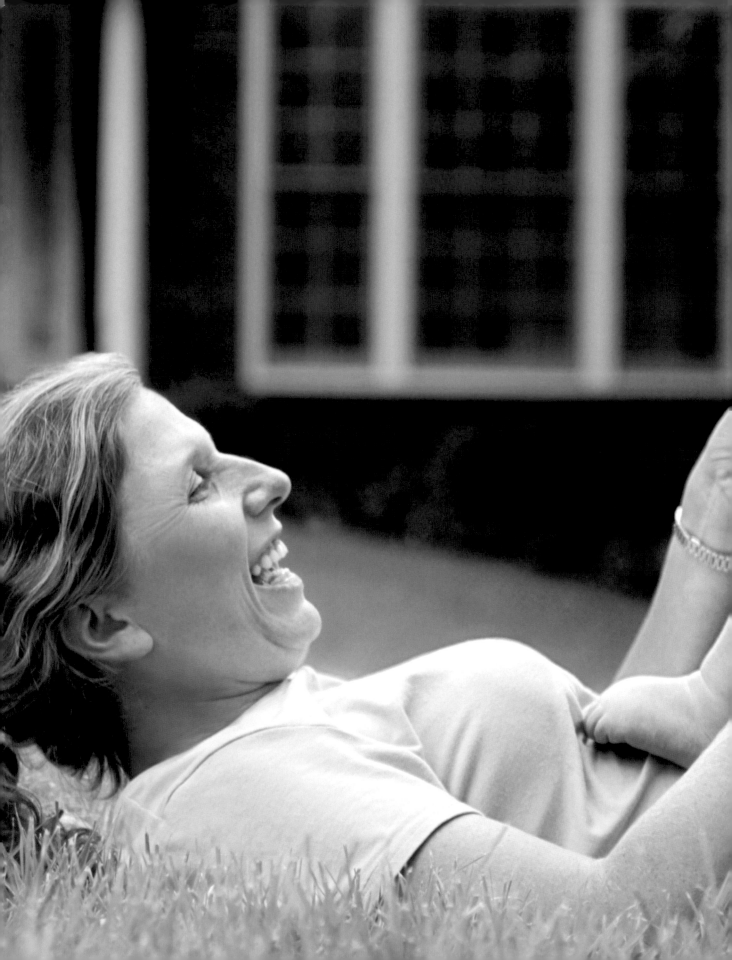

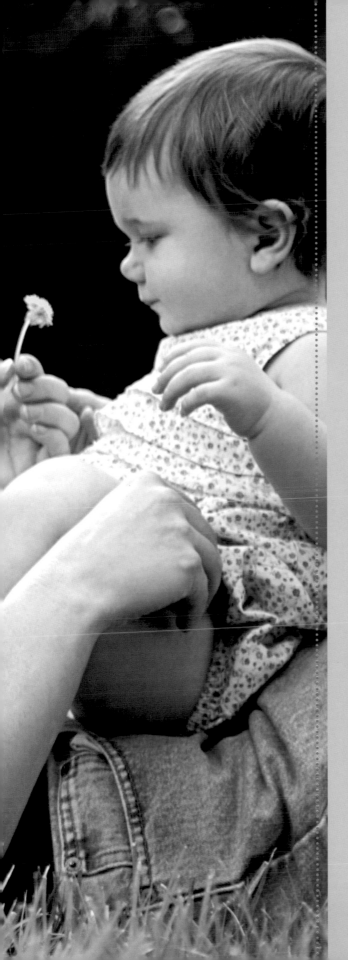

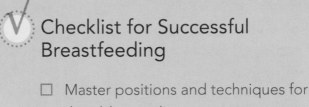

CHAPTER 10

Nursing Your Older Baby or Toddler

✓ Checklist for Successful Breastfeeding

- ☐ Master positions and techniques for the older nursling.
- ☐ Deal with negative comments from others.
- ☐ Dispel myths about nursing an older baby or toddler.
- ☐ Learn to nurse a teething baby.
- ☐ Offer your baby a cup or baby bottle.
- ☐ Feed your breastfed baby solids.
- ☐ Know about nursing during a new pregnancy.
- ☐ Decide when you would like to wean.
- ☐ Figure out the easiest way to wean.
- ☐ Understand how you might feel about weaning.
- ☐ Remember that a child is never too old to nurse.

Breastfeeding your older baby and toddler can be an experience very different from breastfeeding an young baby. But there are many benefits, both physically and emotionally. As the American Academy of Pediatrics (AAP) recommends breastfeeding your baby for at least one year and as long after as you and your baby would like to continue, there are things you need to know.

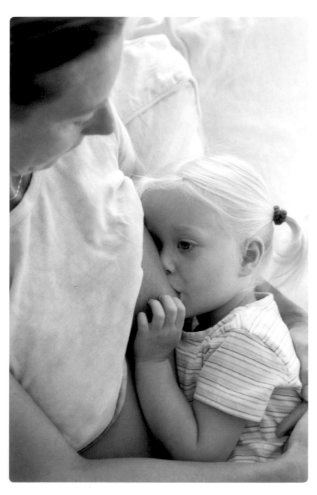

As your child gets older, there are a variety of positions in which she will nurse.

MASTER POSITIONS AND TECHNIQUES FOR THE OLDER NURSLING

Nursing positions for a larger baby or toddler can be interesting. Unlike nursing an infant, you can't just curl the baby up and help her to latch on. While latching should not be an issue with an older baby, where to put your baby on your lap—and, often, how to keep her still—does become an issue.

There are no real rules about how to hold your bigger baby. Your baby will tell you how she wants you to hold her. In fact, now that your baby is an old pro at nursing, you can bet she's going to have something to say on this matter.

Often, the problem isn't about how you hold the baby, but rather how well your baby stays on your lap, no matter how you are holding her. As babies get older, they become multitaskers. Once your baby starts moving around, you'll soon find she can nurse while standing up, sitting down, or lying down. Your baby also probably has a good take on which positions she wants to use when breastfeeding. This can make it difficult for you to get a good hold on your baby, particularly if you recollect how it was to nurse a newborn. Be open to these new positions that your baby creates. Let her lead the way, and go with the flow. If you're flexible, you'll soon see you'll come up with new and creative methods for dealing with your baby's nursing-position antics.

Cope with a Distracted Nurser

When your baby hits the six-month mark, you might notice she's easily distracted while breastfeeding. This might mean ambient noise will cause her to look around during a breastfeeding session. Your baby might be a great nurser until there's another person in the room. Or your baby might want to gaze over at the television while breastfeeding.

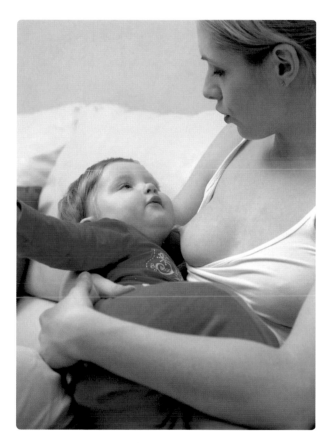

The distracted nurser may nurse for a few minutes or seconds before finding something else to look at during feeding time. While this may be challenging for you, look at it from your baby's point of view.

These nursing interruptions can make life interesting, to say the least. Your breast milk might leak or spray a bit if your baby pops off and on a lot. Some babies even begin to make a game of nursing in this way. Your baby will probably think this is hilarious, while your frustration level may go up.

Be prepared. There might be times when you are out and distracted nursing leads to indiscreet nursing. If that's unacceptable, stop the nursing session. Your baby might put up a fuss, but stay firm and just explain why you are ending the nursing session. You can try again in a few minutes. Many babies will do this a few times before they understand that you mean business.

You can also try to distract your baby by using a breastfeeding cover, wearing an interesting necklace, holding your baby's hand, and so on. For some infants, simple tricks such as these are all they need to refocus on breastfeeding. Other babies need to be taken to a quiet room to nurse, where distractions can be kept to a minimum.

This distractibility might or might not affect how long it takes your baby to eat. As you are trying to nurse your baby, you might have to tack more time on to the breastfeeding session. Then again, you might find that your once leisurely nursling is now a no-nonsense kind of baby who wants to nurse and be finished quickly. Some days, you might find your baby would rather play and explore her world than spend time nursing. Whichever the case may be, know that as babies get older they realize when they are really hungry and will eventually buckle down for a good nursing session!

CHAPTER
10

DEAL WITH NEGATIVE COMMENTS FROM OTHERS

As with any parenting choice you make, there will always be someone there to tell you what to do, when to do it, and why your method of doing it is wrong. When it comes to nursing your baby, comments from the peanut gallery really seem to come out of the woodwork. You can deal with unsolicited advice from others in many ways. You just need to be confident in your breastfeeding choices and be ready to respond when necessary.

Who Are the Comments Coming From?

The first thing you need to figure out is how to deal with the negative talk based on who is making the comments. You would likely handle the situation differently if the comments were coming from a stranger versus your mother. People who know you are probably more likely to say something to you about breastfeeding. This is simply because they have a closer bond with you and feel freer to chime in.

People who do not know you are less likely to say anything within earshot, although sometimes you might overhear comments or pick up on something that travels through the grapevine from a friend of a friend.

But what this issue really comes down to is not who is more likely to say something about your choices, but whose comments are more likely to matter to you. A stranger making a passing remark might incite your anger only momentarily, as you think, "Why did she say that?" whereas you'll probably take your best friend's comments much more to heart.

What Is Prompting the Comments?

You may hear negative things about your choice to breastfeed, particularly if you choose to breastfeed as recommended. Because the art of breastfeeding has been lost in large part, it seems, because many people have something to say about offering your baby cereal at a very young age, weaning after just a few months of breastfeeding, and so on. Before you respond to such comments, think about where they are coming from. Following are some frequent reasons people make comments:

- They do not know the benefits of extended breastfeeding.
- They are curious about breastfeeding, but do not know how to ask.
- They didn't breastfeed for as long as you have.
- They are concerned about you and your baby.
- They have misinformation about breastfeeding.

Basically, all of these possibilities come from an unawareness of the benefits of breastfeeding in general, and extended breastfeeding in particular. People who are commenting on your breastfeeding choices might be working from a framework of no knowledge or, perhaps, misinformation. To help you form your response, you should consider what they do and do not know.

Having a conversation with a good friend or family member can be helpful. Make sure you're in a safe, private space where both of you can talk freely. Explain why you are making the choice to breastfeed your toddler. Talk about the personal reasons and the facts. Then open the floor for honest and respectful questions. Many people do not know the difference between nursing a newborn and nursing an older baby or toddler. Usually this type of open communication is best for both parties.

If this does not work, you have a couple of other options. If the person you're dealing with is a family member or close friend, you could ask the person if he or she would like to attend a breastfeeding support group meeting with you. You could offer the person literature on the benefits of breastfeeding beyond the first six months. If all of this fails, it might be time to agree to disagree and ask that the person simply support you in your decision, even if he or she does not agree with it.

Respond to Critics

Some parents are very sensitive to what others have to say about breastfeeding. Other families really do not pay much attention to what others think. But the truth is that if you are breastfeeding a baby who is older than six months, someone is likely to say something to you.

If you choose to nurse a toddler, people's comments might be even more obvious. Realize that most of these statements stem from misinformation. Don't let other people's lack of breastfeeding knowledge phase you. You can choose to try to correct the misinformation, or simply ignore it.

Choosing to help educate someone is usually a matter of personal opinion. For example, it might be easier for you to educate a friend or family member because you have more access to him or her, and you share more time together. You might also derive more benefit from taking the time to educate these people because they might then become more supportive of you and of breastfeeding.

WOMEN'S WISDOM:

Weaning might sneak up on you. Be mindful of how you and your older child are nursing. Some moms find they simply nurse less and less as time goes on, until before they know it, nursing has stopped. If that's not how you want weaning to happen, pay attention to how your child is nursing. The nutritive and emotional value is still there, so there is no reason to wean just because other people want you to wean. If a medical professional tells you that you have to wean by a certain time (not for medical reasons, but because he or she mistakenly believes the time for your child to benefit from breast milk has passed, ask lots of questions: Why? Why now? Who says so? What do they know? Who can you talk to? Remember, you don't have to take any advice if it's not right for you. You and your child often know better than anyone else.

CHAPTER
10

DISPEL MYTHS ABOUT NURSING AN OLDER BABY OR TODDLER

Everyone has an opinion about everything when it comes to parenting. And breastfeeding for more than six months is an act that seems to stir up a lot of opinions. The problem is that most of those opinions are based on myths. Following are some of the more common myths about breastfeeding a baby beyond the first six months of life. (For more on breastfeeding myths, refer to Appendix A, page 280.)

Myth: Breast Milk Has No Nutritional Value after Six Months

Breast milk always has nutritional value. In fact, in its ever-increasing wonder, breast milk continues to change the longer you nurse. The fat content of breast milk increases as your baby's need for more fats increases in the later half of the first year and beyond.

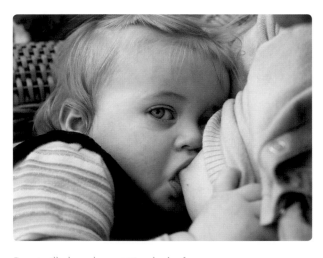

Breast milk always has nutritional value for your baby and provides necessary antibodies geared toward your child's age.

The American Academy of Family Physicians (AAFP), and the American Academy of Pediatrics (AAP), to name a few, agree that one year is the *minimum* for the length of breastfeeding, while the World Health Organization (WHO) believes that two years is the minimum. These important organizations all believe there are nutritional as well as other health benefits to baby and mother—not to mention emotional benefits—from continued breastfeeding.

Myth: If Your Baby Is Still Nursing after a Year, Baby Will Need Braces

According to the article "Breastfeeding is Early Functional Jaw Orthopedics," published in *Functional Orthodontics,* breastfeeding can actually help your baby's facial structures align properly. The muscles required for breastfeeding support proper facial and jaw development. Does this mean your child will never need braces? Not necessarily. But there might be a potential reduction in their use or duration. In any case, breastfeeding is certainly not a cause for needing the aid of an orthodontist. That's more likely a simple case of genetics.

This myth, perhaps, stems from people mistakenly assuming that breastfeeding has negative effects on mouth structure just as bottles and pacifiers can. However, breastfeeding is totally different and more natural, actually helping the development of the face and oral cavity.

Myth: It Is Selfish to Nurse an Older Baby

Breastfed babies are ill less often. They have higher IQs. They have fewer allergies. When a breastfed baby gets ill, he recovers more quickly. These are all well-researched facts, according to many peer-reviewed journals and articles on the benefits of breastfeeding, including the article: "Breastfeeding and Cognitive Development: a Meta-Analysis," published in the *American Journal of Clinical Nutrition*. Breastfeeding is not about being selfish; it's about doing what is natural and feels right for you and your baby. Breastfeeding beyond a year can do both you and your baby good. If it is an important element of your bond and relationship together, you should continue to breastfeed!

Though breastfeeding is not a selfish act, there are excellent benefits for mothers who breastfeed. These can include a reduction in the rates of many cancers, most notably breast cancer. This reduction of risk is related to the length of time a mother has breastfed. So the longer you breastfeed the less chance you have of developing breast cancer.

Myth: You Can't Get Pregnant If You Are Nursing

While breastfeeding can be used as birth control when followed in a very strict method (outlined on page 164), in general you are still able to conceive if you are nursing in an extended fashion. One of the biggest things people do not realize is that nursing a toddler is vastly different from nursing a newborn.

As the amount of time you spend nursing drops, your hormone levels drop and your menstrual cycles return. This can be tied either to the overall amount of time you spend nursing, or longer lengths of time between nursing sessions. Once your period has returned, you have likely returned to your baseline fertility.

Checking for ovulation can help you to determine the best times to get pregnant. You can do this with basal body temperature charting, urine testing, or other fertility measures. Breastfeeding will not interfere with any of these tests.

Myth: Breastfeeding Babies Bite

Breastfeeding babies rarely bite more than occasionally. That is because if they bite down on the nipple, they cannot draw any milk from the breast. Remember, a baby's tongue must extend over his lower gums to get the proper latch; sinking in with his top teeth will not enable a good latch either. And age really has nothing to do with biting. Sometimes babies might accidentally nip lightly if they are falling asleep at the breast and slipping off. Other times they might think it's funny to play and make a game of biting, because they are looking for your reaction. In any case, if your baby does bite, simply pop him off the breast and say "No biting!" firmly. Babies get the idea quickly. Biting problems rarely persist, and babies can go on nursing for a long time, with all of their teeth. (For more on nursing a teething baby, see the section that follows.)

CHAPTER
10

Myth: If Babies Are Old Enough to Ask to Nurse, They Are Old Enough to Wean

All babies ask to nurse. This is something that most people do not realize because they think only about words when they consider someone asking for something. But even your newborn baby has feeding cues that let you know it is time to eat!

Feeding cues change, and so does the breast-feeding relationship in general, as the baby gets older. Just as you would not want your mate to sit down at the dinner table bawling uncontrollably because dinner is five minutes late, you also do not want to see that type of behavior from an older baby or toddler. The polite thing, of course, is to ask for

Sign Language

Using sign language with your baby is an amazing way to help them communicate what they are thinking before they are physically able to speak. Milk is a common sign taught to babies early on. When you nurse your baby you can show your baby the sign for milk, shown below. This way they will learn to ask for milk and not become frustrated. There are many classes that use American Sign Language (ASL) for infants and toddlers, even those who are hearing. This can be a fun and rewarding activity for you and your baby.

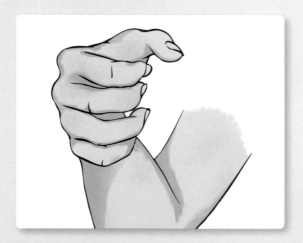
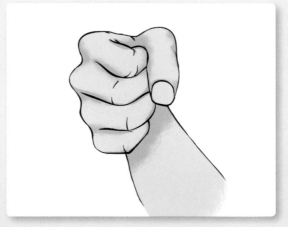

Start with a fist that is slightly open and with the bottom edge of your hand parallel to the floor. Squeeze your fingers gently and repeat to sign "milk."

what you need, and this is exactly what older babies and toddlers learn to do.

Some families try to be nonchalant about breastfeeding in public by using code words. You might hear a toddler or older baby asking for "num nums," "milk," "cuddles," and so on. All families have their own special words for breastfeeding. You might also decide to use sign language. This can help your child say what he wants, before he can even speak. You can use American Sign Language

signs or you can use a sign that your child has made up, as long as you are both in agreement about the meaning of the sign.

Myth: Your Baby Will Never Self-Wean

According to research, babies are programmed to self-wean. The issue becomes that our time table and their internal clocks might be slightly off from one another. The fact is, what babies and toddlers need and what our society tells us about weaning

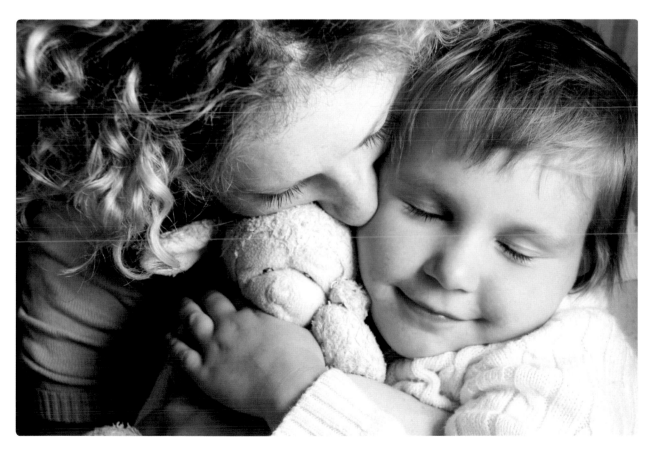

Eventually everyone weans. Following your baby's lead is best for all involved.

isn't the same thing. Most children, when given the choice, would wean between two and a half and seven years of age.

This means that self-led weaning is probably the easiest way to wean. The most important thing to remember is that weaning does not happen overnight. From the moment your baby begins to show interest in solid foods, he is beginning the process of slowly self-weaning in stages. From then on, he will let you know as he gets older when he needs to nurse and when he doesn't. This is all quite normal and part of the natural weaning process. The key is that self-weaning is typically gradual and requires no effort on your part. One benefit of nursing a child is that you can use words to talk about your nursing relationship. You can also begin to teach concepts of patience, respect for others' feelings, and so forth, by helping your toddler understand that he cannot simply throw tantrums and demand to nurse anytime he likes—there are times when he must wait to nurse.

Myth: Breastfeeding Your Older Baby Will Make Him Gay

Breastfeeding is in no way, shape, or form related to a person's sexual orientation. You can't "turn your baby gay" by breastfeeding him for too long. This is true no matter the sex of your baby or the length of time that the two of you decide to have a breastfeeding relationship.

Myth: Nursing a Toddler Will Spoil Him

You simply cannot spoil a baby with love and affection. Spoiling does not come from meeting your baby's needs, but rather with excessive material objects, overindulgence, and no limits. If anything, by responding to your child when it comes to breastfeeding, you are showing him that you value his needs and feelings and, thus, you will help him to become confident and secure.

LEARN TO NURSE A TEETHING BABY

When it comes to their babies, many breastfeeding mothers are concerned about teeth. After all, teeth and sensitive parts of one's body, such as the breasts, just do not seem to mix. Fortunately, a baby or toddler who is actively nursing cannot bite you without first biting herself on the tongue, meaning she most likely won't get as far as biting you. That's not to say that if you are not paying attention you can't get bitten. Here is some advice on nursing your teething baby and toddler.

Teething Basics

Many babies will start the teething process long before they actually get teeth. You might notice an increase in drooling and some general fussiness in your baby at first. In the later stages of teething, you may also be able to see or feel your baby's swollen gums, which might or might not also be reddened. This is a sign that the teeth are emerging.

You are likely to see your baby's first teeth when she is around six months old, although some babies get teeth sooner and some later. Teeth typically break through in pairs, so once you see one tooth, another one usually is not far behind it. The bottom front teeth are typically first, followed by the top four teeth. Molars and incisors come later.

What to Do with a Biter

You have to remember that a baby who bites while nursing is typically not intending to hurt you. Nursing bites are not the same as other bites, which you likely think of as being mean. Biting while nursing is usually about comfort; remember that pressure helps to alleviate pain. It's just that in this case the pressure produces a bite on mom's breast, which is not a good thing.

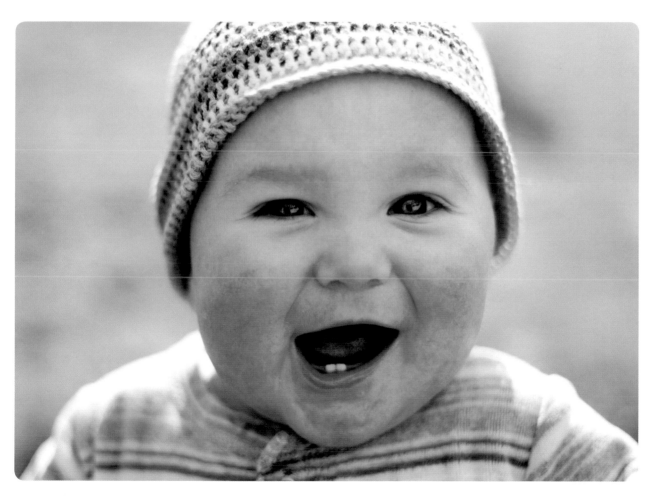

No need to fear a teething baby. Just be mindful and watchful to avoid those teeth.

CHAPTER
10

Proactively, you can try to prevent biting by watching your baby closely during nursing sessions. Most biting occurs as the baby finishes nursing. When actively nursing, the baby's tongue protrudes over the teeth, acting as a barrier between your nipple and the teeth. When babies fall asleep or get lazy, they stop nursing well and pull their tongues back, meaning that there is not a cushion anymore. Ouch!

So watch for signs that your baby is done with a feed. You might notice that she is falling asleep at the breast. You will see that the rate of sucking has rapidly declined. Your baby might stop swallowing breast milk and you might see it begin to roll down her cheek. Or you might notice that your baby is sliding off the nipple. At this point, you should break the suction and pop your baby off the breast. If your baby is not done with the feeding session, she will let you know but will now be awake enough to nurse without letting her tongue drift.

If you do get bitten, you'll probably yelp in pain, which is completely natural and normal. However, your baby might then begin to cry as well. It is almost a comical situation as you then are comforting the person who made you yelp in pain. Remember, your baby is sensitive to you, and to your emotions and actions. Any sudden move or noise and your baby will definitely react. Try not to feel too bad. You really can't do much to prevent babies from being frightened and startled in this way. Hopefully, your reaction will help to make it clear to your baby that she should not bite again!

Stop Baby from Biting

Occasionally, babies bite just to see what will happen. Given that most mothers let out a very surprised yelp when their babies bite, it rarely happens again. The best advice for breaking a baby of the biting habit is to press her into your breast if she bites. This makes her let go. Then end the nursing session and try again later.

OFFER YOUR BABY A CUP OR BABY BOTTLE

A baby bottle is not always required. While no one can say with certainty that nipple confusion won't happen, after the second month you can usually offer a bottle to a baby who is nursing well and has a good milk supply. However, some breastfed babies skip baby bottles altogether. These babies typically go straight to a cup.

As your baby gets older, introducing a cup can be very helpful. Typically, a cup is introduced around the six-month mark. This skill is usually picked up easily with some practice.

When Is the Best Time to Introduce a Cup?

Although six months is typical, you do not have to introduce a cup at this point. Remember, a breast-feeding baby does not need supplements of water or juice. This is true even when solids are introduced. However, some parents are really interested in giving some water or using a cup for breast milk. This is a personal choice. In general, as with many other instances during breastfeeding, watch your baby's cues to determine when to use a cup. Most babies will begin to show interest in cups at some point, and you can proceed accordingly when your baby does.

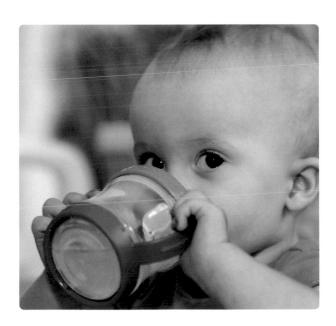

As your baby advances to use a cup, be decisive about what you put in it. Breast milk and water are great options.

What Type of Cup Should You Use?

An overwhelming number of cup types are available. You can use a plastic cup with no lid or a cup with a straw, but that can get really messy with a young toddler! Most parents go with some form of capped cup.

Capped cups might have a straw attached at the top, or they might have a simple spout. This means your baby will need to tip the cup back or suck on the spout to get anything from the cup. Obviously, the benefit to the cap is that there are fewer spills.

Some capped tops have intricate spouts with lots of parts, making the pieces difficult to clean. Be sure you can purchase replacement parts. These cups are often billed as spill-proof. Parents will tell you that "spill-proof" is not always as effective as you would think. The bigger issue is that sometimes spill-proof cups can create pressure on the ears when your baby is drinking. As such, these might not be your best bet.

What Should You Put in the Cup?

There should not be a huge argument about what goes inside the cup. Lots of moms will use the cup as a way to give their baby breast milk when they are not available to nurse. Some families will put water in the cup for a meal.

In general, juice is usually not in the best interest of your baby. Juice contains a lot of calories and sugar, and has been investigated for its role in childhood obesity. Talk with your baby's practitioner before adding juice to your baby's diet. And if you need to give your toddler juice, make sure you limit the amount he drinks each day to no more than 6 ounces (177 ml). Always remember to buy 100 percent juice, as opposed to juice that is mostly sugar.

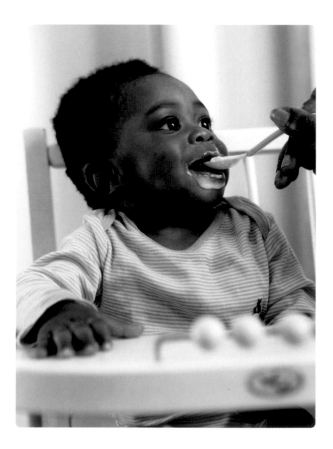

FEED YOUR BREASTFED BABY SOLIDS

The official recommendation is exclusive breast milk until at least six months of age, at which point you can start thinking about introducing solid foods into your baby's diet. The truth is that this is simply a general guideline. Not all babies are ready for solids at the six-month mark. Following your baby's lead with some gentle guidance from your doctor and lactation professional can be very helpful when it comes to reading your baby's cues for eating solid foods.

When to Start Solids

Your baby is incredibly smart. She will show you exactly what you need to know in terms of when to start solids. Here are some of the developmental skills that will indicate that babies are ready to try solids:

- Can sit alone for a few minutes
- Watches you eat with great interest
- Places hands to mouth; might even try to grab food and bring it to mouth
- Does not thrust tongue forward when food is introduced

Feeding your baby solids is a part of the weaning process, but your breast milk is still the main course for a long while.

Watch your baby for signs that she is ready to begin solids. Some babies are ready right near the six-month mark. Others are not ready until closer to the nine-month mark. This is not necessarily a bad thing. Beginning solids too soon can be a problem for allergies in some children. It can also be troublesome if your baby doesn't yet have teeth to eat. So if your baby isn't able to tolerate eating solids just yet, it's best not to force the issue for safety reasons, be it allergy alerts or choking hazards.

How Solids Affect Breastfeeding

There is an intricate dance between solid foods and breastfeeding. In the beginning, solids should not be considered as a replacement for breastfeeding sessions. These first tastes and bites are about getting used to eating solids and digesting them. First meals are also a chance to see what your baby's preferences are. You'll also be able to test for infant allergies, by introducing solid foods one by one to see whether your baby has any adverse reactions to them. Be extremely careful not to reduce the amount of breastfeeding you do when you start solids.

Breastfeeding with Solids

Once you have started solids, you might wonder how you should breastfeed. There should be few changes in the beginning. You should just continue to breastfeed your baby as you did before.

As you progress with solids, your nursing relationship might change a bit. You will want to decide whether it's better to breastfeed before or after you feed your baby the solids. If your baby is extremely fussy and is not likely to settle enough to eat from hunger, nursing before you feed solids is usually best.

Eventually, a feeding with solids will replace a nursing session. This typically happens naturally, without any force from you or your baby. This might frequently be a sit-down meal that your baby shares with the whole family. More often than not, this is either dinner or breakfast.

Need to Nurse When Sick!

If your baby is sick, solids might be the last thing on her mind. Most babies revert to complete nursing when ill. Fortunately, breast milk is often just what a baby needs to feel better. You might also notice that her stools return to what they looked like when she was exclusively breastfed, depending on the length of the illness. This is not worrisome. Breast milk is also great because it is easier to keep down if your baby is vomiting. It can also prevent your baby from becoming dehydrated during vomiting or diarrhea.

CHAPTER
10

For instance, you might be busy making lunches for the day as your baby is sitting in the high chair. You'll get busy with preparing for the next stage of the day. Before you know it, the nursing session that used to happen just after breakfast is suddenly a thing of the past.

As I briefly mentioned earlier in this chapter, the advent of solids is the beginning of weaning. Do not let this fact scare you. Most babies are nowhere near ready to leave breast milk behind. Remember, weaning is a slow process that happens gradually and in stages. This is just the first step. The minimum amount of time suggested to breastfeed is one year for a reason—very few babies willingly wean themselves before this point. In the unlikely event that your baby were to self-wean before one year, you would need to use supplemental breast milk or other alternatives.

You'll learn more about weaning in sections to come, but suffice it to say that the last nursing sessions to end as a child weans are typically nursing sessions that center on sleep or wake cycles. At these times, toddlers use nursing as a chance to prepare and focus for the day—a transition, if you will. These important nursing sessions are about nutrition and comfort. Therefore, they are often the last nursing sessions children let go of because of their dual purpose.

Changes in Bowel Habits

Your baby, when fed only breast milk, has a certain stool habit. You might have gotten used to the unique smell of your breastfed baby's stools (sort of like spoiled milk, but not so offensive overall). Once solids are introduced, you will notice a change. Some babies actually can experience a bit of constipation when they start to eat solids.

You might notice that your baby's stools now smell foul. They also might be less frequent. The color and consistency might change. The amount of change is typically related to how frequently and which type of solids your baby is eating.

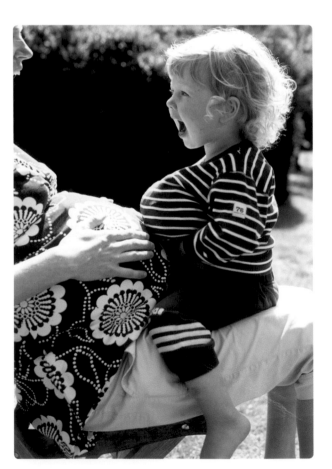

Being pregnant and breastfeeding mixes quite nicely.

You can help to ease your baby's bowel movements, based on both the milk and the food your baby eats. The more your baby nurses, the less likely she is to be constipated. The same is true for many fruits and vegetables: All that fiber prevents babies from being constipated. The opposite is true for meats and refined pastas and grains, including baby cereals. These foods are more likely to cause constipation.

KNOW ABOUT NURSING DURING A NEW PREGNANCY

These days, more and more women are nursing for longer and longer. This means that as they extend the amount of time they nurse their children, it is more likely that they will be nursing during a pregnancy. Nursing during a new pregnancy brings up many thoughts and questions.

The Safety of Nursing during Pregnancy

Nursing during a subsequent pregnancy was done frequently before babies were weaned as early as they have been in the past few decades. The safety of nursing in the average, low-risk pregnancy is well established. In fact, the problems associated with nursing and pregnancy are not really about safety at all, but more about how your nursling will tolerate the changes.

If you are pregnant, let your midwife or doctor know you are breastfeeding at your first prenatal checkup. Be prepared that some might tell you to stop nursing. This recommendation is usually based on lack of information. Some doctors worry about breastfeeding hormone changes causing preterm labor. Others are concerned that a nursling will "steal" important nutrients from the fetus. Before you agree to wean before you and your baby are ready, be sure to ask questions, including:

- Which sources might I look at for information about nursing during pregnancy?

- What are your sources of information for breastfeeding during pregnancy?

- Why must I stop nursing? What is the harm?

Consider talking to other mothers who have nursed during a subsequent pregnancy for advice. They can give you the real scoop on how pregnancy affected their ability to nurse. You can usually find someone through your local breastfeeding group.

Changes in Breast Milk during Pregnancy

Breast milk changes in varying degrees, depending on the individual mother, during pregnancy. Some women notice a lack of milk or a decrease in the amount of milk they produce. Other moms notice only changes in taste, as reported by their nurslings.

If you do not know of anyone locally, there are on-line communities that can help to get you connected to someone who has nursed during pregnancy.

In some cases, breastfeeding is not recommended during pregnancy, and this will vary from woman to woman. You should consult your obstetrician or midwife when in doubt, but they will include mothers who:

- Have a history of preterm labor
- Are carrying more than one baby

How Your Nursling Will React to Pregnancy

Sometimes the first clue that you are pregnant can be the changes in your nursling's breastfeeding habits. This can mean different things to different women. For some, it might mean your current nursling nurses less frequently. Sometimes you might hear complaints that the breast milk tastes different or even about the changes in the quantity of breast milk.

Breast soreness is a frequent symptom of pregnancy, particularly in the early months. If you have previously been nursing without discomfort and suddenly start having sore nipples, there could be many reasons. But if you have dismissed all of the more common reasons for an older nursling to cause pain at the breast, such as teething and yeast, pregnancy hormones might be the culprit.

Toward the end of your pregnancy, your breast milk will begin to change into colostrum. This is in preparation for the new baby. This might also signal to your older child that he no longer wishes to nurse. Some mothers are fine with this decision. If you would prefer that your older child continue to nurse, be sure to talk to him. Talk about the differences in the breast milk and why there are changes. Be sure to let your child know that you, he, and the baby do not have any control over what happens to the milk. It's simply a natural process playing itself out.

Tandem Nursing

"Tandem nursing" describes a mother who is nursing two or more children who are not twins or other multiples. Tandem nursing can happen naturally when you practice child-led weaning. The big question that parents have about nursing two children at the same time are usually about milk consumption. Your breasts will respond to the stimulation from both the new baby and your older nursling. This means you will have enough milk to feed both children.

Mothers who are nursing an older child rarely suffer from engorgement and other problems commonly associated with early nursing as it relates to supply issues. This is because their bodies are already regulating the milk supply for one child, and they are now merely adding another baby to the mix. The contents of the breast milk will stay geared toward the newer baby.

If you are tandem nursing, remember to feed your newborn first, or at least simultaneously. This will ensure that the new baby gets the nourishment he needs first. While it is typically not an issue, this can help to allay your fears, as well as those from your medical professionals and, perhaps, even your family. Nursing the baby first also serves a practical purpose, as you will not be forcing your newborn to wait to eat, and thus, the baby will not become overly hungry and distraught.

Since your older child is less likely to nurse as often as your new baby, it only seems to make sense that your newborn will nurse more frequently. This means you will have at least some feedings alone with only one child. You should consider nursing separately if you are still trying to work out any breastfeeding issues with the new baby. This is also true if your older child is having problems with jealously. After these initial differences are worked out, you can figure out how to enjoy the benefits of nursing simultaneously.

Before the birth of a sibling, explain to your older child that babies can't eat anything but breast milk. Show him that as an older kid, he can also eat table foods, unlike the baby who will thrive only on mommy's milk. Be prepared for some discussions and even negotiations as you go forward with tandem nursing.

You and your older child will really have to figure out what works best for you. But you need to be the one to set up some ground rules. Be clear that the new baby has to be fed first. Continue to remind your older child that this is the only food the baby can take in. Also remind your older child that he must play nicely and be gentle with the baby. This might mean being hands off during the nursing session (think of your hair, clothes, baby's head, etc.). You might also want to talk about how positions for nursing might need to change in the early months when siblings nurse together. Then remind your eldest child that when he nurses alone, he can choose the position in which he would like to nurse.

How long you choose to tandem nurse will depend on your children. Your eldest might lose interest, but not always. Some mothers say that having an older child nurse is helpful in preventing some of the issues that can arise in the early days of

Can Older Children "Unwean?"

If your older child has already weaned, you might be surprised to hear him ask to nurse once a new sibling is born. This is normal. Consider saying yes. Most children are not looking to "unwean"; they simply want to know that you would say yes. It's really not about the actual nursing. If your child accepts the yes and tries to nurse, you will likely find that he does not remember how to nurse or isn't really all that interested.

nursing, such as engorgement. Tandem nursing can also help to ease the transition to having a sibling and even potentially lessen jealousy issues.

Deal with What Others Say about Tandem Nursing

Chances are good that you are not going to see a lot of support for tandem nursing. The best place to look for support will be in your local breastfeeding support group meetings. You might also look for a local toddler nursing group, as it will be the most likely place to find tandem nursing families. If you strike out with finding other local families, you can also look online for support groups.

Your family and friends are probably less inclined to be supportive. Try to remember that this is not necessarily because they are "anti-tandem nursing." It simply might be that they do not know a lot about feeding two babies at one time.

This means you need to take what naysayers believe with a grain of salt. You can try to educate people about the benefits of extended breastfeeding or of tandem nursing, but chances are you will not win many people over. Forget about what others say, and simply work on what's right for you and your family.

For some families, this means they do not really talk about nursing two kids at once. This might mean nursing the older child only at home or in private. Other families are not concerned with other people's beliefs and continue to nurse as they would at home. There is not one right answer.

Just in case, prepare some comebacks for when someone says something. Be ready should a family member, friend, or stranger comment on your tandem nursing. Remember to stop and ask yourself what motivates the person's comments. You never know when someone is asking a legitimate question. It could be someone you might inspire.

What Do the Medical Professionals Say?

The American Academy of Pediatrics (AAP) recommends breastfeeding for a minimum of one year and the World Health Organization (WHO) for a minimum of two years. Neither organization has an age limit on when a child should or must wean. This is because breast milk always has nutritional value. It also has other benefits associated with it, such as antibodies that prevent infection and reduce the likelihood of obesity. There are physical benefits for the mother, as well, including decreased risks of some cancers.

DECIDE WHEN YOU WOULD LIKE TO WEAN

Weaning is truly a slow process for many families. In fact, most women will tell you that they can't pinpoint when it started or even when it ended. Breastfeeding starts out with a bang, but sometimes it slips off into the dark without you even noticing. This is gentle weaning for the mother and the child.

That being said, weaning truly starts the moment your baby is given anything but breast milk. This includes pacifiers and other soothies that prevent your baby from getting breast milk. For most families, this means introducing solids, even though solids are not meant to replace breast milk at first.

Who Decides When to Wean?

When you first decided what your breastfeeding goal was, probably before your baby was even born, you might have thought you had all the answers. As you have gotten involved in your breastfeeding relationship, your goal might have shifted. This can often mean that you want to breastfeed longer than you might have originally thought, or occasionally, less if you have had unexpected circumstances.

Choosing a date, either way ahead of time or in the near future, is called mother-led weaning. This means you have made the decision when to wean. Sometimes mother-led weaning is done for emotional or mental reasons. Perhaps you have simply picked a time and decided to act on it. Very rarely does a mother have medical needs that might require her to wean soon or even abruptly.

Breastfeeding Medicine

If you have been told for any reason that you should wean because of a medical condition, it would be a good idea to get a second opinion. In the past few years, advances have been made in an emerging specialty called breastfeeding medicine. This increasingly recognized new specialty is made up of medical doctors who are committed to preserving the breastfeeding relationship. Unlike the baby's doctor, whose priorities are well-child checks and vaccinations, or the obstetrician, who is concerned with pregnancy and birth, the breastfeeding medicine specialist sees the mother and baby as a pair. The consult centers on a breastfeeding assessment.

The specialist has access to cutting-edge research or information not yet known by your primary care provider, which might preserve your breastfeeding despite a recommendation to wean. You can ask your local breastfeeding support group about a doctor who specializes in breastfeeding medicine or is a member of the American Academy of Breastfeeding Medicine. If your baby is not ready to wean, it is often worth it to find one of these physicians in your area.

CHAPTER
10

Baby-led weaning is different. This means letting your baby decide when to wean. As I already mentioned, this is also typically a slow process. The difference is that you might not notice it as it is happening. For instance, you and your baby might begin to get busy and miss the typical afternoon snack, and before you know it you no longer nurse at that time. This continues to happen until eventually, all breastfeeding sessions are gone. In fact, it might take time before you realize you haven't nursed for a few days.

FIGURE OUT THE EASIEST WAY TO WEAN

As with most things in life, there is an easy way and a hard way to wean. The easy way—weaning gradually by allowing your baby to lead the way—is the best and gentlest way to wean for both you and your baby. The hard way? Well, it's hard and not so gentle, but sometimes it is the only answer for your family for a variety of reasons.

You might be feeling pressure to wean from your baby's doctor simply because he or she has never seen anyone breastfeed beyond the first weeks or months. Perhaps you are battling misinformation or myths in terms of the benefits of breast milk for toddlers and older children. Remember that, barring a history of preterm labor or multiples, there is no need to wean in pregnancy. In these cases, weaning is a decision best made between a mother and her child only.

Steps to Initiate Weaning

The easy way to wean is the slow and gradual method. If weaning is not happening as quickly as you would like, or if you are not seeing any signs of your child's nursing sessions decreasing in frequency or duration, you might take matters into your own hands. The easiest way to start the weaning process is to reduce the number of nursing sessions per day.

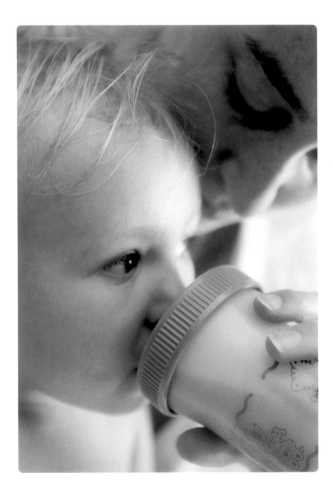

Being able to go from breast to cup is a good idea. Take steps to teach this skill when thinking about weaning.

TIP — Avoid Going Cold Turkey

There are very few reasons to go cold turkey when weaning a child. Doing so can cause you physical pain and discomfort, as well as bring emotional distress for you and your little one. A slower weaning process is usually easier on everyone involved.

To do this, you should identify one nursing session that you would like to drop. Sometimes there is an obvious nursing session that you know your child can easily drop, such as the five-minute session in the afternoon that is not connected to any sleep sessions. Other times, you might not have a time that stands out as a good option, and you just have to choose the best one.

Remove the same nursing session at the same time every day. This will allow your milk supply to adjust. By allowing your body to adjust to dropping one feeding at a time, you can help to prevent problems that can occur with sudden weaning, such as blocked ducts or mastitis. You will want to wait three or four days before removing another feeding. Or perhaps removing just one feeding is where you are ready to stay for now.

CONFIDENCE CUE

You and your child should decide when to wean. Tell naysayers you are confident in your decision. This can be hard if you are hearing a lot of pressure to wean, particularly from family. Sometimes it's not even what relatives say, but how they act. Such judgment is often what leads some women to nurse only at home or in secret. Don't hide! Have confidence that you are not alone in nursing a child who is no longer a newborn.

The trick is to determine what to do in place of the nursing session you remove. If the nursing session was a long, nutritive session, a snack is in order. Sometimes it can be a good idea to offer a snack and then nurse for just a minute or two, instead of the full nursing session. Other times, you might choose to go cold turkey with that session.

CHAPTER
10

If you remove breast milk feedings, ensure that your child is getting enough calories and the appropriate nutrients from replacement foods. Some families choose to replace nursing sessions with cups of either cow's milk, rice milk, or soy milk for toddlers over the age of one year, whereas other families substitute meals. Cow's milk is not a requirement for good health. In fact, many children have problems with dairy. If your baby is younger than one year of age, you should check with your pediatrician for what you should substitute in place of the nursing session. There are more options than you might believe.

How Long Will Weaning Take?

To determine how long weaning will take, first look at the number of nursing sessions your child has per day. Multiply that number by the four to seven days it will take to reduce each session. So, if your child is currently nursing six times per day, it will probably take between twenty-four and forty-two days to wean (6 × 4 = 24; 6 × 7 = 42), depending on your body and your little one. The best answer is to proceed according to your and your child's needs. Remember, it might take varying lengths of time to eliminate each session. For example, your child might give up an afternoon session in the three-to-four-day range, but she will probably hold on to a pre-bed nursing session for longer.

Prevent Breast Problems When Weaning

Sometimes weaning can cause physical problems. The most common physical issues that mothers face during the weaning process are:

- Plugged ducts
- Mastitis (breast infection)
- Pain
- Engorgement

These symptoms can usually be reduced greatly, or even eradicated, with a slow weaning process. If you start to feel engorgement, this can be a signal that your body is weaning too quickly. Try to slow down a bit and see if your engorgement eases up.

Do not make the mistake of adding a pumping session to relieve pain from engorgement. Pumping and other forms or breast stimulation will only encourage your body to make more milk. Some mothers recommend lining your bra with cabbage leaves at night to help signal your body to dry up your breast milk. There are also some commercial products that claim to be weaning aids. However, there is no good medicinal solution to aid you in drying up your breast milk. Try to wear a tight bra to ease discomfort. You might also try some over-the-counter pain relievers.

Your baby might also experience some negative symptoms associated with weaning. The most common physical reaction will be changes in bowel habits. This is frequently a combination of the lesser amount of breast milk and the foods you have substituted for the breast milk. Water and fiber can go a long way toward get a child's bowels moving. Exercise is also helpful.

Occasionally, you might see some food allergies as well. If you notice rashes, a runny nose, or other obvious signs, talk to your pediatrician for advice about dealing with food allergies.

UNDERSTAND HOW YOU MIGHT FEEL ABOUT WEANING

Breastfeeding is not just a physical process; it also comes with a lot of emotional ties attached to it. So when it comes time to think about weaning, it should not surprise you that your emotions can run high as well. Remember, there are no right or wrong answers. In the end, you need to make the decision that is acceptable to your family alone. But also be sure you are allowed to have those feelings.

Weaning When You Do Not Want to Wean

Rarely, something will happen that will cause you to wean before you are ready. It might be that your baby has suddenly seemed to stop nursing, you or your baby have had a drastic illness, or for some other reason. In this case, you might have lots of feelings, some of which could be conflicting.

First things first: Ask yourself, "How do you know it is really weaning?" Short of being told to wean, accepting that information, and moving forward, how can you be sure your child is really weaning? If you are assuming it is weaning because your baby is not nursing, perhaps it is not weaning, and only a nursing strike. Babies often have temporary nursing strikes when they are ill.

Before assuming your child is weaning, be sure that you have worked through all of the suggestions for dealing with a nursing strike. These can look a lot like weaning sometimes, but they might not be. Misreading the cues of a nursing strike can lead to weaning that neither you nor your baby wanted.

TIP **Be Adaptable**

Nothing says that weaning has to happen in a certain way for you and your child. You can change your method of weaning at any point during the process. If one way is not working for you as you had hoped, think about your options and reconsider.

Self-Care Tips

Watch your breasts for signs of engorgement as breastfeeding slows. If you feel fullness or pain, you might need to pay more attention. You can accidentally have problems with plugged ducts and the like if you are not mindful. Remember to massage any smaller plugged ducts and even apply warm compresses. It doesn't happen all the time, but it is more likely to happen with sudden weaning.

CHAPTER
10

When it is not your choice, weaning can be very difficult to deal with for many moms. You might be particularly disappointed if you were unable to reach the original goal you set up early in your breastfeeding life, perhaps even before your baby was born. It can be particularly upsetting when you are not able to take part in the decision about when weaning occurs.

Know that it is okay to feel upset. You might need time to grieve the loss of something very special to you. Ask yourself what you will miss about nursing. For many mothers, what they will miss most is the snuggling time. Remember that breastfeeding is not the only way to snuggle and be close to your child (although it certainly makes it easier), because each time you feed the baby you can ensure that you and your baby have quiet, snuggling time that does not include breastfeeding.

You might also be surprised that you feel fine with the decision to wean. Perhaps you are relieved. This revelation might surprise you, even upset you. It has nothing to with whether you are a good mother. So avoid the trap of feeling guilty for not feeling guilty. There is plenty of guilt to go around in motherhood; there's no need to borrow any.

Weaning When You Want to, but Baby Doesn't

You might have decided to wean because you have met your goal. (Congratulations!) You might have decided to wean due to an illness or medication, social pressure, breastfeeding challenges, or many other reasons.

Once you have decided to wean, your next step is to decide how you want to wean. You will want to determine what is best for your baby and your body. Consider your child's age, the duration of breastfeeding, what alternative comfort measures you can use in place of nursing, and any medical or nutritional issues that you might need to address.

Nursing for the Last Time

It might be difficult to pick the last nursing session if you are the one making the choice. But if this is the weaning method you have chosen, be sure to give yourself the time to enjoy it and reflect on your nursing relationship. Perhaps you have overcome a lot of struggles to get to this point. Maybe you've met a big goal for yourself.

It's okay to feel ambivalent during the last nursing, and even after. You might even tear up or cry. This can be quite common, and not something you should worry about. It is the normal expression of your love for your baby and wanting to do what is best for both of you.

It can also be normal to nurse your baby and be happy. Perhaps you are glad to be done with nursing. Perhaps you are just elated about reaching your goal.

Nighttime is typically the last nursing session to be given up, though it may or may not work that way for your baby.

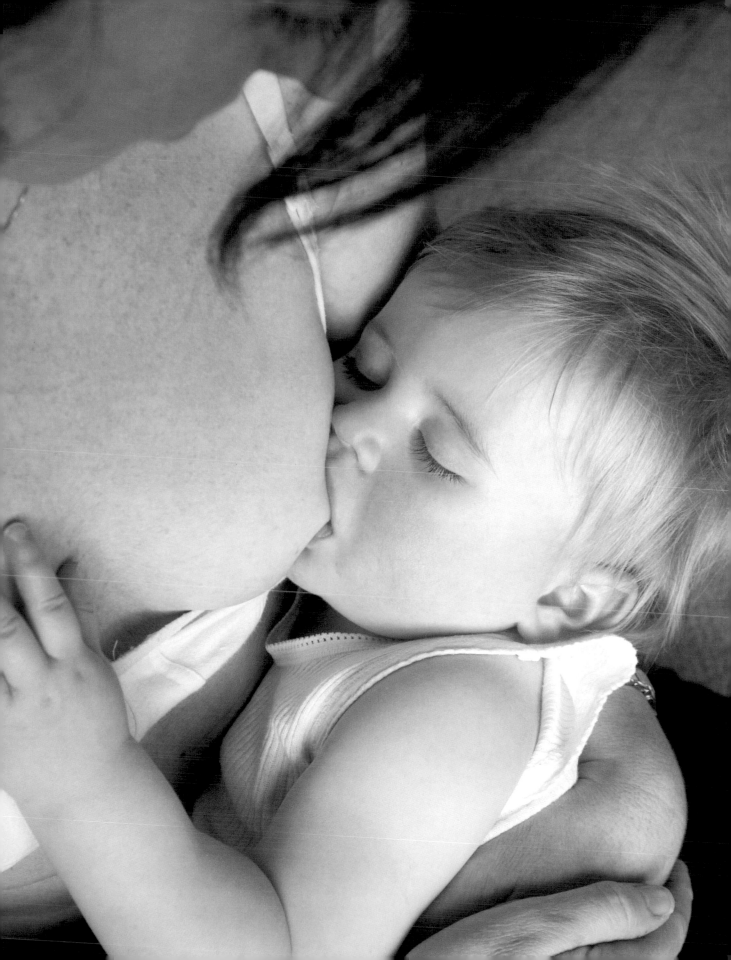

Partial and Nighttime Weaning

As children get older, moms who do not want their children to wean may sense that it might be necessary to set some limits on the nursing relationship. At these times, partial and nighttime weaning methods can be good options. For instance, partial weaning can work well for moms who work. As toddlers get older, moms might choose to stop pumping during the day, but continue to nurse their kids when they are at home. Nighttime weaning can be a possibility for toddlers who wake up often and continually want to nurse during the night. If excessive nighttime waking becomes too much of a disturbance to everyone's sleep, moms can set limits by gradually teaching their little ones that mommy milk has to go to sleep at night. As an option, moms might allow their children to nurse before going to bed and then again some time closer to the morning, while instead offering a water cup for wakings in between.

You can also use redirection to help prevent your child from asking to nurse. For example, if you know that right before naptime your child will want to nurse, do something else. Create a different ritual. Before your toddler can even ask, scoop him up and sit on the couch with a book. Snuggle up close and read before naptime. This method works particularly well when you sense your child might not really need to nurse and could easily be satisfied with something else.

You might also use counting as a way to encourage weaning. This means your child can nurse, but only for a certain amount of time. It might be one minute or five minutes. You set the time. This can be another way to wean gently, even if it does take more time.

Another alternative is to have someone else do a bedtime ritual with your child. Have your partner get your little one ready for bed. Your child can ask dad to nurse, but it's not going to work. You might go out grocery shopping, take a bath, or do whatever works for your family. But simply being unavailable is sometimes enough of a distraction to help your child move through to bedtime and other activities without nursing.

Breastfeeding Affirmation

My baby and I know how long to breastfeed.

Remember that just as breastfeeding is a natural instinct you are taught to do, you might need to work out weaning with your heart and your mind as well. Most families prefer gentle weaning. This combination of love and facts will help you to find the best solution for you and your family.

Gentle Weaning Techniques

Weaning should occur as gently as possible. One method that can be mother-and-child centered is what's called the "don't offer, don't refuse" approach. This means you do not offer the breast to your child. But if your child asks you to nurse, you do not refuse. This allows you both to have some say in the process, and allows your child to tell you when he really needs to nurse.

REMEMBER THAT YOUR CHILD IS NEVER "TOO OLD" TO NURSE

When we think of breastfeeding we think of babies. Mothers struggle to nurse until their babies are at or beyond their first birthday, and very few manage to make it that far. While it is becoming more common to see women nursing toddlers in public, the few women who admit to nursing toddlers are still few and far between.

Breastfeeding is not something that is limited by time or to a certain age of your child. There are sustained benefits nutritionally, immunologically, and emotionally as breastfeeding continues. There is no question about these benefits.

You may find that you have people tell you that your child is too old to nurse. This is one of the bigger stumbling blocks that families face when deciding when to wean their child. This is, however, a personal decision between you and your child.

Dr. Katherine Dettwyler has spent a great deal of time studying breastfeeding. In her studies, she has found that the natural span of breastfeeding is between about two and half and seven years. Her work can be found at www.kathydettwyler.org.

So the bottom line is that if you and your child are happy in your breastfeeding relationship, then there is no reason to stop nursing simply because of a specific age.

The truth is that there is not an age that is too old to be nursing. The American Academy of Pediatrics (AAP) says it best: "Breastfeeding should continue as long as is mutually desired. The nutritional benefits are always present, at any age. The immunological benefits are still there. And the emotional bonds of breastfeeding stay with a child forever. There is nothing wrong with breastfeeding the older child, and many reasons that are right about it."

CHAPTER
10

APPENDIX A:
BREASTFEEDING MISCONCEPTIONS

In this appendix you will find answers to questions people ask you or myths people may tell you about breastfeeding. Just flip through these common breastfeeding myths and find the answer. Then share your newfound knowledge.

Myth: Breastfeeding hurts.

Breastfeeding does not have to hurt. Breastfeeding can feel weird or strange at first because it is not something you have ever done. But pain means there is something wrong. Sore nipples are the most common pain experienced when breastfeeding. This is most likely due to a problem with the position your baby is in while breastfeeding. Talking to a lactation counselor or consultant can be particularly helpful to ensure that you and your baby have a great position and latch. This will go a long way toward preventing pain or curing any pain that you are experiencing.

Myth: You should wash your breasts before each feeding.

While you are breastfeeding, avoid putting anything on your nipples other than water and your baby. Soaps and lotions can dry out the natural oils in your skin. Your baby might also ingest whatever you put on your nipples. Plain water when bathing or showering is sufficient for cleaning your breasts.

Myth: Toughening your nipples is a good idea.

Toughening your nipples was something our grandmothers were taught to do. Back then, you were supposed to take a washcloth and rub your nipples vigorously. The goal was to cause enough irritation so that the skin would toughen up, much like your feet do after a long summer of being barefoot. This does not work. All it does is make your nipples hurt, and it can cause damage. It does not prevent nipple pain when breastfeeding—teaching your baby proper latch solves that problem.

Myth: When you first breastfeed you should feed your baby for only fifteen minutes per side to prevent pain.

Whatever the time limit placed, this statement is still a myth. You do not need to feed your baby for any set number of minutes on any side. Your baby should be a good judge of how long he needs to eat. Remember, the milk-ejection reflex and amount of milk coming out per minute varies widely from mother to mother. And all babies nurse at different rates. Some babies are very efficient nursers, and fifteen minutes would be way too long for them. Other babies require much longer lengths of time to do the same job, making fifteen minutes too short for them to be adequately fed. Pain is not caused by the length of time your baby stays on your nipple.

Myth: Your breasts are too small to breastfeed.

People often equate the amount of milk with the size of the container. The container, in this instance, would be your breasts. Small breasts are not an issue when it comes to breastfeeding. This is because the amount of milk is relative to the level of demand from your baby, rather than the amount of fatty tissue you have, which is what determines the size of the breast.

Myth: Your breasts are too big to breastfeed.

Larger breasts can be culprits in making breastfeeding a bit more complicated, particularly when your baby is tiny. But simply having large breasts is no reason not to breastfeed. The internal plumbing is the same. You just need to be aware of ways to position your baby so that you can see how he is feeding and be sure he can get a good latch without having to hold all of your breast tissue constantly. With some practice, this can be easy to do.

Myth: Your nipples are too large to breastfeed.

Big nipples and little mouths can be an interesting combination in the first few weeks of breastfeeding. Fortunately, most babies seem to take the size of the nipple in stride. Remember, your nipple is not supposed to look like something on the end of a baby bottle. With good positioning and conditioning your baby to open wide, you will have your little one nursing well in no time.

Myth: Your nipples are too flat to breastfeed.

Flat or inverted nipples are not horrible issues for many women. In fact, a good suction from your baby is often enough of a cure. Some babies are more hesitant to latch when their mothers have flat or inverted nipples. You can try to "evert" the nipple on your own just prior to feeding to encourage your baby as he is learning to breastfeed. stSome tools of the trade do the same thing—the only difference is the cost, and using your hands versus using a piece of plastic. Some mothers also have a lot of luck using a breast pump just prior to feeding.

Myth: You can't breastfeed if you have had breast surgery.

While some women who have had breast surgery will find it more difficult to breastfeed, that is not the case for every woman. You will need to get your records from your surgeon for a more complete picture, but even then, you cannot be sure until you have given your body a chance to make milk with the hormones and changes that giving birth brings. Be sure to talk to your lactation professional prior to giving birth and immediately afterward to stay on top of your needs.

Myth: You had a breast reduction, so you can't breastfeed.

While a breast reduction should have no bearing on whether you can breastfeed, it might have something to do with how much milk you supply. Depending on the type of surgery you had and when your surgery was done, you might be able to achieve a full milk supply with no issues. Being aware of what the issues are and how to tell what type of a milk supply you have will be the key to your success.

Myth: You have breast implants, so you can't breastfeed.

Breast implants should not have much of an effect on your ability to breastfeed. Certain older surgeries could have caused issues because of the types of incisions made, but those are fewer and farther between. You might, however, experience some of the issues that go along with large breasts and small babies. Simply keep an eye on your milk supply and be attentive to positioning.

Myth: Your baby is too small to breastfeed.

Small babies can be an issue when it comes to breastfeeding. If your baby is small and premature, he might have some difficulties with sucking and swallowing as well as other issues. This might mean you need to wait for a period of time to begin breastfeeding. If this is the case, you would simply build your supply, do a lot of skin to skin with your baby, feed your baby expressed breast milk with an alternative feeding device, and add breastfeeding in once your baby can tolerate it.

Myth: Your baby is too big to breastfeed.

Some people will take a look at your baby and declare him to be too big to breastfeed. Perhaps they do not believe your body will make enough milk to stimulate a large enough supply to feed a huge baby, or simply because it will be hard to hold him. Fortunately, your baby is growing so well because you are feeding him well. His size has nothing to do with how much or how little milk you make.

Myth: You have twins, so you won't make enough milk.

Many mothers are able to nurse twins without batting an eye. The key to breastfeeding twins successfully is to start on the right foot as soon as possible. If you and your babies are separated, get a pump, and go early with it. Do not sweat having two babies—your breasts got the note about there being two of them, and your body can build up a supply accordingly!

Myth: You can't breastfeed if you take medication.

This one is mostly a myth, though certainly some medications you cannot or should not take while nursing. However, most of the common medications taken by women of childbearing age are safe for use in nursing. If you are curious about a particular medication, have your pediatrician or OB look it up in the current breastfeeding and pharmacology literature to see if it is safe. If it isn't, check to see if there is another similar drug that is safe. Sometimes you might need to take a drug for a very short period of time. You can then choose to pump and dump the breast milk during that period.

Myth: If you get an infection you need to quit breastfeeding.

Infections are a part of life. Most antibiotics are safe for use when breastfeeding; just ask your doctor. If you are experiencing a breast infection, also known as mastitis, you will want to be sure that you are breastfeeding. To stop breastfeeding will worsen this condition. You do not need to toss your breast milk if you have mastitis.

Myth: Breastfeeding women get breast infections a lot.

Some women will breastfeed and have a breast infection, and some women seem to get more than others. However, this is not the normal cycle of things for breastfeeding women. Most mothers will never get breast infections while nursing.

Myth: If you need surgery you will have to quit nursing.

Medications are the reason most mothers will quit breastfeeding because of surgery. Again, check with your doctors to see which medications you will be given and how long you would need to pump and dump, if at all. Simple, outpatient surgeries rarely require weaning.

Myth: Breastfeeding is beneficial for only the first few weeks.

The nutritional benefits of breast milk are amazing. Your baby receives exactly the right amount of calories, proteins, and fats throughout the day. In fact, your breast milk changes to meet the needs of your baby. So the breast milk you make at one week is very different from the breast milk you make at one month or even one year. Your milk also changes throughout the day. There is always nutritional value to your breast milk. There is also the added benefit from the immune-system boost your baby gets.

Myth: Young (or older) mothers do not make enough milk to feed their babies.

Your age at the time of birth will not affect your ability to breastfeed. What might occasionally effect your breastfeeding abilities are your health status and your nutritional status. Be sure to talk to your practitioners and lactation professional about the things you will need to keep an eye out for when it comes to nursing.

Myth: If you breastfeed, your husband or partner will feel left out.

Breastfeeding is the one thing that someone else cannot do for you. Your partner can participate in many other lovely baby-care activities, including playing with your baby, snuggling, bathing, and caring in a general manner. It is not necessary to give bottles, even with breast milk, to make your partner feel like he is a part of the process. There will be plenty of time for your partner to help feed the baby down the road, once the baby is ready to eat solids!

APPENDIX B:
RESOURCES FOR BREASTFEEDING SUPPORT AND BEYOND

BLOGS

Blacktating

http://blacktating.blogspot.com

Elita is the mother to a wonderful toddler boy who is still nursing. She was inspired to create the Blacktating blog because of her passionate commitment to breastfeeding. What started as a side project to keep her occupied while on maternity leave has become her second baby. This blog is for all the moms out there, particularly women of color, who are breastfeeding their babies. Hopefully you will find good information, support, and a sense of community here while you're breastfeeding, whether for a day, a week, a month, or years!

Mama Knows Breast

http://mamaknowsbreast.com

Andi Silverman, author of a book with the same title, shares her insights on breastfeeding from a personal and professional perspective.

Motherwear's Breastfeeding Blog

http://breastfeeding.blog.motherwear.com

The Motherwear Breastfeeding blog started out as a part of this company's clothing website. The blog is written in a thorough manner and covers a variety of topics. There are lots of fun stories to share as well as some great giveaways!

Permission to Mother

http://permissiontomother.blogspot.com

A doctor and lactation consultant, Dr. Denise Punger talks about the real-life benefits of nursing, including candid accounts of nursing her own children.

BREASTFEEDING EDUCATION

Videos by Dr. Jack Newman

www.drjacknewman.com

Dr. Jack Newman is a pediatrician and breastfeeding guru. He has traveled the world, helping mothers to breastfeed. His collection of videos and handouts is amazing and can be viewed for free on his website.

Best for Babes

www.bestforbabes.org

This website provides an interesting look at breast-feeding education—with a new spin.

La Leche League International

www.llli.org

Here you'll find educational handouts, discussions, information on support groups in your area, and more. This service organization is dedicated to helping mothers breastfeed, whether for a day, a month, a year, or longer. They are trained, certified volunteers who have help lines, Internet resources, and local chapters with meetings, and other help.

SPECIAL ISSUES IN BREASTFEEDING

Low Milk Supply

www.lowmilksupply.org

This site helps mothers who have low milk supplies for various reasons, including breastfeeding after a breast reduction and more.

Breastfeeding After Reduction

www.bfar.org

Breastfeeding after a breast reduction involves many intricate issues. This website provides facts and personal stories.

BREASTFEEDING SUPPORT AND LACTATION PROFESSIONALS

About Breastfeeding

http://breastfeeding.about.com

Here you'll find the latest news and informative articles on breastfeeding written by an IBCLC and mother.

Baby Friendly USA

www.babyfriendlyusa.org

This is the certifying organization that decides whether hospitals are breastfeeding friendly. How does your hospital rank?

Got Mom?

www.gotmom.org

This website provides a look at breastfeeding and resources from the American College of Nurse Midwifery.

International Lactation Consultants Association (ILCA)

www.ilca.org

You can use ILCA's site to find a board-certified lactation consultant (IBCLC).

Ask Lenore

http://asklenore.info

This site is about expanding your family through adoption and other alternatives, and it has an extensive section on adoptive breastfeeding.

Nursing Mothers Council

www.nursingmothers.org

This organization provides free phone counseling for mothers in the United States as well as local visits for mothers who live in California. All services are provided by mothers who have breastfed, some of whom are trained as lactation professionals.

Kelly Mom

http://kellymom.com

The KellyMom site is written by IBCLCs for mothers. It includes lots of great information on breastfeeding, addressing the simple and the not-so-simple issues alike.

Making More Milk by Diana West, IBCLC, and Lisa Marasco, MA, IBCLC

This book provides an in-depth look at what can cause low breast milk supply and how to overcome it.

BREAST PUMPS

Ameda

www.ameda.com

Avent/Phillips

www.avent.com

Medela

www.medela.com

Hygeia

www.hygeiababy.com

PumpMoms

http://groups.yahoo.com/group/pumpmoms

This group is dedicated to women who pump full- or part-time for their babies. It is an open group for mothers who fit into this category, and it is a very supportive community.

Human Milk Banking Association of North America

www.hmbana.org

This site details the process for donating breast milk or requesting breast milk and explains the process of freezing and storing breast milk.

Prolacta Human Breast Milk Fortifier

www.prolacta.com

Sometimes premature infants need to have their feedings jam-packed with calories. Until recently there was no human milk version, but now you can ask for Prolacta.

CESAREAN RECOVERY

International Cesarean Awareness Network (ICAN)

www.ican-online.org

ICAN offers online and local support groups for those who have had a cesarean birth.

DAYCARE

About Child Care

www.childcare.about.com

Here you'll find informational articles on choosing a daycare and working with your provider.

MOTHERS' HEALTH

American Academy of Breastfeeding Medicine

www.bfmed.org

Here is where you will find the professional organization dedicated to physicians and the support and study of breastfeeding. Has your baby's physician signed the pledge?

American Academy of Family Physicians

www.familydoctor.org

This helpful website has a lot of information that is geared toward the health of the whole family, from newborns and upward.

American Academy of Pediatrics (AAP)

http://aap.org

This is the official organization of U.S. pediatricians. Here you can find all of their official recommendations.

Medications and Mother's Milk by Dr. Thomas Hale

This book is the mainstay for practitioners and mothers alike when researching medications and their breastfeeding safety for babies.

My Pyramid

www.mypyramid.gov

This website gives you basics on your nutritional needs after you provide information, including your breastfeeding status. This will help to ensure that you are meeting your daily nutritional needs.

PARENTING

Mothering Magazine

www.mothering.com

This magazine is all about mothering and parenting in general. It is written from a more holistic style than most parenting magazines.

Stay-at-Home Parents

http://stayathomeparents.about.com

Join other stay-at-home mothers to discuss life as well as read informative articles on everything from managing your home to raising your kids.

Work-at-Home Moms

http://workathomemoms.about.com

This informative site talks about how to run a business from home while managing the kids.

PREEMIES

About Preemies

http://preemies.about.com

Read stories from other parents who successfully breastfed in the NICU. They share their tips and tricks as well as other information on premature babies from birth forward.

March of Dimes

www.marchofdimes.com

This is a complete resource from pregnancy through birth with a special emphasis on keeping healthy in pregnancy, preventing premature birth, and caring for your preterm baby, including the benefits of breastfeeding.

MULTIPLES

About Multiples

http://multiples.about.com

Looking at life with twins or more? This site has informative articles as well as a discussion area meant to help parents support each other in the journey.

National Organization for Mothers of Twins Clubs

http://nomotc.org

This organization is designed to help mothers of twins and other multiples find and support each other. You can search for local clubs as well as look through the numerous resources.

Mothering Multiples by Karen Kerkoff Gromada

This provides a great look at the last days of pregnancy, early parenting, and life with multiple babies. This is the most informative book on realistically feeding your babies and getting by without being overwhelmed.

POSTPARTUM

DONA International (formerly Doulas of North America)

www.dona.org

Interested in finding a postpartum doula for some help at home? This is the largest certifying agency for postpartum doulas. The site can give you a list of postpartum doulas in your area.

International Cesarean Awareness Network (ICAN)

www.ican-online.org

ICAN provides local and online support groups for women recovering from cesarean section as well as those planning for a vaginal birth after a cesarean (VBAC) or a repeat cesarean section.

The Birth Survey

www.thebirthsurvey.com

Once you have given birth, log on to The Birth Survey to have a chance to talk about your labor and birth. You can also rate the care you received prenatally and during birth. This is a free service.

Laughter and Tears
by Elisabeth Bing and Libby Coleman

This provides a gentle look at how life after having a baby can be amazing and frightening all at once.

This Isn't What I Expected
by Karen Kleiman and Valerie Raskin

This provides a realistic look at life as a new parent.

The Everything Mother's First Year Book
by Robin Elise Weiss, LCCE

A guide to finding yourself as a mother during your baby's first year.

Eat Well, Lose Weight While Breastfeeding **by Eileen Behan**

Learn how to lose weight safely while breastfeeding.

The Everything Guide to Postpartum Care **by Megan Francis**

This guide can help you get back on your feet after having a baby and discusses everything, from the physical to the emotional, vaginal to cesarean.

Essential Exercises for the Childbearing Year
by Elizabeth Noble

This is an easy guide to follow for simple and effective exercises that you can do before, during, and after you give birth.

POSTPARTUM DEPRESSION

Postpartum Support International

www.postpartum.net

This site will provide you with information on the signs and symptoms of postpartum mood disorders and help you to get in touch with local resources.

SLEEP

Sleeping with Your Baby
by Dr. James McKenna

This takes a look at baby sleep science, including a historical look at co-sleeping, co-sleeping benefits, and how to have a safe co-sleeping experience.

The No Cry Sleep Solution
by Elizabeth Pantley

This book is a favorite among new parents. It discusses various methods to help you and your baby get more sleep in the gentlest approach possible. It includes stories from many families with a variety of sleeping arrangements. There is something for everyone in this book.

Helping Baby Sleep
by Anni Gethin and Beth MacGregor

This book marries current research with a practical approach to helping your baby sleep. Gone are the days of simply being told what to do. Here is a way to understand why things work and do not work for infants. The book also offers practical and sound ways to deal with sleep issues.

NURSING PRODUCTS

Bébé au Lait
www.bebeaulait.com

Bravado Bras
www.bravadodesigns.com

Expressiva
www.expressiva.com

La Leche League International Clothing
www.llliclothes.com

Medela, Inc.
www.medela.com

MoBoleez
www.moboleez.com

Motherhood
www.motherhood.com

Mother Wear
http://motherwear.com

EMPLOYERS AND BREASTFEEDING

The Business Case for Breastfeeding
www.womenshealth.gov/breastfeeding/
programs/business-case
Here, employers can find facts about how breast-feeding benefits the whole company, a tool kit on making your recommendations to employees, and other resources including the ability to order a free tool kit.

Working It Out: Breastfeeding at Work
www.llli.org/Law/LawEmployment.html
Here is a look at how to approach your employer about breastfeeding and pumping, and convincing them to help.

BREASTFEEDING ADVOCACY

Birth Activist
www.birthactivist.com
This site will give you something to think about. Everything is related to breastfeeding and birth. It lets you speak up and have your voice heard on parenting issues directly affecting you.

World Breastfeeding Week
www.worldbreastfeedingweek.org
Celebrated the first week of August, this celebration has a different theme each year. Join us next year!

International Baby Food Action Network

www.ibfan.org/

This website provides a list of the baby food manufacturer's code of marketing—a list of things that makers of baby formula can and can't say about their products, according to the World Health Assembly, also known as the International Code of Marketing Breastmilk Substitutes.

World Alliance for Breastfeeding Action

www.waba.org.my/

WABA works to protect and promote breastfeeding worldwide.

Sources: **Vital Nutrients for Infant Health** (page 138)

www.kellymom.com; www.drspock.com; www.foodconsumer.org

ABOUT THE AUTHOR

ROBIN ELISE WEISS, B.A., I.C.C.E.-C.P.E., C.D. (DONA), F.A.C.C.E., L.C.C.E., C.L.C. knows a thing or two about breastfeeding. Her eight children, including a set of twins, were all breastfed. Personally dealing with many of the challenges and joys of breastfeeding lead Weiss to help other mothers with their breastfeeding goals. As a pregnancy and parenting expert, Weiss has written over ten books to help families have safe and satisfying experiences. You can find her on the Internet where she is the pregnancy guide at About.com (pregnancy.about.com) as well as her personal website, robineliseweiss.com. Drop by and read more on the subject or ask questions and get support for all of your breastfeeding and parenting needs.

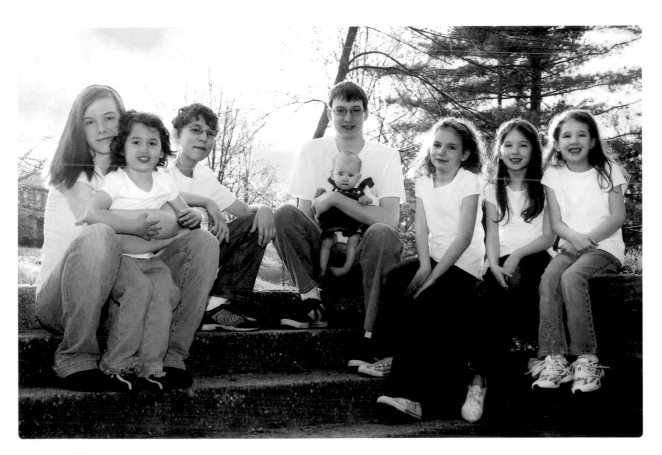

Photo: Laura Kline

ACKNOWLEDGMENTS

Writing a book can be a lot of fun, mixed with a lot of blood, sweat, and tears. Many people assisted me in this journey. I'd like to thank Dr. Denise Punger for her great technical advice; Andrea Mattei for her editing and knowledge of the subject matter; Betsy Gammons and Jill Alexander for keeping me on track; and Barb Doyen for her support. Without these ladies, this project would not be the beautiful book it is today.

An additional group of women also supported me as I wrote. They acted as fact checkers, cheerleaders, and word counters. These people let me bounce ideas off of them while I was writing. Many thanks to them, including Ashley Benz, Teri Shilling, Marci Yesowitch Hopkins, Pat Predmore, Diane Graf, Deanna Godman, Heather Levinson, Stacie Walker, Sharon Muza, Juliet Dietsch, Angela Garvin, Nicole Aldridge, Amy Goforth, Faye Rothberg, and Dawn Olmo.

And my acknowledgments would not be complete without thanking the people who gave me plenty of hands-on time with the topic of breastfeeding, pumping, and the like. In the course of my life, I have spent more than eighteen years nursing, pumping, or tandem nursing. I have had the joy of nursing singletons and twins. I even had a baby who had so many difficulties that she never came to breastfeed, but I provided her with my breast milk by pumping for her for more than eighteen months. So thanks go out to Hilary, Benjamin, Isaac, Lilah, Owen, Clara, Ada, and Noa for providing me with hands-on learning experience with the art and science of breastfeeding and everything that goes along with it! A huge thanks to my mother-in-law, Alyse Weiss, for breastfeeding when it wasn't popular and for being a great support system when it came to encouraging breastfeeding. And, of course, to my husband, Kevin, who was very supportive; a great combination of sweet and tough love while I nursed our children and beyond.

PHOTOGRAPHER CREDITS

INDEX

FURTHER READING

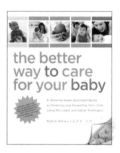

The Better Way to Care for Your Baby

Robin Elise Weiss, L.C.C.E., C. D.

ISBN–13: 978-1-59233-420-9

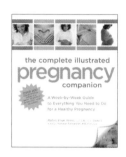

The Complete Illustrated Pregnancy Companion

Robin Elise Weiss, L.C.C.E., C. D. (DONA) with Dr. Marcello Pietrantoni, M.D.

ISBN–13: 978-1-59233-358-5

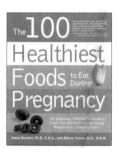

100 Healthiest Foods to Eat During Pregnancy

Jonny Bowden, Ph.D, C.N.S. and Allison Tannis, M.S., R.H.N

ISBN–13: 978-1-59233-400-1

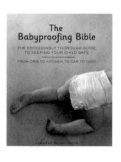

The Babyproofing Bible

Jennifer Bright Reich

ISBN–13: 978-1-59233-248-9

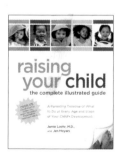

Raising Your Child: The Complete Illustrated Guide

Jamie Loehr, M.D., and Jen Meyers

ISBN-13: 978-1-59233-376-9

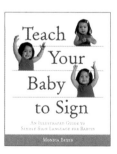

Teach Your Baby to Sign

Monica Beyer

ISBN-13: 978-1-59233-273-1